Recent Progress in Orthopedics

Recent Progress in Orthopedics

Editor: Johan Saunders

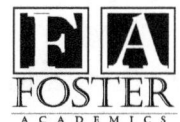

www.fosteracademics.com

www.fosteracademics.com

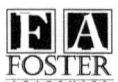

Cataloging-in-Publication Data

Recent progress in orthopedics / edited by Johan Saunders.
    p. cm.
Includes bibliographical references and index.
ISBN 978-1-63242-581-2
1. Orthopedics. 2. Musculoskeletal system--Wounds and injuries. I. Saunders, Johan.
RD731 .R43 2019
616.7--dc23

Foster Academics,
118-35 Queens Blvd., Suite 400,
Forest Hills, NY 11375, USA

ISBN 978-1-63242-581-2 (Hardback)

Contents

Preface

The purpose of the book is to provide a glimpse into the dynamics and to present opinions and studies of some of the scientists engaged in the development of new ideas in the field from very different standpoints. This book will prove useful to students and researchers owing to its high content quality.

Orthopedics is a branch of surgery that develops surgical interventions for the treatment of musculoskeletal disorders. The treatment of musculoskeletal trauma, degenerative diseases, tumors, spine diseases, etc. is dealt within orthopedics. Knee and shoulder arthroscopy, laminectomy, lumbar spinal fusion, hip replacement, etc. are some of the common surgical procedures. Orthopedic physical therapy is a vital procedure involved in the diagnosis, management and treatment of orthopedic disorders and injuries. It is also concerned with rehabilitation for patients who have undergone orthopedic surgery or trauma like strains, sprains, etc. This book is a compilation of chapters that discuss the most vital concepts and emerging trends in the field of orthopedics. The various studies that are constantly contributing towards advancing technologies are examined in detail. In this book, using case studies and examples, constant effort has been made to make the understanding of the difficult concepts of orthopedics as easy and informative as possible, for the readers.

At the end, I would like to appreciate all the efforts made by the authors in completing their chapters professionally. I express my deepest gratitude to all of them for contributing to this book by sharing their valuable works. A special thanks to my family and friends for their constant support in this journey.

Editor

Conversion of external fixation to internal fixation in a non-acute, reconstructive setting

T. Monni · F. F. Birkholtz · P. de Lange ·
C. H. Snyckers

Abstract The aim of the study is to determine the outcomes in patients who underwent conversion from an external fixator to an internal fixation device. This is a retrospective review of 18 patients (24 limbs) who underwent conversion from external to internal fixation. The patients had external fixators applied for traumatic bone defects or congenital deformities. Conversion to internal fixation was performed for reasons of patient dissatisfaction with external fixation, pin track sepsis, persistent non-union or refracture. The complexity of cases was graded using Paley's level of difficulty score. Patients were either converted acutely or delayed. Internal fixation devices were either intramedullary nails or plate and screws. Outcome was regarded as excellent if the patients were fully weight-bearing and pain-free on a mechanically well-aligned limb and without need for further surgery: good if the patient required subsequent surgery to achieve union and poor if irreversible complications occurred. Acute conversions (fixator removal and introduction of internal fixation device at same surgery) were done in 19 limbs and delayed conversion (interval between fixator removal and internal fixation) in 5. In the acute group, 17 limbs (89.4 %) had at least a good outcome, 16 of these limbs had an excellent result. Two limbs (10.6 %) had a poor result and required amputation. Both cases were after acute conversion to intramedullary nails; the original presenting diagnosis was of an infected non-union of the tibia and both had Paley scores above 7. In the delayed conversion group, all limbs (100 %) had at least a good outcome, with 4 limbs (80 %) having an excellent result. The mean external fixator time was 185 days (61–370). Both the cases with poor outcomes had longer external fixation times. This series supports the practice of conversion of external fixation to internal fixation with the majority of patients attaining good results. It identifies that plate devices appear to produce fewer deep sepsis complications, as compared to intramedullary nails, particularly when the original presenting diagnosis is a septic non-union.

Keywords External fixation · Internal fixation ·
Conversion · Limb reconstruction · Scoring system ·
Consolidation phase

Introduction

Despite the versatility of distraction osteogenesis in limb reconstruction surgery, prolonged external fixation is uncomfortable for the patient and has associated complications [1, 2, 8, 9, 14]. Methods to decrease frame time have been developed; these include lengthening over a nail [3, 4, 7, 11, 15] and lengthening with submuscular plating [5, 6, 12] from which patients have shown improved comfort and recovery of joint range of motion. The risk of combining external and internal fixation is deep infection. This is documented to be 3–15 % [11, 13]. There is no consensus as to which internal fixation method, when used after external fixation, leads to better results.

Rozbruch et al. [16] suggested that the reaming through the regenerate enhances bone healing but was concerned

T. Monni · P. de Lange · C. H. Snyckers
Steve Biko Academic Hospital, Pretoria, Gauteng, South Africa

T. Monni (✉) · P. de Lange · C. H. Snyckers
Department of Orthopaedics, University of Pretoria,
Pretoria, Gauteng, South Africa
e-mail: tonimonni@hotmail.com

F. F. Birkholtz
Private Practise, Netcare Unitas Hospital,
Pretoria, Gauteng, South Africa

over the infection risk with use of intramedullary nails. He felt it important to pay special attention to the placement of external fixator pins to avoid contact between the nail and the pin sites. His reported deep infection rate was 2.5 %. He went on to investigate the technique of lengthening then plating. He found a decreased frame time but no deep infections [17]. Uysal et al. [10] believed that both the endosteal and periosteal blood supplies are preserved with this technique. However, Rozbruch et al. [17] did note a high incidence of varus deformity.

The literature is limited on the subject of sequential use of internal fixation after external fixation in post-traumatic limb reconstruction and deformity correction. The technique would decrease frame time in the treatment for post-traumatic bone loss and non-unions as well as deformity corrections and prove valuable but has the risk for complications.

Materials and methods

This is a retrospective case series on 18 patients (24 limbs) who underwent sequential conversion from external to

internal fixation in the period 2007–2011. All patients who underwent distraction osteogenesis for traumatic bone loss, sepsis or for the correction of deformities and had internal fixation applied prior to union or regenerate consolidation were included. There were no specific exclusion criteria.

Patients were grouped according to the timing of conversion from external to internal fixation as well the type of internal fixation used. The following groups were defined:

1. The acute conversion group consisted of patients who underwent removal of the external fixator device and insertion of internal fixation at the same surgical procedure. The operation also consisted of debridement of the external fixation pin tracks and careful placement of the internal fixation device with care to avoid contact with the previous external fixation pin sites.

2. The delayed conversion group consisted of patients who underwent separate procedures for removal of external fixation and placement of the internal fixation device. Debridement of external fixation pin tracks was done during the first procedure. Stability in the interval between procedures was achieved by various

Table 1 Paley's level of difficulty score [4]

Points scored	0	1	2	3
Age	5–19	20–29, 0–4	30–50	>50
Complexity of correction of deformity at level of lengthening	None	Angulation >5° <20° Rotation >10° <30° Translation <50 % or change of mechanical axis 1–3 cm	Angulation ≥20° Rotation ≥30° Translation ≥50 % or change of mechanical axis >3 cm	Combination of deformities at one level or multilevel deformity
Other levels of treatment in same bone	None	1 Additional level, mild complexity	1 Additional level, moderate complexity	1 Additional level, severe complexity or ≥addition
Associated tibial lengthening (cm)	None	1–3	3.1–6	>6
Instability of joint	None	Grade I—mild instability: anteroposterior instability of knee with end point. Shenton's line not broken	Grade II—moderate instability: anteroposterior instability of knee without end point. Shenton's line broken but reducible	Grade III—fixed subluxation or dislocation
Fixed flexion deformity of knee (°)	0	1–5	6–20	>20
Flexion of knee (°)	>120	100–120	65–99	<65
Osteoarthrosis of joint	None	Marginal osteophytes, subchondral sclerosis	Narrowing of joint space	Loss of joint space (bone on bone)
Quality of bone	Normal	Ollier's disease, mild osteoporosis, non-union	Radiation, neurofibromatosis, osteogenesis imperfecta	Osteonecrosis, infection
Quality of soft tissue	Normal	Spastic, obese, muscular	Fibrotic, post-radiation, small open wound	Tissue necrosis, infection, large open wound
Medical problems and medications	None	Smoking, hypertension, rheumatoid arthritis or other systemic arthritis	Diabetes, haemophilia, sickle cell anaemia, mild immunosuppression, bone-inhibition medication	Moderate immunosuppression, anti-metabolic chemotherapy

Table 2 Patient data

Group	Case	Presenting problem	Management (ex-fix days)	Conversion (delay days)	Conversion	Outcome	Paley score
Plating delayed	1	Atrophic non-union humerus	TSF reconstruction (159)	TSF delay to ORIF (12)	Refracture, second debridement	Pin track sepsis	8
	3	Valgus deformity correction femur	TSF deformity correction (70)	TSF delay to ORIF (35)	Pin tracks infected debrided	Good	6
	4	Varus deformity correction femur	TSF deformity correction (70)	TSF delay to ORIF (35)		Good	6
	9	Septic non-union	Ilizarov, cement spacer, bone graft (238)	Ilizarov to ORIF (28)	Pin tracks curetted	Good	6
Plating acute	5	Lengthening femur defect 7 cm	Ilizarov—LRS lengthening (242)	LRS acute ORIF	Repeat debridement, bone graft and ORIF	Non-union	9
	6	Segmental fracture tibia mal/non-union	Ilizarov reconstruction (221)	Ilizarov to ORIF	Pin tracks excised	Good	7
	7	Bow leg deformity L	TSF and deformity correction (29)	TSF to ORIF	Pin tracks excised	Good	5
	8	Bow leg deformity R	TSF and deformity correction (29)	TSF to ORIF		Good	5
	11	Atrophic non-union femur	LRS, corticotomy, bone transport (266)	LRS to ORIF	Pin tracks excised	Good	6
	12	Non-union distal tibia	Ilizarov deformity correction (218)	Ilizarov to ORIF	Pin tracks curetted	Good	7
	15	Lengthening femur defect 5 cm	LRS, corticotomy (97)	LRS to ORIF	Distraction device	Good	6
	16	Lengthening femur defect 5 cm	LRS, corticotomy (91)	LRS to ORIF	Pin tracks excised	Good	6
	18	Bow leg deformity L	TSF and osteotomy deformity correction (33)	TSF to ORIF	Pin tracks curetted	Good	4
	19	Bow leg deformity R	TSF and osteotomy deformity correction (33)	TSF to ORIF	Pin tracks curetted	Good	4
	23	Segmental fracture tibia mal/non-union	TSF reconstruction	TSF to ORIF	Pin tracks curetted	Good	6
	24	Oligotrophic non-union tibia	TSF reconstruction	TSF to ORIF	Pin tracks curetted	Good	6
Nail delayed	14	Comminuted tibia fracture, distal 1/3	Ilizarov, corticotomy, lengthening (281)	Ilizarov to nail (4)	Pin tracks curetted	Good	6
Nail acute	2	GA III B tib fib, non-union, shortened 5 cm	TSF reconstruction and plastics (370)	TSF acute nail	Delayed amputation (142)	Amputation	9
	10	Septic non-union femur	LRS, corticotomy, bone transport (266)	LRS to nail	Bone transport 12 cm	Good	6
	13	Septic non-union distal tibia	Trulok, corticotomy, bone transport (126)	Trulok to nail	Pin tracks excised	Good	5
	17	Segmental tibial fracture	TSF reconstruction and plastics (90)	TSF acute nail	Pin tracks curetted	Good	5
	20	GA III B tibial fibula	TSF reconstruction and plastics (218)	TSF acute nail	Delayed amputation (93)	Amputation	7
	21	Open fracture radius	TSF reconstruction (61)	TSF acute nail	Pin tracks curetted	Good	5
	22	Open fracture ulna	TSF reconstruction (61)	TSF acute nail	Pin tracks curetted	Good	5

methods including traction, plaster of Paris and functional braces. This was individualized according to site and stability. This interval varied and the secondary procedure was performed when the surgeon deemed the pin tracks to be healed with no infection.

The internal fixation devices were either intramedullary nails or plates and screws.

An available scoring system to allow for sample description or classification was not identified. We chose to adopt Paley's level of difficulty score for femoral

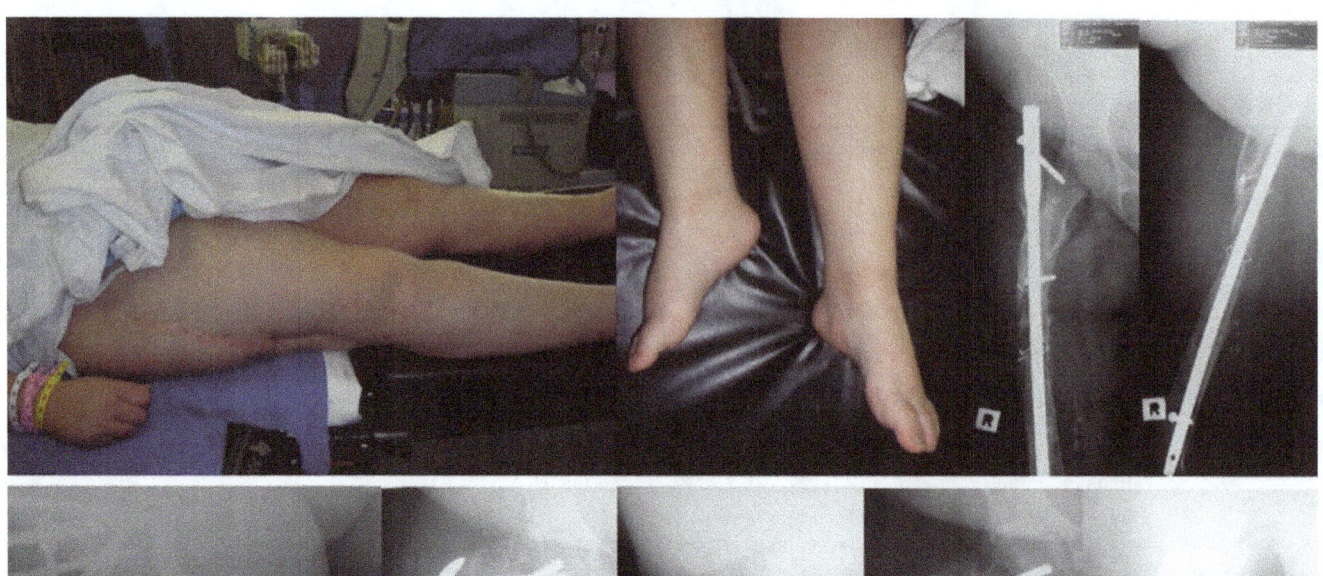

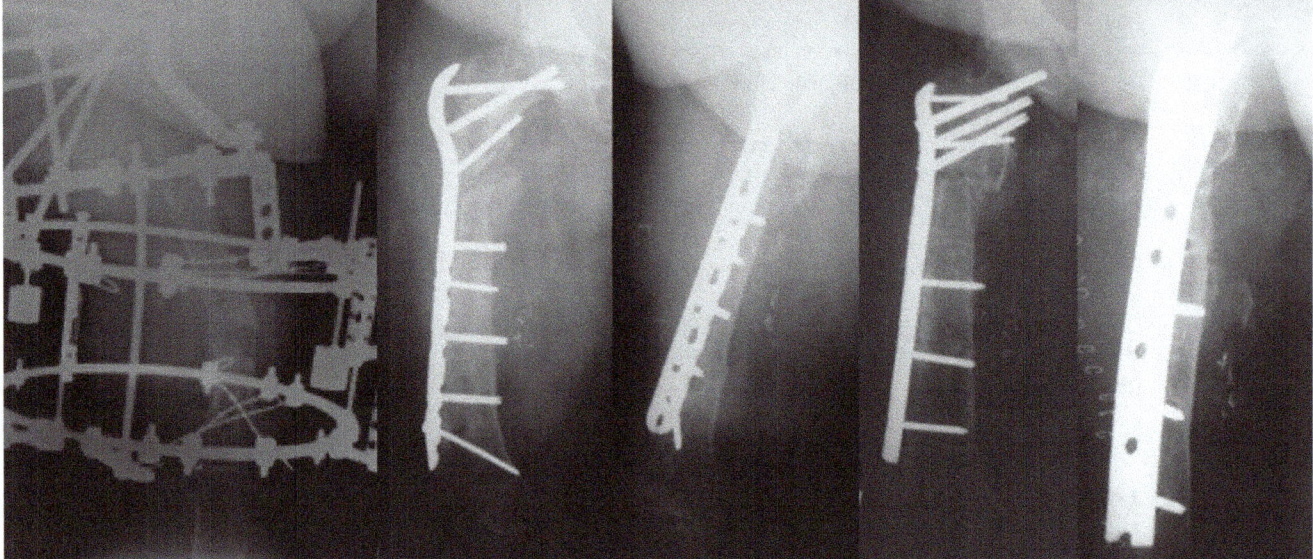

Fig. 1 A 31-year-old female presented with a subtrochanteric non-union and a 12-cm leg length discrepancy after 14 previous surgeries. This reconstruction (Paley's level of difficulty 9) required a second procedure (internal fixation and bone graft) to promote union after the initial conversion procedure (original frame time 242 days)

lengthening in which 11 variables are separately evaluated and include not only host and local factors but also the complexity of correction (Table 1).

This classifies the cases into 3 categories:

1. Mild; 0–6 points
2. Moderate; 7–11 points
3. Severe; >12 points

These scores were used to determine the level of difficulty of these cases as well as the possible relationship between a high score and complications. The outcome measure was based on a combination of function, alignment and need for further intervention: this is considered excellent if the patients were fully weight-bearing and pain-free on a mechanically aligned limb without need for further surgery; good if the patient required more surgery to achieve union; and poor if irreversible complications occurred.

No statistical analysis was performed as the numbers reported are small. Descriptive statistics are used.

Results

The mean age of the patients was 32 years (range 22–39). There were 11 males and 7 female patients. The aetiology was divided into 18 post-traumatic causes and 6 development-related abnormalities. Distraction osteogenesis was used for limb lengthening in 7 cases, for the reconstruction of bone defects or non-unions in 10 cases and for deformity corrections in 7 cases. Patient data are summarized in Table 2.

The reasons for conversion to internal fixation included dissatisfaction with the period in external fixation for 11 cases, persistent pin track infections in 8 cases, docking site-related problems in 4 cases and a refracture in one patient. The mean external fixator time was 185 days (61–370). Using the criteria described earlier, 20 limbs (83.3 %) had an excellent result, 2 patients had a good result (requiring further surgery to achieve union) and two with poor results (8.4 %).

Both patients with poor results had requested amputations for persistent painful septic non-unions. These cases had prolonged frame time (280–370 days) and had high scores using Paley's level of difficulty (7, 9) (Fig. 1).

Acute conversion was done in 19 limbs and delayed conversion in 5 of the 24 limbs. Although 17 limbs (89.4 %) in the acute conversion group had a good outcome (16 limbs of which with an excellent result), two limbs (10.6 %) had a poor result and required amputation. No deep infections were encountered in the acute conversion to plate fixation group. However, both amputations were after acute conversion to intramedullary nails after initial treatment for tibial septic non-unions. All cases in the delayed conversion group had a good outcome with the 4 limbs (80 %) having an excellent result. The number of cases in this group is small; the single delayed conversion to an intramedullary nail had no complications.

Discussion

This retrospective case series provides some support for the strategy of conversion from external to internal fixation. The number of complications was low, considering the severity of these cases, with an average Paley's level of difficulty score of 6 (moderate). Plate fixation had a lower complication rate in the acute conversion group in comparison with intramedullary nails. This concurs with the findings of Rozbruch et al. [16, 17]. These authors also encountered a higher infection rate with the use of intramedullary nailing following external fixation lengthening (LATN) when compared to plating following lengthening (LAP). Our two amputations in this case series suggest that acute conversion to an intramedullary nail should be avoided when converting an external fixator to internal fixation if the original problem was a septic non-union. As

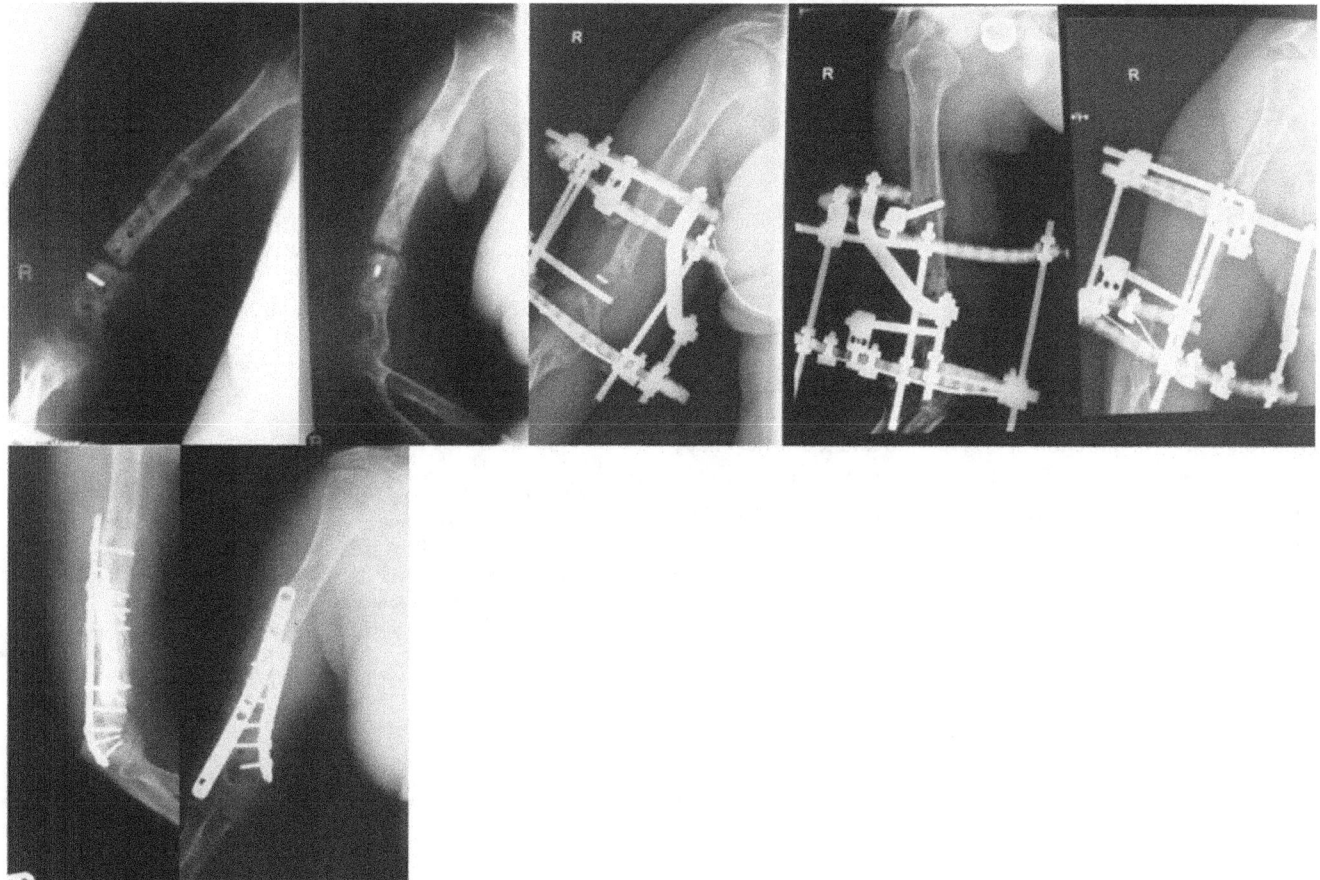

Fig. 2 A 41-year-old female presented with an atrophic non-union of the humerus (Paley's level of difficulty 8) which was managed with both Ilizarov and TSF frames (frame time 159 days) before being plated. The procedure was performed after a delay to allow secondary debridement for persistent pin track sepsis

to whether this risk is attenuated when there is a delay between fixator removal and nail introduction requires further study with a larger sample (Fig. 2).

Infection remains a problem during prolonged external fixation and is a risk when the method of fixation is changed to internal fixation. The average follow-up in this study was 20 months with a shorter minimum follow-up period; thus, the infection rates quoted in this case series have to be interpreted with some caution as occult sepsis may not be excluded conclusively. Another shortcoming in this study is that initial pin track infections prior to conversion were treated empirically and culture and sensitivity results unavailable. As both amputations were due to persistent infection, knowledge of pre- and post-conversion bacteriology may have provided further information in terms of risk factors and reasons for conversion failure.

The heterogeneity of patients in a reconstructive setting and the small sample in this case series makes it difficult to weigh the impact of medical comorbidities on outcome. We found the Paley level of difficulty score in femoral lengthening helpful as a system to quantify the additive nature of these negative effects. However, the system of scoring has to be validated further or be evolved to a more comprehensive limb reconstruction scoring system.

Conclusion

Complex reconstruction surgery on limbs based on the technique of distraction osteogenesis will entail prolonged periods of external fixation. There will be, due to the nature of complexity of cases, a need for conversion to internal fixation owing to reasons of patient non-compliance, failure to progress in treatment or persistent complications with continued use of the external fixator device. This series supports the practice of conversion and identifies that plate devices appear to produce fewer deep sepsis complications, particularly when the original presenting diagnosis is a septic non-union.

References

1. Paley D (1990) Problems, obstacles and complications of limb lengthening by the Ilizarov technique. Clin Orthop 250:81–104
2. Fischgrund J, Paley D, Suber C (1994) Variations affecting time to bone healing during bone lengthening. CORR 301:31–37
3. Kristiansen LP, Steen H (1990) Lengthening of the tibia over an intramedullary nail, using the Ilizarov external fixator: major complications and slow consolidation in 9 lengthenings. Acta Orthop Scand 70:271–274
4. Paley D, Herzenberg JE, Paremain G, Bhave A (1997) Femoral lengthening over an intramedullary nail: a matched-case comparison with Ilizarov lengthening. J Bone Joint Surg Am 79-A:1464–1480
5. Oh C, Kim J, Choi J, Min W, Park B (2009) Limb lengthening with a submuscular locking plate. J Bone Joint Sur Br 91-B:1394–1399
6. Iobst CA, Dahl MT (2007) Limb lengthening with submuscular plate stabilization: a case series and description of the technique. J Pediatr Orthop 27:504–509
7. Simpson AH, Cole AS, Kenwright J (1999) Leg lengthening over an intramedullary nail. J Bone Joint Surg Br 81:1041–1045
8. Maurer DJ, Merkow RL, Gustilo RB (1989) Infection after intramedullary nailing of severe open tibial fractures initially treated with external fixation. J Bone Joint Surg Am 71:835–838
9. Linh HB, Feibel RJ (2009) Tibial lengthening over an intramedullary nail. Tech Orthop 24:279–288
10. Uysal M, Akpinar S, Cesur N, Hersekli MA, Tandogan RN (2007) Plating after nailing: technical notes and preliminary clinical experiences. Arch Ortop Trauma Surg 127:889–893
11. Brewster MBS, Mauffrey C, Lewis AC, Hull P (2010) Lower limb lengthening: is there a difference in the lengthening index and infection rates of lengthening with external fixators, external fixators with intramedullary nails or intramedullary nailing alone? A systematic review of the literature. Eur J Orthop Surg Traumatol 20:103–108
12. Oh CW, Song HR, Kim JW, Choi JW, Min WK, Park BC (2009) Limb lengthening with a submuscular locking plate. JBJS Br 91-B:1394–1399
13. Sun XT, Easwar TR, Manesh S, Ryu JH, Song SH, Kim SJ, Song HR (2011) Complications and outcomes of tibial lengthening using the Ilizarov method with or without a supplementary nail. JBJS Br 93-B:782–787
14. Sabhawal S, Green S, McCarthy J, Hamby RC (2011) What's new in limb lengthening and deformity correction? JBJS Am 93-A:213–221
15. Kocaoglu M, Eralp L, Kilicoglu O, Burc H, Cakmak M (2004) Complications encountered during lengthening over an intramedullary nail. JBJS Am 86-A:2406–2411
16. Rozbruch S, Kleinman D (2008) Limb lengthening and then insertion of an intramedullary nail. CORR 466:2923–2932
17. Harbacheuski R, Fragomen A, Rozbruch S (2012) Does lengthening and then plating (LAP) shorten duration of external fixation? Clin Orthop Relat Res 470:1771–1781

2

Repositioning of the humeral tuberosities can be guided by pectoralis major insertion

Alec Cikes · Étienne Trudeau-Rivest ·
Fanny Canet · Jonah Hébert-Davies ·
Dominique M. Rouleau

Abstract In complex proximal humerus fractures, positioning of the tuberosities can be a challenge. This study demonstrates the constant angle between the pectoralis major (PM) and the medial lip of the bicipital groove (BG) on the horizontal axial plane. This angle can be used to determine the rotation, as well as the positioning of the tuberosities, when planning a hemiarthroplasty or a reconstruction. Thirty-one shoulder MRIs were reviewed by three independent observers. The measurements were taken by superposing the axial cut of the proximal humerus, at the level of the distal bicipital groove, and the cut at the top of the PM insertion. By aligning the centers of rotation, we could determine the arcs of rotation between the insertion of the PM and the lips of the medial and lateral bicipital groove (MBG and LBG). Both angles were compared in terms of reliability, reproducibility, and precision. The mean PM–MBG angle was 3.7° [standard deviation (SD) 14.7°] and 27.4° (SD 14.4°) for the PM–LBG angle. We obtained good and very good intra-class correlation coefficient (ICC) results for inter- (0.675) and intra-observer (0.793) reliabilities on the medial angle, plus excellent results for the lateral angle (inter-observers 0.962 and intra-observer 0.895). This study demonstrates that the repositioning of humeral tuberosities can be guided by pectoralis major insertion. This will help achieve proper positioning of the metaphysis in relation to the diaphysis during surgery for complex proximal humerus fractures.

Keywords Shoulder · Pectoralis major · Bicipital groove · MRI · Tuberosity · Proximal humerus fracture

Introduction

Proximal humerus anatomy varies substantially between individuals and even from side to side in the same individual [1]. Therefore, accurate knowledge of the osseous anatomy is very useful in the reconstruction of complex fractures [2]. Recent literature has identified standard values for tuberosity height in open reduction and internal fixation (ORIF) as well as implant height in shoulder arthroplasty [3–6]. While some recommend putting shoulder hemiarthroplasty in 20 degrees of retroversion for fractures [7], finding proper rotation in ORIF is challenging. While humerus rotation can be assessed reliably by computerized tomography (CT scan), as in this case of humeral malunion (Fig. 1), no intra-operative method is described.

Proximal humerus fractures are the third most frequent type of osteoporotic fractures [8], and surgical success depends on correct tuberosity positioning and healing [9]. Malposition of the tuberosities can lead to impingement and decreased range of motion [3, 9, 10]. As stated by Murray [11], establishing the rotation of metaphysis on the diaphysis is the last step of the reduction after controlling translation. There are two goals for reduction: The greater tuberosity height should be 5 mm lower than the top of the humeral head [12], and on the axial plane, both tuberosities

A. Cikes · É. Trudeau-Rivest · F. Canet · J. Hébert-Davies ·
D. M. Rouleau (✉)
Hôpital du Sacré-Cœur de Montréal (HSCM), 5400 Gouin
Ouest, Local C-2095, Montreal, QC H4J 1C5, Canada
e-mail: dominique_rouleau@yahoo.ca

A. Cikes
Synergie-Medical Center, Rue du Grand-Pré 2B, 1007 Lausanne,
Switzerland

É. Trudeau-Rivest · J. Hébert-Davies · D. M. Rouleau
University of Montreal, 2900 Boulevard Edouard-Montpetit,
Montreal, QC H3T 1J4, Canada

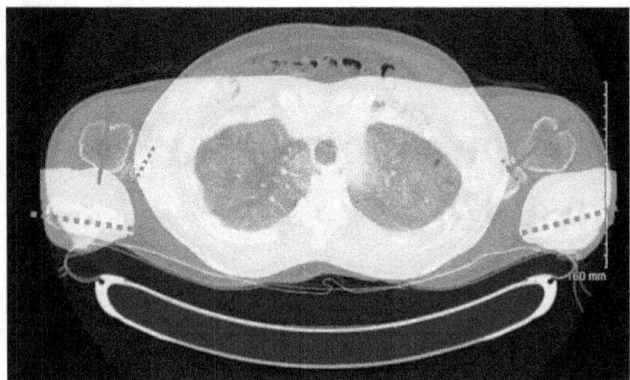

Fig. 1 Example of malposition of a humeral subcapital fracture leading to later glenohumeral osteoarthritis

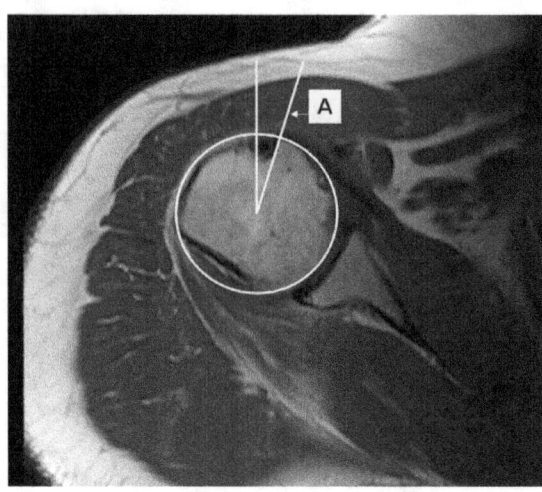

Fig. 2 Axial cut of the proximal humerus at the level of the distal bicipital groove. *Line A* is drawn from the center of rotation to the medial lip of the bicipital groove at the level of the inferior insertion of the subscapularis muscle

should have even heights and be on either side of the bicipital groove [13].

Our study's primary objective was to demonstrate the presence of a constant angle between the pectoralis major (PM) insertion on the humeral shaft and the bicipital groove (BG) in the axial plane. This angle could be used to determine the rotation and positioning of the tuberosities because even in Neer IV fractures, the fracture line between lesser and greater tuberosity rarely involves the bicipital grove [14, 15]. Two different angles will be compared: medial lip of the bicipital groove to PM insertion and lateral lip to PM insertion.

Our hypothesis is that the mean medial angle (PM–MBG) is less than 10 degrees, the lateral angle (PM–LBG) is greater than 10 degrees, and that these angles are reliable. The ideal landmark would present good inter- and intra-observer reliabilities, be the smallest possible, and show minimal variability.

Materials and methods

The protocol was as follows: A database of randomly selected shoulder magnetic resonance imaging (MRIs) was reviewed by a musculoskeletal radiologist to confirm inclusion–exclusion criteria and to identify those that included the entire pectoralis major insertion that was needed for the study. All skeletally mature patients with all types of pathologies not affecting the anatomy of the humerus were included, but all MRIs performed for proximal humerus fractures, pathologies of the pectoralis major, or any other abnormality affecting bony anatomy (previous surgery, infection, tumor or dysplasia) were excluded. Thirty MRIs were deemed necessary, following the recommendations by Harrison and et al. [16], and because no established values exist for the measurements needed (from the distal most level of the insertion of the subscapularis at

the distal bicipital groove and at the top of the PM insertion). There was no power study. Finally, all measurements were taken once, by three different observers, and they were then repeated in a separate setting by two of the three previously mentioned observers, blinded and in a different order, to evaluate intra-observer reliability.

Measurement criteria

Measurement was taken by superimposing two axial cuts of the proximal humerus: one at the distal most level of the insertion of the subscapularis at the distal bicipital groove, and one at the top of the PM insertion. The center of rotation for each cut was defined as the center of a fitted circle applied on the axial cut. Then, two lines were drawn: the first (line A) from the center of rotation to the medial lip of the bicipital groove (Fig. 2), and the second (line B) from the center of rotation to the medial aspect of the PM proximal insertion (Fig. 3). The angle formed by these two lines was measured (Fig. 4). This angle was named "the rotation arc between the pectoralis major and medial bicipital groove" (PM–MBG). Another angle was measured in the same fashion using the lateral lip as the reference line and was named PM–LBG. Both angles were compared in terms of reliability, reproducibility, and precision.

All measurements were taken using a specialized validated software (SliceOMatic, Tomovision, Magog, QC, Canada).

Statistics

Descriptive statistics were used to define the PM–MBG angle and PM–LBG angle. The Mann–Whitney test was

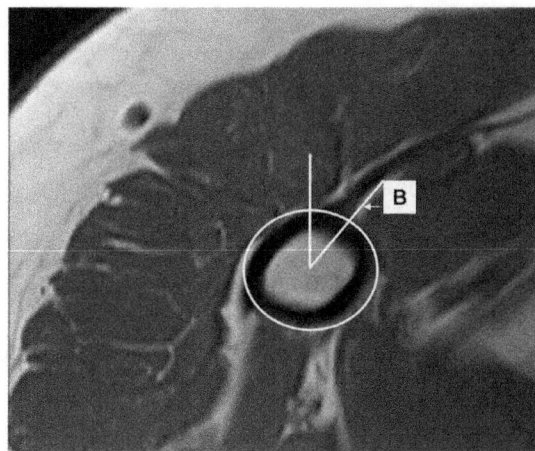

Fig. 3 Axial cut of the proximal humerus at the level of the top of the PM insertion. *Line B* is drawn from the center of rotation to the medial aspect of the PM proximal insertion

used to compare mean PM–BG angles between males and females as our groups contained less than 20 subjects. Inter- and intra-observer reliabilities were tested using intra-class correlation coefficient (ICC) with the following standard classification: ICC 0.61–0.75 = good, ICC 0.76–0.9 = very good, and ICC > 0.91 = excellent.

Results

A total of 31 MRIs were reviewed with a mean patient age of 54 years (25–86, SD 14).There were 15 males and 16 females, and the left shoulder was evaluated in 22 cases.

The mean PM–MBG angle was 3.7° (SD 14.7°), and the mean PM–LBG angle was 27.4° (SD 14.4°). The medial lip

of the biceps gutter was the closest to the pectoralis major insertion.

There was no statistically significant difference in the PM–MBG angles between males and females ($p > 0.3$) for all angles tested with the Mann–Whitney test. There was good inter-observer correlation and reliability for the medial angle with a mean ICC of 0.675 (range 0.368–0.846), and it was excellent for the lateral angle with an ICC of 0.962 (range 0.926–0.982) (Table 1). We also obtained very good intra-observer correlation and reliability, with ICC values of 0.897 and 0.793 for observers one and two (PM–MBG).

Discussion

Ideally, proximal humerus fractures are treated by anatomic reduction using fracture lines as reference points. However, achieving this can be particularly complicated in four-part fractures with comminution. After restoration of the proximal humerus, it can be hard to assess and restore humerus rotation: too much retroversion will decrease internal rotation and affect functionality. Inversely, creating too much anteversion will decrease external rotation. Figures 1 and 5 are examples of cases of secondary arthritis with malunion in excessive retroversion. Malrotation can also cause problems in the fixation of the proximal humerus as the plate should be just lateral to the bicipital groove to be able to lie distally between the pectoralis major insertion and deltoid insertion.

Tuberosity positioning after surgery of a proximal humeral fracture is the key to a good clinical outcome [14]. Final tuberosity malposition is correlated with unsatisfactory results such as superior migration of the prosthesis,

Fig. 4 Schematic representation of the superposition of both axial cuts with PM–MBG and PM–LBG angles

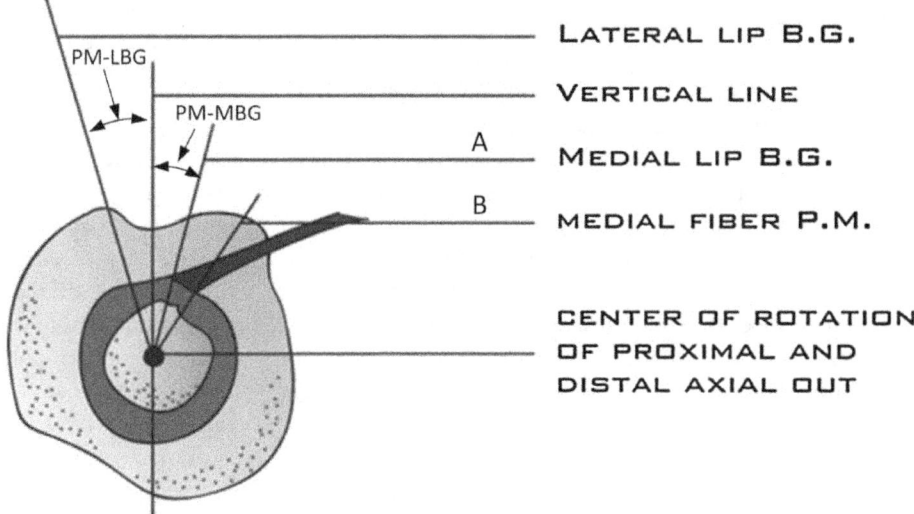

Table 1 Results—inter-observers and intra-observer ICCs for PMMBG and PMLBG measurements

Reliability	Evaluators	Angle	ICC (95 % CI)
Inter-observer	Evaluators 1, 2, 3	PMMBG	0.675 (0.368–0.846)
		PMLBG	0.962 (0.926–0.982)
Intra-observer	Evaluator 1	PMMBG	0.897 (0.895–0.899)
		PMLBG	0.895 (0.890–0.898)
	Evaluator 2	PMMBG	0.793 (0.570–0.900)
		PMLBG	0.898 (0.799–0.949)

ICC intra-class correlation, *CI* confidence interval

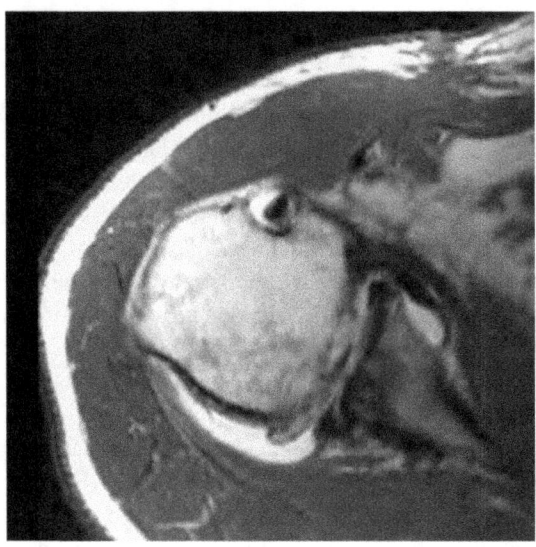

Fig. 5 Secondary osteoarthritis in a case of severe malrotation

stiffness, weakness, and chronic pain [9]. Furthermore, tuberosity malposition and migration is linked with poor functional results because of the modified lever arm of glenohumeral abduction [17, 18].

The purpose of this study was to identify the presence of a reliable angle between the pectoralis major (PM) insertion on the humeral shaft and the bicipital groove (BG). Our results confirm that the medial aspect of the bicipital gutter is relatively parallel with the insertion of the pectoralis major proximal insertion. While it is a reliable measurement, the lateral edge should not be used to guide rotation because it is not in line with the tendon insertion. While there is a certain amount of variability, it is important to remember that the precision of angle measurements on MRI is much greater than on actual bone. Because an MRI allows more precise measurements, it thus gives a value of what the rotation should be and a fair estimate for the surgeon intra-operatively.

Therefore, we recognize that our study might not describe a perfect measurement method for MRI

evaluation; however, we feel that this angle (PM–BMG) is useful intra-operatively for evaluating rotation. While a previous study exists evaluating rotator cuff insertions for tuberosity reduction, questions can be raised about its reproducibility [3]. Both the bicipital groove and the pectoralis major tendon are easily identifiable in open shoulder surgery and are thus ideal candidates for anatomic landmarks. Our measurements showed both good inter- and intra-observer reliabilities, demonstrating that this angle (PM–BMG) is reliable. This landmark is particularly useful in complex and comminutive fractures such as a fracture dislocation or a Neer IV fracture that are classically treated by open deltopectoral approach.

By using this anatomic marker, malposition could be avoided. Using these findings and others previously described [11], we can now devise an evidence-based protocol for the reduction in fragments in Neer IV complex proximal humeral fracture (three- and four-part fractures) in cases of open reduction and internal fixation (ORIF):

1. Exposing the humeral head by tuberosity mobilization and rotator interval opening.
2. Restoring the humeral head to 20 degrees [6] retroversion and 130 degrees of neck angle, with temporary fixation of the head to the glenoid with small smooth K-wires.
3. Reducing the tuberosities around the humeral head (the rotation will be determined by rotator cuff tensioning) [9].
4. The GT needs to be 5 mm lower than the humeral head [12].
5. The height of the humeral head is then adjusted 5.5 cm [19] from the pectoralis major proximal fiber with temporary wire and sutures.
6. Finally, the rotation of the proximal humerus in relation to the diaphysis is corrected to adjust the medial bicipital gutter to the medial insertion of pectoralis major fibers.
7. Definitive fixation of fragments is performed.

Conclusion

Our study demonstrated that, in normal shoulders, the medial edge of the bicipital groove is relatively parallel to the insertion of the pectoralis major tendon. These two easily identifiable bony landmarks can then be used to evaluate rotation during osteosynthesis even in very severe fractures. Further studies are needed to determine whether this method is as applicable as we believe it to be in an operative setting. Nevertheless, it remains a useful adjunct for surgeons performing ORIF on complex proximal humerus fractures.

Acknowledgments No financial support was received for this study. We thank Dr. Danielle Bédard, Radiologist.

References

1. DeLude JA, Bicknell RT, MacKenzie GA, Ferreira LM, Dunning CE, King GJ et al (2007) An anthropometric study of the bilateral anatomy of the humerus. J Shoulder Elbow Surg 16:477–483
2. Neer CS 2nd (1970) Displaced proximal humeral fractures. I. Classification and evaluation. J Bone Joint Surg Am 52:1077–1089
3. Hromadka R, Kubena AA, Pokorny D, Popelka S, Jahoda D, Sosna A (2010) Attachments of muscles as landmarks for implantation of shoulder hemiarthroplasty in fractures. J Shoulder Elbow Surg 19:130–136. doi:10.1016/j.jse.2009.03.023
4. Kontakis GM, Damilakis J, Christoforakis J, Papadakis A, Katonis P, Prassopoulos P (2001) The bicipital groove as a landmark for orientation of the humeral prosthesis in cases of fracture. J Shoulder Elbow Surg 10:136–139
5. Hempfing A, Leunig M, Ballmer FT, Hertel R (2001) Surgical landmarks to determine humeral head retrotorsion for hemiarthroplasty in fractures. J Shoulder Elbow Surg 10:460–463
6. Angibaud L, Zuckerman JD, Flurin PH, Roche C, Wright T (2007) Reconstructing proximal humeral fractures using the bicipital groove as a landmark. Clin Orthop Relat Res 458:168–174
7. Balg F, Boulianne M, Boileau P (2006) Bicipital groove orientation: considerations for the retroversion of a prosthesis in fractures of the proximal humerus. J Shoulder Elbow Surg 15:195–198
8. Hirzinger C, Tauber M, Resch H (2011) Proximal humerus fracture: new aspects in epidemiology, fracture morphology, and diagnostics. Unfallchirurg 114:1051–1058. doi:10.1007/s00113-011-2052-4
9. Boileau P, Krishnan SG, Tinsi L, Walch G, Coste JS, Mole D (2002) Tuberosity malposition and migration: reasons for poor outcomes after hemiarthroplasty for displaced fractures of the proximal humerus. J Shoulder Elbow Surg 11:401–412
10. Krishnan SG, Bennion PW, Reineck JR, Burkhead WZ (2008) Hemiarthroplasty for proximal humeral fracture: restoration of the Gothic arch. Orthop Clin North Am 39:441–450, vi. doi:10.1016/j.ocl.2008.05.004
11. Murray IR, Amin AK, White TO, Robinson CM (2011) Proximal humeral fractures: current concepts in classification, treatment and outcomes. J Bone Joint Surg Br 93:1–11. doi:10.1302/0301-620X.93B1.25702
12. Takase K, Imakiire A, Burkhead WZ Jr (2002) Radiographic study of the anatomic relationships of the greater tuberosity. J Shoulder Elbow Surg 11:557–561
13. Huffman GR, Itamura JM, McGarry MH, Duong L, Gililland J, Tibone JE et al (2008) Neer Award 2006: biomechanical assessment of inferior tuberosity placement during hemiarthroplasty for four-part proximal humeral fractures. J Shoulder Elbow Surg 17:189–196. doi:10.1016/j.jse.2007.06.017
14. Foruria AM, de Gracia MM, Larson DR, Munuera L, Sanchez-Sotelo J (2011) The pattern of the fracture and displacement of the fragments predict the outcome in proximal humeral fractures. J Bone Joint Surg Br 93:378–386. doi:10.1302/0301-620X.93B3.25083
15. Tamai K, Ishige N, Kuroda S, Ohno W, Itoh H, Hashiguchi H et al (2009) Four-segment classification of proximal humeral fractures revisited: a multicenter study on 509 cases. J Shoulder Elbow Surg 18:845–850. doi:10.1016/j.jse.2009.01.018
16. Harrison DE, Harrison DD, Cailliet R, Janik TJ, Holland B (2001) Radiographic analysis of lumbar lordosis: centroid, Cobb, Trall, and Harrison posterior tangent methods. Spine 26:E235–E242
17. Rietveld AB, Daanen HA, Rozing PM, Obermann WR (1988) The lever arm in glenohumeral abduction after hemiarthroplasty. J Bone Joint Surg Br 70:561–565
18. Boileau P, Walch G (1999) Shoulder arthroplasty for fractures: problems and solutions. In: Springer (ed) Shoulder arthroplasty. Springer, Heidelberg, pp 297–314
19. Torrens C, Corrales M, Melendo E, Solano A, Rodriguez-Baeza A, Caceres E (2008) The pectoralis major tendon as a reference for restoring humeral length and retroversion with hemiarthroplasty for fracture. J Shoulder Elbow Surg 17:947–950. doi:10.1016/j.jse.2008.05.041

3

Femoral supracondylar focal dome osteotomy with plate fixation for acute correction of frontal plane knee deformity

Sherif Ahmed El Ghazaly[1] · El-Hussein Mohamed El-Moatasem[1]

Abstract Focal dome osteotomy (FDO) allows deformity correction without secondary translational deformity. The purpose of this study was to evaluate the degree of correction and knee functional outcome after correction of frontal knee deformity using femoral supracondylar FDO fixed with plate and screws. A prospective study included 12 consecutive cases of femoral frontal plane deformity that underwent correction using supracondylar focal osteotomy fixed by plate and screws. Average age was 27 years, while mean follow-up was 2.1 years. Functional assessment was done using the Hospital for Special Surgery (HSS) knee score. The HSS knee score improved from 85 to 96.8 points. Desired correction was achieved in all cases. Postoperative mechanical axis analysis on long film and scanogram showed no secondary deformity. The overall postoperative mechanical axis was at 3.2 mm medially (range 2–5 mm). Autogenous bone graft was not used in any case, and uneventful osteotomy union was achieved at a mean of 13.8 weeks. Minor complications were encountered in two cases. There were no implant failures or reoperations. Supracondylar FDO of the femur with plate fixation is a reproducible technique that can produce full correction of distal femoral frontal plane deformity, while avoiding creating a secondary deformity. Knee function was improved with good patient satisfaction.

Keywords Knee valgus · Varus knee · Frontal knee deformity · Focal osteotomy · Femoral osteotomy · Dome osteotomy

✉ Sherif Ahmed El Ghazaly
sherifghazaly@hotmail.com;
sherif_ghazaly@med.asu.edu.eg

[1] Orthopedic Department, Al-Demerdash Hospital, Ain Shams University, Abbassia Square, Abbassia, 11381 Cairo, Egypt

Introduction

Frontal plane knee deformity may be idiopathic or secondary to trauma or osteomalacia. Tibio-femoral premature arthritis can occur from single compartment loading with patellofemoral arthritis in valgus knees. An angular correction by wedge corrective osteotomy is the standard treatment. Some drawbacks of the wedge osteotomy are limb length discrepancy, a mismatch of fragment ends created by osteotomy and the need for translation of the distal fragment. Circular bone cuts allow deformity correction without introducing a length discrepancy, mismatch or need for segment translation. A dome osteotomy (DO) is a cylindrical osteotomy [1, 2], with the corresponding bone cuts rotating around the central axis of the cylinder [3]. No bone is resected, and this avoids a length discrepancy. Brackett [4] described a dome osteotomy of the proximal femur to treat an ununited fracture of the femoral neck. A focal dome osteotomy (FDO) allows deformity correction while avoiding the need to produce a translation at the osteotomy in order to realign the proximal and distal axes [2, 3, 5]. We hypothesized that a FDO and plate fixation may be used in the distal femur to ensure full deformity correction without a secondary deformity and with maximal contact at the osteotomy, which allows improved healing and function.

Materials and methods

From July 2010 until December 2012, a prospective observational study was conducted of 12 cases on frontal knee deformity treated using a supracondylar FDO. Inclusion criteria were frontal plane deformity causing mechanical axis deviation, mechanical lateral distal femoral angle (mLDFA) below 84° or above 95° (Fig. 1), normal

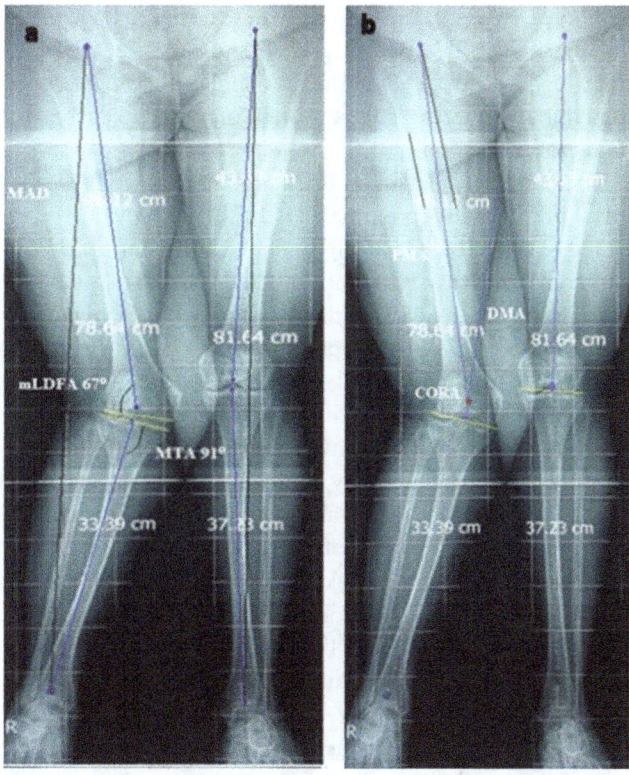

Fig. 1 a Preoperative planning (case 2) showing lateral mechanical axis deviation with normal mMPTA 91° and mLDFA 67° so the patient had genu valgum of femoral origin; **b** CORA was determined by intersection of the proximal mechanical axis (PMA) (a line 7° valgus to the anatomical axis, extending from the centre of the hip) and the distal mechanical axis (DMA), which was measured at a mLDFA of 88° (the contralateral knee was taken as the normal)

medial proximal tibial angle (MPTA) and anterior knee pain (retropatellar and/or joint line). Cases with combined femoral and tibial deformity were excluded.

There were seven males and five females with average age 27 years (range 16–38). The study was reviewed and approved by the university ethical committee. All patients gave their informed consent. There were nine valgus knees and three varus knee deformities with five knees showing radiological evidence of arthritis. Causes of deformity were traumatic (four), idiopathic (six) and osteomalacia (two cases).

Preoperative planning

All patients had antero-posterior long-limb films and a CT scanogram. Mechanical femoro-tibial angle (mFTA) was measured on long-limb films, while scanograms were used to confirm mechanical axis deviation (MAD) using the mal-alignment test and to define the magnitude of deviation. MAD was measured in millimetres from the knee centre. For every patient, the magnitude of femoral deformity was defined via the mLDFA, while the centre of rotation of angulation (CORA) was radiologically defined (Fig. 1). The preoperative MAD ranged from 86 mm lateral to 20 mm medial. The average preoperative mFTA was 18.5° in cases of valgus deformity and 18° in varus cases. The average angular deformity was 11.5° (range 8–19) and mLDFA 75.2° (range 67°–82°) in valgus cases; 25° (range 24°–26°) and mLDFA 102° (range 100°–104°) in varus cases (Table 1).

Table 1 Demographic, preoperative and postoperative alignment data for all patients

No.	Varus/valgus	Age	Sex	m F-T angle preop	m F-T angle postop	Deformity angle	Angle corrected	Preop mLDFA	Postop mLDFA	Preop MAD	Postop MAD
1	Val	16	M	15	5	8	10	82	93	+48 mm	−3 mm
2	Val	30	F	26	6	19	20	67	87	+86 mm	−2 mm
3	Val	32	M	18	7	11	11	76	91	+54 mm	−5 mm
4	Var	38	M	18	6	25	24	102	94	−20 mm	−3 mm
5	Val	17	F	15	5	8	10	79	93	+49 mm	−3 mm
6	Val	32	F	18	5	11	13	75	94	+56 mm	−4 mm
7	Val	35	M	19	7	12	12	77	91	+54 mm	−3 mm
8	Var	28	M	17	5	24	22	100	93	−19 mm	−3 mm
9	Val	34	M	21	6	14	15	72	90	+56 mm	−4 mm
10	Var	24	F	19	4	26	23	104	93	−20 mm	−3 mm
11	Val	22	M	17	5	10	12	75	93	+55 mm	−3 mm
12	Val	21	F	18	6	11	12	74	88	+53 mm	−2 mm
Mean	–	27 (16–38)	M:7	Val:18.5	Val:5.75	Val: 11.5	Val: 12.77	Val:75.2	Val:91	Val:56.75	Val:3.25
			F:5	Var:18	Var:5	Var:25	Var:23	Var:102	Var:94	Var:20	Var:3

Operative procedure

Patients received general anaesthesia and were operated in the supine position. A second generation cephalosporin was given at induction. A pneumatic tourniquet was applied and inflated to 350 mmHg. The C-arm was positioned in order to obtain a clear view of the distal half of the femur. Two markers were placed at the mid-inguinal point corresponding to the femoral pulse and at the mid-ankle position. Using a 15- to 20-cm lateral incision and posterolateral approach, the vastus lateralis was elevated from the lateral intermuscular septum. The lateral and anterior femoral cortices in the supracondylar area were exposed. A blunt-tipped Hohmann retractor was placed medially exposing the anteromedial cortex, and a second wide retractor was placed subperiosteally posterior to the distal femur to protect the vascular bundle (Fig. 2). At the selected site (metaphyseal area, 1 finger breadth above the medial femoral condyle), a circular line was drawn using electrocautery. A 2.5-mm drill bit and drill sleeve were used to create drill holes along the circular line, just penetrating the posterior cortex. The holes were created close to each other to ensure a smooth circular shape. The osteotomy was convex superior, creating a FDO (Fig. 2a). A ¼ in. osteotome was then used to connect the

drill holes, except at the corners, where a curved bone gauge was used (Fig. 2b). Before completing the osteotomy, the plate to be used for fixation (7–8 holes femoral buttress condylar or humeral "T" plate) was contoured to the desired degree of correction.

The plate was placed on the lateral cortex, and two drill holes immediately proximal to the osteotomy site were drilled and tapped. Carefully under C-arm control, a ½ in. osteotome was used to finalize the osteotomy medially, taking care not to advance the osteotome too far medial or too far posterior. With the plate in position and fixed with two screws, the osteotomy was completed slowly by osteoclasis. The leg was manipulated into varus or valgus according to initial deformity, until the knee joint line was horizontal and the deformity clinically corrected. The distal femoral fragment rotated along the osteotomy and was aligned under the plate. Deformity correction and overall limb alignment were checked under C-arm; an electrocautery cord was placed from the femoral head marker to the mid-ankle marker, and the knee was viewed to ensure that this line was brought in the knee centre or just lateral to the medial tibial spine. According to plate type, plate fixation was completed using 2–3 fully threaded cancellous screws (Figs. 2d, 3).

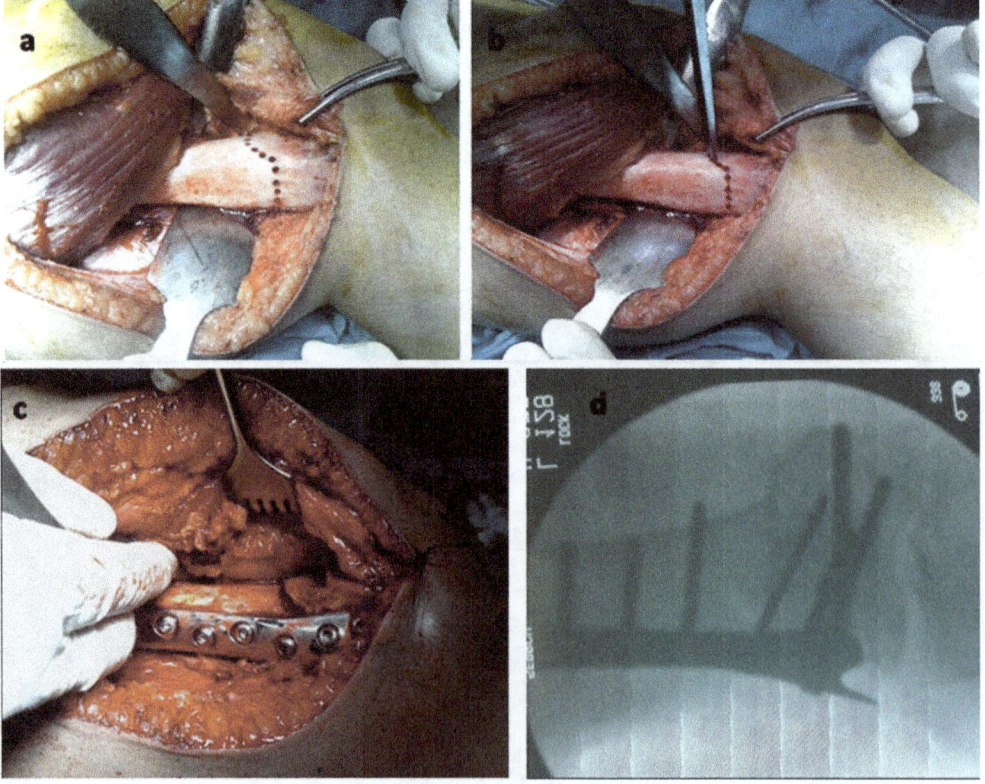

Fig. 2 **a** Intraoperative photo showing exposure of the supracondylar region of the femur and drilling of the planned dome osteotomy; **b** intraoperative photo showing connecting the predrilled holes using the osteotome; **c** intraoperative photo showing correction of deformity and plate and screw fixation; **d** intraoperative fluoroscopy showing correction of deformity, minimal translation and plating

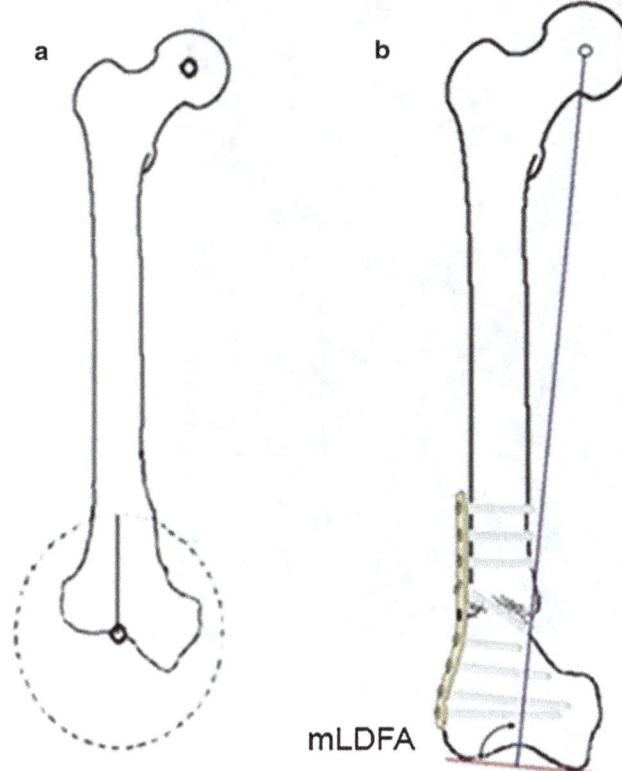

mLDFA

Fig. 3 **a** Schematic drawing showing the CORA-based planning of focal dome osteotomy; **b** drawing showing correction of deformity using focal dome osteotomy, minimal translation and plating with one screw transfixing the osteotomy

All patients followed the same rehabilitation protocol: gradual progress of return of knee range of motion and function by knee flexion and extension and quadriceps exercises beginning from third postoperative day. Ambulation was allowed using two axillary crutches, but no weight-bearing was permitted for the first 3 weeks. This was followed by toe-touch walking for 2 weeks, and at 5 weeks, one axillary crutch was used for the next month with gradual transition to full weight-bearing.

Results

The average follow-up was 2.1 years (range 1.6–2.5) years with regular monthly follow-ups. The patients were assessed using the Hospital for Special Surgery (HSS) knee score preoperatively, at 6 months and at final follow-up. Data were collected regularly into a special data collection sheet, entered into a computer for analysis and presented in the form of mean and ranges.

All osteotomies united uneventfully (Fig. 4). The mean time to union was 13.8 weeks (range 12–16). The preoperative limb malalignment was corrected, and the desired correction was achieved in all cases (Fig. 5). The average angular correction for valgus deformities was 12.77° (range 10°–20°) and 23° (range 22°–24°) for varus deformities. In valgus deformities, the mechanical axis improved from an average preoperative value of 56.75 mm laterally to an average of 3.25 mm medially; the improvement for varus deformities was from 20 mm medially to 3 mm. The overall postoperative mechanical axis was at 3.2 mm medial to the centre of the knee (range 2–5 mm). Postoperatively, the mean mLDFA was 91° in valgus cases and 94° in varus cases (Table 1).

The mean preoperative HSS score was 85, and this improved to 96.8 at final follow-up. Patients were satisfied with the procedure. Two complications are reported: a case of superficial wound infection which improved on oral antibiotics and one patient complaining of local irritation of the iliotibial band over the end of a buttress condylar plate. This patient used warm packs and anti-inflammatory

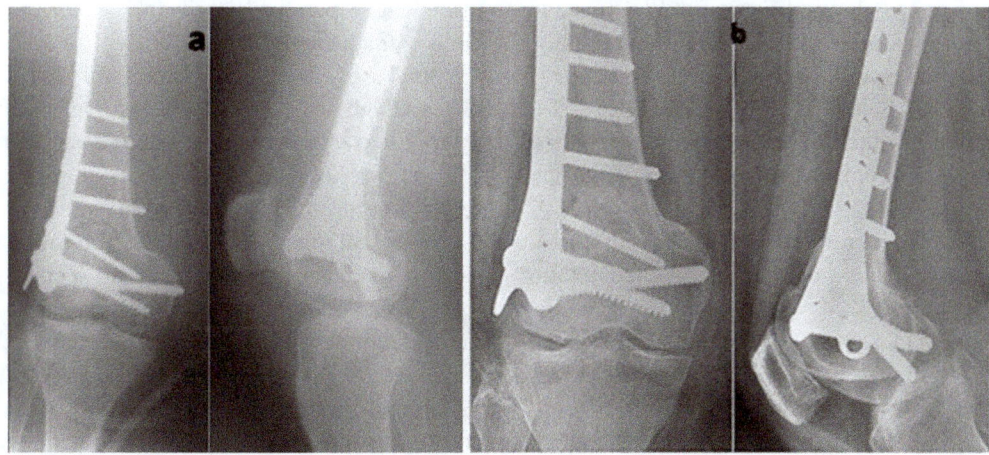

Fig. 4 **a** X-ray of the distal femur showing full correction of deformity and plating. This patient had osteoarthritis; **b** X-ray 6 months postoperative showing full union

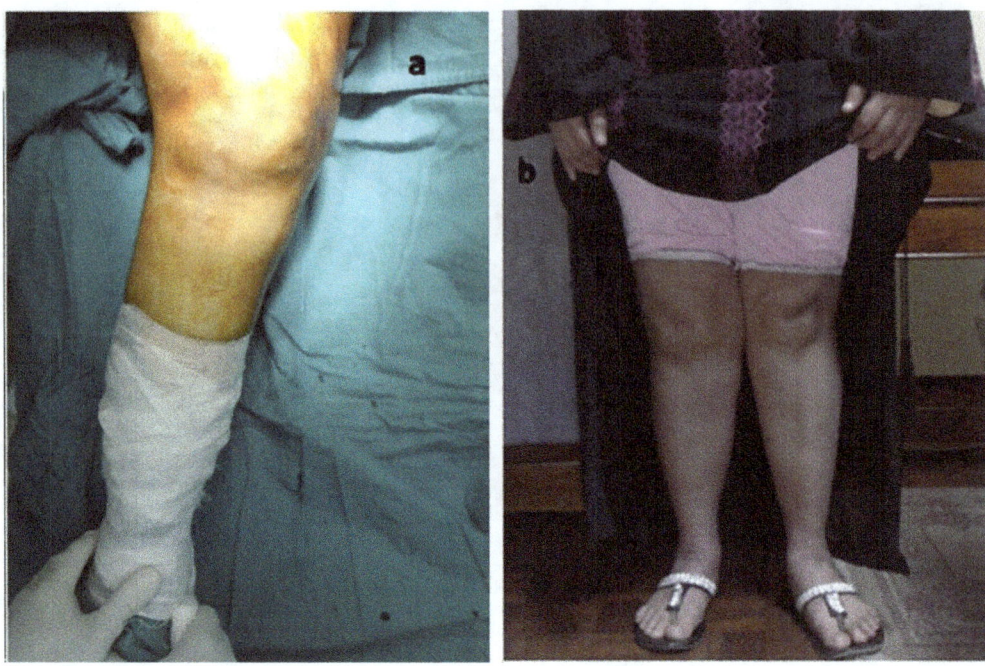

Fig. 5 a Intraoperative photo showing severe genu valgum before correction; **b** clinical photo of the same case, 19 months later, showing full correction

medication until plate removal. There were no cases of implant failure, and no cases required secondary intervention for union of the osteotomy.

Discussion

Realignment osteotomy aims to correct limb alignment and may influence knee osteoarthritis [6]. Assessment of overall limb alignment was with the mechanical axis, while realignment of the knee was judged through correction of the joint orientation line. Deformity correction in the coronal plane may be achieved using wedge osteotomy or the DO [7]. According to Paley and Tetsworth [8, 9], DO is a cylindrical osteotomy with corresponding bone cuts, which rotate around the central axis of a circle. When this central axis corresponds with the CORA, this is called a FDO and correction of the deformity can be attained without translation of the bone axes [8, 9]. In our series, the preoperative radiographic planning showed the CORA to be at the knee joint or femoral condyle level in all cases. Using this CORA as the centre of a circle, the planned arc upon which the DO was created was based on the centre of this circle ensuring a FDO. Full correction was attained with minimal translation of the distal bone fragment (Fig. 3). Only cases with isolated femoral deformity were included for this observational series.

The dome osteotomy was chosen instead of a wedge osteotomy to avoid limb shortening in closing wedge

corrections or a delayed union with more restrictive weight-bearing in opening wedge corrections (absent bone contact). The DO provides a large surface and maximizes bone contact, thereby ensuring optimal healing. Multiple drill holes followed by a low-energy osteotomy produces small bone spikes that interdigitate at the osteotomy after acute deformity correction; this can be compressed for added stability, reducing segment motion during osteotomy fixation and reducing the stress on the plate and screws. This caters for early partial weight-bearing, which was started at 3 weeks.

The DO allows high degrees of correction in the coronal plane. This was seen at preoperative planning and confirmed intraoperatively and on postoperative radiographs. Unlike Gugenheim and Brinker [6] who fixed the osteotomy using a retrograde femoral nail, we chose to use plates which are easily contoured. Deformity correction of up to 20° was accomplished with ease, and the osteotomy site remodelling resulted in an absence of secondary femoral deformity, which facilitates arthroplasty later.

Some authors describe an antero-medial approach, separating the vastus medialis and a medial knee arthrotomy [10]. We prefer the lateral approach as being more familiar and allows for an iliotibial band release, which is usually tight in valgus knees. The DO is technically demanding as performing the osteotomy as an arc needs care and precision to maintain the circular contour to ensure perfect segment rotation and bone contact and avoid inadvertent propagation. Gugenheim and Brinker [6] have described a percutaneous technique. We chose an open technique, which facilitates precision under direct vision and simpler plate fixation. Fixation of supracondylar osteotomies has been described using angled blade-plates, angle-stable plates or intramedullary nails [7, 11]. Wang and Hsu [12] chose to fix the osteotomy with a 90° angled blade-plate. We used a buttress condylar plate or "T" plate, avoiding the cost of more expensive or modern implants while retaining the ability to contour the plate (before osteotomy) to reach the desired correction. In adolescents, the antero-posterior dimensions of the distal femur are not large enough to place a condylar buttress plate, but we found the "T" plate suitable for fixation. Placing three screws in the distal segment and one transfixing, the osteotomy gave sufficient stability until osteotomy union. We found a transfixing screw important for all cases and provided the added stability as described by Wang and Hsu [12]. The "T" plate is a relatively weak implant in comparison with the condylar buttress plate, but we found it performed well for the selected cases and did not encounter implant failure.

Alternative techniques involve a lateral incomplete open-wedge osteotomy with use of spacer plates [7]. Some limitation of deformity correction is encountered by the limited ability to open a large wedge without need for bone grafts; this is in contrast to the greater versatility and rotational capacity of dome osteotomy.

We have used this technique to correct a coronal knee deformity in two patients near skeletal maturity with the average age 16.5 years unlike the work by Gugenheim and Brinker [6] who were not able to use their technique for skeletally immature patients. In one case (aged 16 years), the T plate was placed proximally such that no screws crossed the physis. In the other case (17 years), the plate was placed in the usual position and the screws distal to the osteotomy passed across the physis in effect fusing it.

In contrast to previous studies where the osteotomy was fixed using an external fixator [5], we have used plates and screws to avoid tethering of the quadriceps, pin track infections, loosening and the use of a cumbersome device. In a comparative study of internal versus external fixation for distal femoral osteotomies, Seah et al. [13] found no significant differences and concluded that the fixation method should be left to the discretion of the surgeon. This work coincides with the work of Wang and Hsu who used 90° blade-plates and screws for osteotomy fixation; the use of femoral condylar buttress or "T" plates is, in our view, easier and requires a less difficult after-care period.

Watanabe et al. [5] have stated that a DO with internal fixation cannot correct angulation precisely due to a difference in the centres of the deformity and that of the osteotomy. The current work has shown that, using the CORA method, executing a FDO for an epiphyseal CORA

and realigning the mechanical axis to the knee centre can achieve deformity correction even when fixed using plate and screws.

Wang and Hsu [12] have reported an improvement in patellar tracking in patients with severe patellofemoral arthritis, which persisted to the time of the latest follow-up. Patellar tracking is improved because this corrective osteotomy effectively reduces the "Q" angle. To ensure proper patellar tracking after such osteotomy, it is important to avoid internal rotation of the distal femoral segment. The patients in this series noted an improvement in anterior knee pain.

The most common complications following corrective angular osteotomies are non-union and failure of fixation [12]. To achieve union, good bone apposition and stable fixation are required [12]. In our series, the use of plate and screws provided the required rigid fixation and allowed full union. We found no technique-related complications or peroneal neuropathy even after correction of high degrees of valgus deformity (>25°), in accordance with work by Gugenheim and Brinker [6], while Watanabe et al. [5] reported one case of transient peroneal neuropathy. Occasionally, mild under-correction may occur if careful planning and execution of surgical steps are not followed. This is in accordance with work by Gugenheim and Brinker [6], who reported no complications other than a single non-union and a single case of under-correction.

The limitations to this study are the small number of cases, and it is an observational study. There is no comparative cohort. Future studies involving a larger numbers of cases and those comparing the use of plates with an external fixator may be useful.

Conclusion

This work shows that an acute angular correction of a distal femoral deformity by FDO, via a postero-lateral approach, can be used to correct either a varus or valgus knee deformity. This is achieved without muscle violation and has the added benefit of using a standard plate and screw fixation device, which is available in most hospitals worldwide. Rigid plate fixation and the absence of muscle division allow for an accelerated rehabilitation programme with early restoration of knee motion and function.

References

1. Hankemeier S, Paley D, Pape HC, Zeichen J, Gosling T, Krettek C (2004) Knee para-articular focal dome osteotomy. Orthopade 33(2):170–177
2. Paley D (2002) Osteotomy concepts and frontal plane realignment. In: Herzenberg JE (ed) Principles of deformity correction, 1st edn. Springer, Berlin, p 112

3. Paley D (2002) Hardware and osteotomy considerations. In: Herzenberg JE (ed) Principles of deformity correction, 1st edn. Springer, Berlin, p 300

4. Sundaram NA, Hallett JP, Sullivan MF (1986) Dome osteotomy of the tibia for osteoarthritis of the knee. J Bone Joint Surg (Br) 68(5):782–786

5. Watanabe K, Tsuchiya H, Sakurakichi K, Matsubara H, Tomita K (2008) Acute correction using focal dome osteotomy for deformity about knee joint. Arch Orthop Traum Surg 128(12):1373–1378

6. Gugenheim JJ, Brinker MR (2003) Bone realignment with use of temporary external fixation for distal femoral valgus and varus deformities. J Bone Joint Surg 85-A(7):1229–1237

7. Heervarden RJV, Wymenga AB, Freiling D, Staubli AE (2008) Indications-planning-surgical techniques using plate fixators. In: Lobenhoffer P, Heervarden RJV, Staubli AE, Jakob RP (eds) Osteotomies around the knee, 1st edn. Thieme Medical Publishers, New York, p 147

8. Paley D, Tetsworth K (1992) Mechanical axis deviation of the lower limbs: preoperative planning of uniapical angular deformities of the tibia or femur. Clin Orthop 280:48–64

9. Paley D, Tetsworth K (1992) Mechanical axis deviation of the lower limbs: preoperative planning of multiapical frontal plane and angular bowing deformities of the femur and tibia. Clin Orthop 280:65–71

10. Heervarden RJV, Wymenga AB, Freiling D, Staubli AE (2008) Indications- Planning- Surgical Techniques using plate fixators In: Lobenhoffer P, Heervarden RJV, Staubli AE, Jakob RP (eds) Osteotomies around the knee, 1st edn. Thieme Medical Publishers, New York, p 153

11. Strecker W (2006) Corrective osteotomy of the distal femur by retrograde nailing. Euro J Trauma 32(1):83–95

12. Wang JW, Hsu CC (2008) Distal femoral varus osteotomy for osteoarthritis of the knee. Surgical technique. J Bone Joint Surg Am 88(Suppl 1):100–108

13. Seah MKT, Shafi R, Fragomen AT, Rozbruch SR (2011) Distal femoral osteotomy: is internal fixation better than external? Clin Orthop Relat Res 469(7):2003–2011

4

The role of soft-tissue traction forces in bone segment transport for callus distraction

A force measurement cadaver study on eight human femora using a novel intramedullary callus distraction system

Konstantin Horas[1] · Reinhard Schnettler[2] · Gerrit Maier[2] · Gaby Schneider[3] · Uwe Horas[4]

Abstract Callus distraction using bone segment transport systems is an applied process in the treatment of bone defects. However, complications such as muscle contractures, axial deviation and pin track infections occur in the treatment process using the currently available devices. Since successful treatment is influenced by the applied distraction force, knowledge of the biomechanical properties of the involved soft tissues is essential to improve clinical outcome and treatment strategies. To date, little data on distraction forces and the role of soft-tissue traction forces are available. The aim of this study was to assess traction forces generated by soft tissues during bone segment transport using a novel intramedullary callus distraction system on eight human femora. For traction force measurements, bone segment transport over 60-mm femoral defects was conducted under constant load measurement using 40- and 60-mm bone segments. The required traction forces for 60-mm bone segments were higher than forces for 40-mm bone segments. This study demonstrates that soft tissues are of relevance biomechanically in bone segment transport. The size of the bone segment and the selection of the region for osteotomy are of utmost importance in defining the treatment procedure.

Keywords Traction force measurement · Soft tissues · Callus distraction system · Intramedullary · Distraction osteogenesis · Bone defect treatment

Introduction

The technique of callus distraction for the treatment of bone defects started at the beginning of the nineteenth century [1]. Despite significant improvements, the treatment of large bone defects remains challenging in many ways. Callus distraction can be accomplished either through extramedullary systems (EMS) such as the Ilizarov method or through totally implantable intramedullary distraction systems (IMS) [2–5]. External fixators in EMS are poorly accepted by patients, frequently resulting in pain, stiffness, irritation and pin track infections [6]. The overall clinical utility for EMS is poor [7]. Even though IMS avoid the problem of pin track infections and are preferred in maintaining quality of life, they are not widely used as the existing models are still limited in terms of function and control [8]. It is known that a series of biological and mechanical elements, most of them not fully understood, are involved in the distraction process. Essential information on variables such as the best velocity of distraction, the traction forces involved in the transport process and whether or not the position of the osteotomy is of relevance is lacking [9].

In order to improve on existing models and develop a novel callus distraction systems (CDS), basic biomechanical knowledge regarding traction forces involved in bone segment transport (BST) is needed. A better

✉ Konstantin Horas
konstantin.horas@sydney.edu.au

[1] Bone Research Program, ANZAC Research Institute, University of Sydney, Gate 3 Hospital Road, Concord 2139, Australia

[2] Department of Trauma Surgery/Laboratory of Experimental Trauma Surgery, Justus-Liebig-University, Rudolf-Buchheim-Str. 7, 35392 Giessen, Germany

[3] Institute of Mathematics, Goethe-University, Robert-Mayer-Str. 10, 60325 Frankfurt, Germany

[4] Department of Orthopaedic and Trauma Surgery, Kliniken des Main-Taunus-Kreises GmbH, Kronberger Str. 36, 65812 Bad Soden, Germany

understanding may help reduce frequent complications such as muscle contractures, axial deviation and traction injury to vessels and nerves but would also allow modifying the treatment regimen. There are little data on forces in callus distraction systems. Previous studies measured distraction forces either in complicated or in using inaccurate systems ignoring frictional force; many were conducted in animal experiments having less relevance for human callus distraction [10–14]. Whether the predominant part of the force is generated by the viscoelasticity of the soft tissues or by the callus itself, is uncertain.

The overall force required for BST consists of several different load components [9, 15, 16]. All adherent structures of the transporting bone segment such as tendons, fasciae and muscles generate a force due to the distraction of the soft tissues. Another component of the overall traction force is directly related to the callus and the new forming bone tissue of the regenerate. The tissue reproduction in callus distraction is stimulated by traction, and the process is known as distraction osteogenesis [17]. A percentage of the force can be attributed to the displacement of the tissue blocking the bone defect and some is directly related to the measuring system itself. Precise knowledge on the applied forces involved in the treatment process is fundamental. The data are diverse in the literature on the overall force required for callus distraction but also the distribution of forces. This study aims to measure the mechanical forces applied by the soft tissues in BST over the whole period of distraction using a novel intramedullary CDS.

Materials and methods

Bone segment transport (BST) over a 60-mm femoral defect was conducted on eight human femora (four cadavers) under constant load measurement. For that purpose, a 40-mm bone segment on the right femur and a 60-mm bone segment on the left femur were generated on each cadaver. All cadavers were frozen to a temperature of −18° Celsius exactly 48 h after *exitus letalis* and defrosted for a period of 24 h prior to the experiment. Each cadaver was carefully selected, and none had a history of bone injury or any musculoskeletal disease that could have had an impact on the measurement.

The novel CDS used in this experiment comprise an intramedullary nail with transverse interlocking screws and an in-line mechanism, with a threaded rod and a threaded rod spindle sitting on top, which produces the connection between the bone segment and the threaded rod (Fig. 1) [18]. A longitudinally slit interlocking nail keeps the defective area open throughout distraction (Figs. 2, 3). The bone segment is moved in the direction of the desired

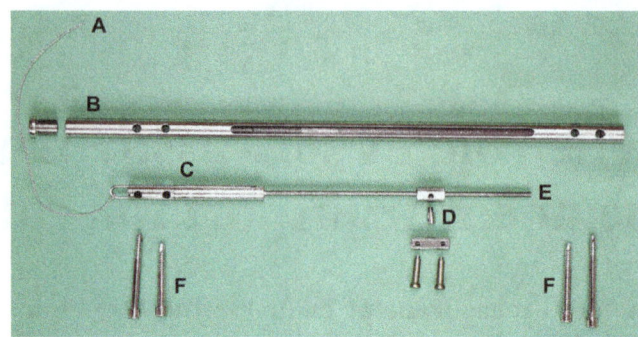

Fig. 1 Individual components of the CDS: *A* traction wire, *B* nail, *C* mechanics, *D* threaded rod spindle, *E* threaded rod, *F* interlocking screw

callus distraction by rotating the threaded rod in a specific way. This rotation is achieved by the mechanism converting a traction force produced by a connected wire into a translational movement. In order to move the wire and trigger the mechanics for BST, a traction force is generated by pulling on the connected wire with a load cell being interposed to measure the generated amount of force (Fig. 4). For clinical application, the traction wire was designed to be fixed to the tibial tubercle, and BST is conducted by generating a traction force on the wire by flexion of the knee joint.

Implantation

In order to avoid damage to the surrounding tissues of the femur, a medial approach was chosen to generate the 60-mm bone defects. The CDS were implanted into the femur via a standard retrograde transarticular nailing in the supine position. Proximal locking of the CDS was carried out in an anterior/posterior direction in the peritrochanteric region of the femur and distal transverse locking in a lateral to medial direction. Bone segments for transport were produced via a minimal lateral approach and osteotomy directly distal to the insertion of adductor brevis muscle at the linea aspera in such a way as to preserve as much of the periosteum as possible. Each bone segment was then connected to the intramedullary CDS using two transcortical screws.

Measurement

For calibration and measurement of the traction force, a servohydraulic testing machine (PSA 40KN Schenk, Germany) and a load cell (PCE MA001, Germany) for an effective range up to 1000 Newton were used. For data record and physical checks, BMLab 200 V.2. software was utilised. Prior to traction force measurement, forces generated by the CDS itself were measured using the

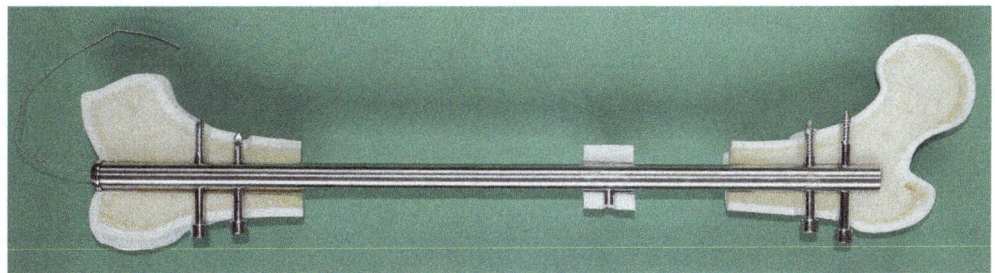

Fig. 2 CDS implanted into the femur (anteroposterior view): the traction wire is connected to the fully inserted mechanics

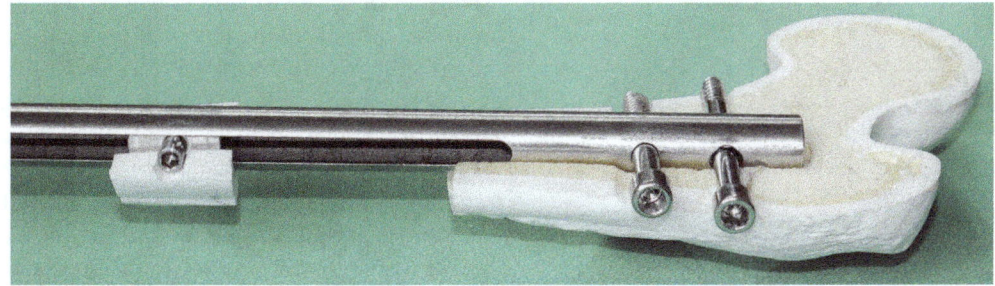

Fig. 3 CDS implanted into the femur with bone segment connected to the threaded rod (lateral view)

load cell. These frictional forces were then subtracted from the measured loads further in the experiment. For traction force measurement, the CDS were released every 15 s, leading to a transport distance of 0.25 mm per release. Records of the measurements were made every 2 mm of transport distance from the beginning of distraction to closing at the docking site. For inspection and validation of the running system and the transporting bone segment, radiographs (AP and lateral) were taken throughout the experiment using an X-ray C-Arm (Siemens, Germany).

Results

All bone segments were transported to the docking site without any complications. During continuous force recordings and radiographic validation, no mechanical obstacles of the system were observed. The total amount of measurements on each of the eight femora varied from 27 to 32 measurements accounting for a transport distance of 53–64 mm. Traction forces showed the same curve progression and the same force pattern in all of the eight femora (Fig. 5). The recorded force data in the graph can be divided into three different groups. After a short period (0–10 mm transport distance) of relatively steep increase in force, traction force increased roughly linearly with distance (10–50 mm). At 50–60 mm transport distance, the recordings showed a rapid increase in forces up to a maximum of 444.5 N.

For further analysis, we focused on the intermediate part of the graph in Fig. 5 in which the force increased linearly with distance and compared the different bone fragment sizes (Fig. 6). We used simple linear regression in order to describe the parameters of the linear increase in force. The resulting estimates of slope and of mean force at two exemplary values of 20 and 40 mm transport distance are given in Table 1. The estimated slope and the mean force required at 20 mm and 40 mm transport distance were larger in 60 mm than in 40 mm bone segments.

Due to the small number of cadaveric specimens, we omitted statistical tests of significance. However, we investigated potential relationships between the slope of the regression and several demographic variables. No clear relation of age, weight and body mass index to traction force was visible.

Discussion

Leong et al. [15] were the first to report distraction loads in humans using an EMS consisting of Steinmann pins and a distraction frame in 1979. In this study, the authors described a time-dependent viscoelastic behaviour of stretched tissues during limb lengthening (LL). Although Aronson et al. agreed that an increase in distraction loads might be due to elastic tissue resistance, they hypothesised that a large portion of the distraction load was generated by the callus itself [10]. This was supported by a study by Younger et al. [12] investigating femoral forces during LL

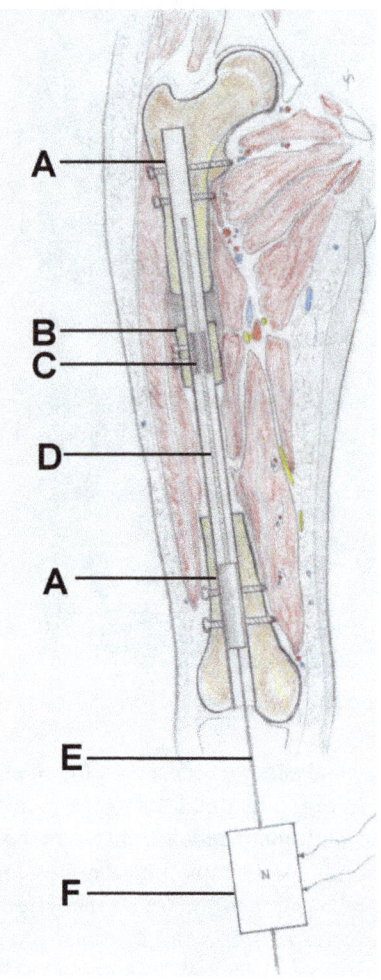

Fig. 4 Schematic of the CDS implanted into the femur. *A* nail, *B* bone segment, *C* threaded rod spindle, *D* threaded rod, *E* traction wire, *F* load cell. By pulling on the load cell connected to the distal wire, bone segment transport is conducted and the required traction force can be measured simultaneously

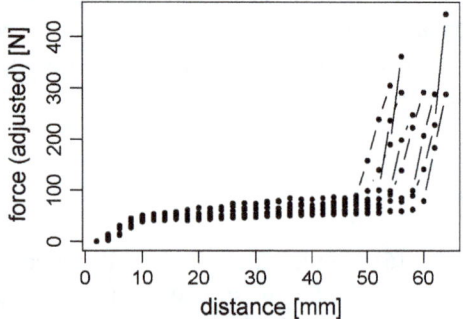

Fig. 5 Adjusted force measurement for 40- and 60-mm bone segment transport in eight human femora. *Each curve* represents one bone segment to be transported within one femur

in children. They suggested that the presence of an inelastic callus in LL mainly affects the magnitude and increase in force. In contrast, Wolfson et al. [19] indicated that traction forces are generated by the soft tissues of the leg from

passive stretch or muscular activity. Simpson et al. [11] supported this theory in their studies on LL comparing forces in patients with post-traumatic shortening to patients with congenitally short limbs. They found a noticeable difference in force between these two groups. In particular, patients with congenitally short limbs developed higher peak forces due to the resistance of the soft tissues. Also known, as indicated by Forriol et al. [14], is that callus properties do not vary substantially while LL is performed. In their opinion, the behaviour in force pattern is likely due to the mechanical properties of the soft tissues. Contrastingly, Brunner et al. [13] suggested that the percentage of muscle and soft-tissue forces of the total force measured in their study on BST in sheep was very low.

There are two existing theories for the generation of the main forces measured in callus distraction: some authors suggest that bone segment transport forces cannot be attributed to the soft tissues, whereas others believe that the soft tissues play a decisive role in force generation. The present study indicates that soft tissues are of relevance in BST biomechanically. As this study was performed on human cadavers, no callus formation was possible, and therefore, no callus-related force was included in the measurements. In contrast to the studies mentioned above, frictional forces of the distraction system were measured prior to the experiment and were subtracted from the resulting data later in the experiment leaving the final force data representing that solely generated by all adherent structures of the bone segment and by the tissues blocking the bone gap. The three-part curve progression shown in the results is interpreted as follows: the initial increase in force can be related to soft-tissue tension from implantation of the CDS (0–10 mm); the subsequent almost linear increase with distance represents the distraction force generated by the soft tissues (10–50 mm); and the rapid increase in force at the end of the transport distance can be related to the soft tissues blocking the bone gap and the impact of the bone segment at the docking site. Forces for 60-mm bone segments were higher throughout the whole period of BST, indicating that a higher amount of adherent tissues had been involved in the transport process (Fig. 6).

As with any cadaveric test set-up, this study has some limitations. Measurements in cadaveric specimens eliminate active muscle forces, which limits the documentation of generated forces to an observation of passive forces solely. As the CDS were released every 15 s to generate a transport distance of 0.25 mm per release until impact of the bone segment at the docking site, this would contrast to the clinical situation where the speed of segment transport is around 1 mm per day allowing some time for the soft tissues to relax between transport intervals. As the soft tissues in our experimental set-up were given 15 s to adapt after each release, it is likely that the viscoelasticity of the

Fig. 6 Adjusted force measurement for bone segment transport in four human cadavers using a 60-mm bone segment (**a**) and a 40-mm bone segment (**b**)

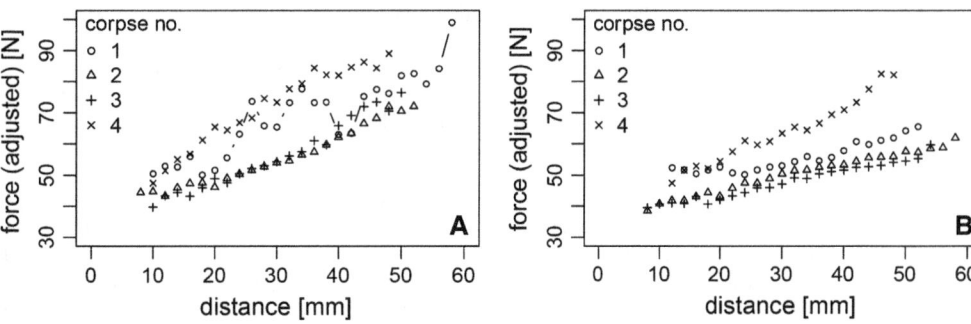

Table 1 Summary of ordinary linear regression of the data given in Fig. 5

Cadaver	Slope (N/mm)		Mean force (N) estimated from linear regression			
			At 20 mm transport distance		At 40 mm transport distance	
	60 mm	40 mm	60 mm	40 mm	60 mm	40 mm
1	0.73	0.35	57.9	51.5	73.4	58.5
2	0.68	0.43	48.9	45.0	62.5	53.4
3	0.88	0.39	47.6	43.5	65.2	51.4
4	1.01	0.89	62.3	54.9	83.2	72.8

For each cadaver, the slope of the regression line and the estimated value at 20 and 40 mm transport distance are given. The estimated slope and the mean force required at 20 and 40 mm transport distance were larger in 60 than in 40 mm bone fragments

soft tissues maintains some resistant force that falsely increases the total amount of force measured. Despite these limitations, we believe that these findings are of value for clinicians designing the treatment regimen. The study shows that transport forces for 60-mm bone segments were higher than transport forces for 40-mm segments, which will have less adherent soft tissues. For this reason, not only the size but the site of the bone segment has to be taken into consideration while defining the treatment procedure.

This is the first described force measurements using an IMS, and there are no previous studies for comparisons to be made. In a similar study presented by Baumgart et al. [16], the force curve progression demonstrated the same pattern of behaviour as in the current authors' subjects. However, as there are no data available on traction forces for BST in living humans measured in IMS, no exact conclusion of the amount of force generated by the soft tissues contributing to the overall force is possible. Despite this, the data above suggest that forces generated by the soft tissues contribute to the overall forces involved in BST.

Conclusion

This study is a first approximation of a force measurement in human cadavers using an IMS. We showed that soft tissues are of relevance in BST and for this reason the amount of force required for BST depends on the size and the localisation of the bone segment to be transported. The findings of this study are of value for the improvement of currently available CDS and might contribute to a reduction in complications in the treatment of bone defects.

Acknowledgments We thank M. Menzel for his assistance in biomechanical experiments and C. M. Zehendner for helpful comments on the manuscript.

Informed consent Written informed consent from the donors was obtained prior to their inclusion in this study.

References

1. Wiedemann M (1996) Callus distraction: a new method? A historical review of limb lengthening. Clin Orthop Related Res 327:291–304
2. Ilizarov GA (1989) The tension-stress effect on the genesis and growth of tissues. Part I. The influence of stability of fixation and soft-tissue preservation. Clin Orthop Related Res 238:249–281
3. Hankemeier S, Pape HC, Gosling T, Hufner T, Richter M, Krettek C (2004) Improved comfort in lower limb lengthening with the intramedullary skeletal kinetic distractor. Principles and preliminary clinical experiences. Arch Orthop Trauma Surg 124(2):129–133
4. Guichet JM, Deromedis B, Donnan LT, Peretti G, Lascombes P, Bado F (2003) Gradual femoral lengthening with the Albizzia intramedullary nail. J Bone Joint Surg Am 85-A(5):838–848
5. Betz A, Baumgart R, Schweiberer L (1990) First fully implantable intramedullary system for callus distraction—intramedullary nail with programmable drive for leg lengthening

and segment displacement. Principles and initial clinical results. Chirurg 61(8):605–609

6. Sun XT, Easwar TR, Manesh S, Ryu JH, Song SH, Kim SJ et al (2011) Complications and outcome of tibial lengthening using the Ilizarov method with or without a supplementary intramedullary nail: a case-matched comparative study. J Bone Joint Surg Br 93(6):782–787

7. Schiedel FM, Pip S, Wacker S, Popping J, Tretow H, Leidinger B et al (2011) Intramedullary limb lengthening with the Intramedullary Skeletal Kinetic Distractor in the lower limb. J Bone Joint Surg Br 93(6):788–792

8. Burghardt RD, Herzenberg JE, Specht SC, Paley D (2011) Mechanical failure of the Intramedullary Skeletal Kinetic Distractor in limb lengthening. J Bone Joint Surg Br 93(5):639–643

9. Gardner TN, Evans M, Simpson H, Kenwright J (1998) Force-displacement behaviour of biological tissue during distraction osteogenesis. Med Eng Phys 20(9):708–715

10. Aronson J, Harp JH (1994) Mechanical forces as predictors of healing during tibial lengthening by distraction osteogenesis. Clin Orthop Relat Res (301):73–79

11. Simpson AH, Cunningham JL, Kenwright J (1996) The forces which develop in the tissues during leg lengthening. A clinical study. J Bone Joint Surg Br 78(6):979–983

12. Younger AS, Mackenzie WG, Morrison JB (1994) Femoral forces during limb lengthening in children. Clin Orthop Related Res 301:55–63

13. Brunner UH, Cordey J, Schweiberer L, Perren SM (1994) Force required for bone segment transport in the treatment of large bone defects using medullary nail fixation. Clin Orthop Related Res 301:147–155

14. Forriol F, Goenaga I, Mora G, Vinolas J, Canadell J (1997) Measurement of bone lengthening forces; an experimental model in the lamb. Clin Biomech 12(1):17–21

15. Leong JC, Ma RY, Clark JA, Cornish LS, Yau AC (1979) Viscoelastic behavior of tissue in leg lengthening by distraction. Clin Orthop Related Res 139:102–109

16. Baumgart R, Kuhn V, Hinterwimmer S, Krammer M, Mutschler W (2004) Tractive force measurement in bone transport—an in vivo investigation in humans. Biomed Tech 49(9):248–256

17. Aro HT, Chao EY (1993) Bone-healing patterns affected by loading, fracture fragment stability, fracture type, and fracture site compression. Clin Orthop Related Res 293:8–17

18. Horas U (2006) A novel internal callus distraction system. In: Leung KTG, Schnettler R, Alt V, Haarman H (eds) Practice of intramedullary locked nails. Springer, Berlin, pp 199–210

19. Wolfson N, Hearn TC, Thomason JJ, Armstrong PF (1990) Force and stiffness changes during Ilizarov leg lengthening. Clin Orthop Related Res 250:58–60

5

Limb reconstruction in Ollier's disease

S. S. Madan[1] · K. Robinson[1] · P. D. Kasliwal[1] · M. J. Bell[1] · M. Saleh[1] ·
J. A. Fernandes[1]

Abstract We present our experience of lengthening and correction of complex deformities in the management of patients with Ollier's dysplasia (multiple enchondromatosis) from 1985 and 2002. All patients were under 18 years with a minimum follow-up time of 2 years (mean 9.6 years, range 2–15 years). There were a total of ten patients of which seven were male and three female. The mean age at presentation was 10.7 years (range 5–17 years; SD 3.7 years). The total length gain was 42.3 mm (range 30–110 mm; SD 28.9 mm). The number of days in external fixation was 164.8 days (range 76–244 days; SD 42.9 days). The bone healing index was 32.5 days/cm (18–50 days/cm; SD 10.3 days/cm). Patients with Ollier's disease have limb length inequality and angular deformities and require multiple reconstructive procedures owing to a high incidence of recurrence. We identified a tendency for the osteotomy to prematurely consolidate and advise the latency period after surgery to be 4–5 days and for distraction to proceed at a faster rate.

Keywords Ollier's dysplasia · Ollier's deformity · Ollier's limb reconstruction

Introduction

In 1889, Ollier described a condition of multiple, typically unilateral enchondromas associated with deformity of the extremities [1]. Multiple enchondromatosis or Ollier's disease is an uncommon, nonhereditary disorder. The number of bones affected can vary greatly, with the phalanges, femur, and tibia most likely affected. As there is a tendency for unilateral involvement, asymmetry from limb length discrepancy and angular deformity is apparent. Limb length discrepancies may be in the range of 10–25 cm by maturity. Deformity and enlargement of fingers may impair normal function. Forearm abnormalities such as bowing, limited rotation, and ulnar deviation of the hand may also be evident [2].

The affected bones show numerous islands of cartilage in close proximity to the physis, resulting in growth inhibition. Eventual malignant transformation into chondrosarcoma has been reported to occur in 20–33 % of those patients affected [3–5].

The abnormalities in bone are more extensive than the physical examination would suggest. On plain radiographs, long bones are affected with radiolucent longitudinal streaks that involve the metaphysis and extend into the diaphysis. The cortex overlying the enchondroma is usually thin, and calcification within the lesion is common [2].

We present our experience of lengthening and correction of deformities in patients with Ollier's dysplasia.

✉ J. A. Fernandes
James.Fernandes@sch.nhs.uk

[1] Department of Trauma and Orthopaedic Surgery, Sheffield Children's NHS Foundation Trust, Western Bank, Sheffield S10 2TH, UK

Methods

This is a retrospective review of patients treated in the limb reconstruction department from 1985 to 2002. All patients who underwent correction and lengthening or were still monitored in that period were included in the study. Data were collected included the dates of operation and removal of fixator, length achieved, deformities corrected, the type of fixator used, and technique of osteotomy and lengthening. All complications resulting from the treatment were documented. Pin site infections were graded as described by Gordon et al. [6].

The osteotomies were performed percutaneously. The osteotomies were metaphyseal or diaphyseal (proximal or distal) close to the metaphyseal diaphyseal junction. Multiple drill holes were made in the near and far cortex, which were then connected by an osteotome. Completion of the osteotomy was confirmed by intraoperative imaging. There is controversy over lengthening through the affected segment of bone involved in Ollier's disease [6]; in this series, the osteotomy was carried out through pathological bone at the site of the deformity.

The lengthening process was started 5–7 days after application of the frame. An average of four quarter turns were done for 1 mm of lengthening per day and one full turn four times a day for angular corrections. This rate was kept constant as long as regenerated bone continued to form progressively along with distraction. All patients were instructed in daily pin site care, which was simply by showering daily [7]. All patients participated in physical therapy daily until they were discharged and twice a week thereafter. Walking was encouraged to help to improve circulation and fitness of the patient [8]. The hospitalization period lasted between 7 and 10 days until patients were familiar with the distraction or correction regime and were mobilizing comfortably full weight bearing with crutches. The ankle was maintained in a plantigrade position with a dynamic splint or a bolt-on foot piece connected to the distal tibial ring.

After the desired length was achieved, the fixator was retained until there was cortical continuity visible on three sides as seen on AP and lateral views of the regenerate. The fixator was dynamized or removed in stages commonly to stimulate consolidation of the regenerate. After removal of the frame, the tibia was protected in a below knee cast for 4–6 weeks and, for the femur, a cast brace for the same length of time. The mean follow-up was 9.6 years (range 2–15 years).

Results

There were a total of 10 patients of which seven were male and three female. The mean age at presentation was 10.7 years (5–17 years). The main problems that patients presented with were limb length inequality and deformities in the lower limbs. Only one patient required surgery for forearm involvement (Table 1). The femur and tibia were affected mostly. Eight of the ten patients had reached skeletal maturity. The total number of operative procedures was 38 major primary procedures on the limbs and over 40 minor secondary procedures. The average length gain was 42.3 mm (30–110 mm; SD 28.9 mm). The number of days

in external fixation was 164.8 days (76–244 days; SD 42.9 days). The mean bone healing index (BHI) was 32.5 days/cm of length gained (18–50 days/cm; SD 10.3 days/cm); (Table 1). One patient required a single procedure that was performed before skeletal maturity, and another declined further surgery after one procedure. The remaining had multiple surgical procedures. A monolateral external fixator was used in 22 procedures, Ilizarov ring fixators in seven cases, and Sheffield ring fixators in two cases. In two procedures, an intramedullary nail was used for fixation. Six segments had bifocal lengthening or correction, and the rest had monofocal reconstruction (Figs. 1, 2, 3).

The majority of patients had deviation of the mechanical limb axes from the presenting angular deformities. The malalignment was addressed during the lengthening process to produce a limb mechanical axis within 10 mm of normal and corrected angular deformity within 5 ° of normal.

Two knees in two patients developed subluxation that was corrected with hinged Ilizarov frames. Four knees had reduced motion by 30–40 %, and six ankles had reduced motion in either direction by 30 % at the latest follow-up. This was particularly seen in the patients who had long limb lengthening. Valgus deformity developed in four knees and five ankles after lengthening that was corrected with the fixator in situ. None developed subluxation at the hip during rehabilitation nor lost joint range of motion at this site.

The major complication was premature healing of the osteotomy (3) and a recurrence of deformity and leg length inequality (15). Premature healing necessitated a manipulation under anaesthesia and osteoclasis or a decision taken to stop lengthening. Rapid or premature healing was avoided by reducing the latency period before lengthening and proceeding at a faster rate than when lengthening for other conditions. One patient suffered with a fracture of the tibia after removal of the frame, and this was treated nonoperatively. Pin site infections were identified in 27 fixators. Eleven of these were each grade I and grade II. Four were grade III of which two required admission in the hospital for IV antibiotics. Only one patient had a grade IV infection. Persistent joint stiffness occurred in two knees after a long lengthening of the limb. Regenerate formation was complete for all patients (Figs. 1, 2, 3).

Discussion

Limb reconstruction in Ollier's disease is complex because the abnormal islands of juxtaphyseal cartilage cause both growth inhibition and angular deformities. Limb length discrepancy is progressive and requires several episodes of

Table 1 Patient data of those with Ollier's disease who underwent limb reconstruction at our hospital

Case	Gender	Age at operation	Side	Bone	EF	EFT (days)	Lengthening (mm)	BHI	Complications
1	M	5	R	Femur	LRS	174	80	22	Joint stiffness, premature healing
		5	R	Tibia	LRS	119	30	39.6	Premature healing
		6	R	Tibia	LRS	151	75	20	Valgus
		10	R	Tibia	LRS	76	0	Cr'n	Premature healing
		12	R	Femur	LRS	232	53	43.7	Valgus
		12	L	Femur	LRS	139	0	Cr'n	Joint stiffness
		17	L	Tibia	Ilizarov	111	0	Cr'n	
		17	R	Femur	LRS	184	45	40.8	Joint stiffness infection
2	M	15	L	Femur	LRS	167	40	41.7	
3	M	8	R	Tibia	LRS	151	57	26.5	
		13	R	Femur	LRS	105	50	21	
		16	R	Tibia	Bifocal LRS	124	44	28	
4	F	8	L	Femur	LRS	194	110	17.6	
		11	L	Femur	Bifocal LRS	208	66	31.5	
		15	L	Femur	LRS	158	0	Cr'n	
		15	L	Tibia	Ilizarov	192	50	38	
		16	L	Femur	LRS	191	0	Cr'n	
5	M	6	R	Femur	LRS	116	50	23.2	
		9	R	Femur	Bifocal LRS	194	40	48.5	
		13	R	Tibia	Bifocal Ilizarov	236	0	Cr'n	
		13	L	Tibia	SRF	236	0	Cr'n	Fracture after fixator removal
6	F	130	L	Femur	Bifocal LRS	188	60	31.3	
7	M	8	L	Femur	Bifocal LRS	123	0	Cr'n	
		12	L	Femur	LRS	200	40	5	
8	M	9	R	Forearm	LRS	118	41	28.7	
9	M	5	L	Tibia	Ilizarov	244	0	Cr'n	
		9	L	Femur	Ilizarov	172	0	Cr'n	
		10	L	Tibia	SRF	137	0	Cr'n	
		10	L	Femur	LRS	137	0	Cr'n	
10	F	7	L	Femur	Ilizarov	166	0	Cr'n	
		7	L	Tibia	Ilizarov	166	0	Cr'n	

EF external fixator, *EXT* external fixation time, *BHI* bone healing index, *LRS* limb reconstruction system, *SRF* Sheffield ring fixator

limb lengthening and axis correction. Traditional methods addressing the effects of Ollier's disease include curettage, bone grafting, osteotomies, and internal fixation. These techniques do not address the problem of length discrepancy fully [6]. The majority of the affected bone segments in this series required repeated lengthening or deformity correction in childhood. Shapiro [9] reviewed 21 patients with Ollier's disease retrospectively. He showed angular deformities were common; 80 % of the affected femora had significant varus or valgus angulation in the distal part, and 42 % of the affected tibiae had a proximal or distal deformity. The apex of the angulation when present, as was

seen in this series too, was metaphyseal with the concavity on the side that was more extensively involved by the enchondroma. Osteotomies were done to correct angulation in the group reported by Shapiro as was the case in this study. Deformity arising in the distal femur required repeat osteotomies to achieve correct alignment by skeletal maturity. Diaphyseal lengthening was done on six occasions, once in the femur and five times in the tibia and fibula, with good results. There were 14 episodes of correction and 17 episodes of segment lengthening in our 10 patients.

Chew et al. [10] described a high incidence of varus angulation in the lower femur in Ollier's disease; eight of a

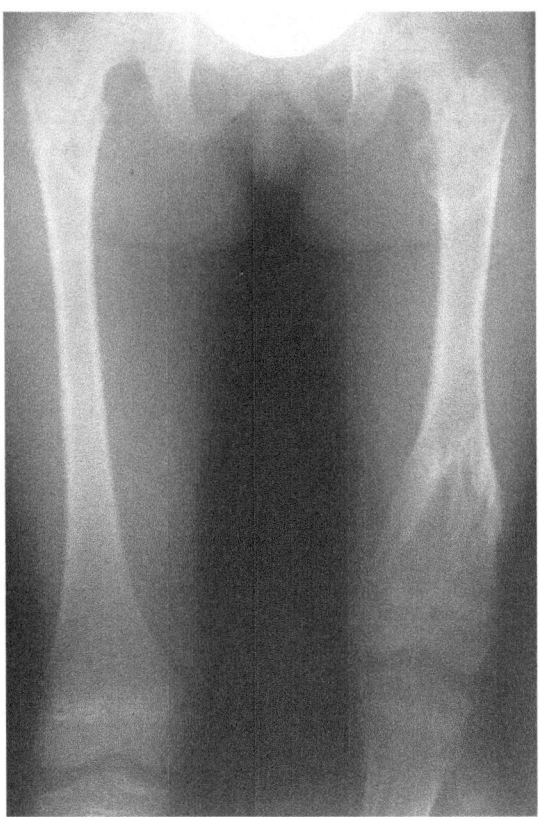

Fig. 1 Radiograph showing *left* femur enchondroma in a child with Ollier's disease

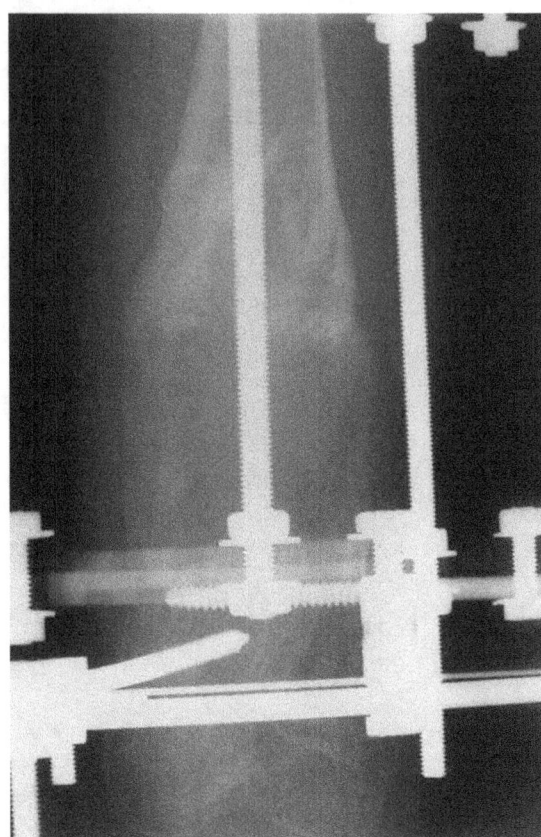

Fig. 2 Radiograph of deformity correction of tibia using external fixation

total of 14 patients had this deformity. Märtson et al. [11] described a case of varus deformity in the femur and valgus deformity in the tibia. The femur was lengthened by 22 cm, and the tibia by 10 cm. No complications were reported. There were five cases of genu varum and six of genu valgum in our group of patients.

D'Angelo et al. [12] used both Wagner's and the Ilizarov method for correction of limb length discrepancy. The latter was more reliable in terms of mechanical hold and correcting severe deformities, producing bone regenerate of excellent quality even in major lengthening procedures. Their results were obtained by adapting the Ilizarov method to the features of the altered bone structure. We found the Ilizarov fixator to be versatile in correcting malalignment with long limb lengthenings. The soft tissues caused problems during treatment but found both Ilizarov and Sheffield ring fixators to be versatile in controlling soft tissue tension, leading to a preference for using ring fixators in the latter part of this study.

Baumgart et al. [13] identified complications when using external fixation. Typically, bone in Ollier's disease is relatively soft, so external fixator pins may cut out resulting in the premature removal of the fixator. Watanabe et al. [14] identified bone weakness in their patients with Ollier's disease. They adapted their procedures that included

adding more wires or half pins to secure the bone; we did not come across this problem in our patients.

Curran et al. [15] reported eight paediatric patients who underwent nine simultaneous ipsilateral femoral and tibial lengthenings with the Ilizarov external fixator. Four complications in three patients occurred as a result of the lengthening process. Three of the complications involved soft tissue contractures, which were successfully treated with one additional surgical procedure, whereas the fourth complication involved poor bone regeneration and required bone grafting and additional immobilization. We performed three femur and tibia angular deformity corrections simultaneously and did not record the above complications; one of these segments (the tibia) underwent a 5-cm lengthening. There is a preference to perform contralateral simultaneous correction and single-segment lengthenings rather than ipsilateral double-segment procedures in our patients to avoid these potential complications.

There were no complications reported by Tsuchiya et al. [16] who also used the Ilizarov method to treat three paediatric patients with Ollier's (age range 6–12 years). Their total length gain was 40.6 mm (38–44 mm in the tibia). Three patients with premature healing, one with delayed union, and one with early union were identified by

Fig. 3 a (Anteroposterior) and **b** (lateral), the corrected femur of an Ollier's patient

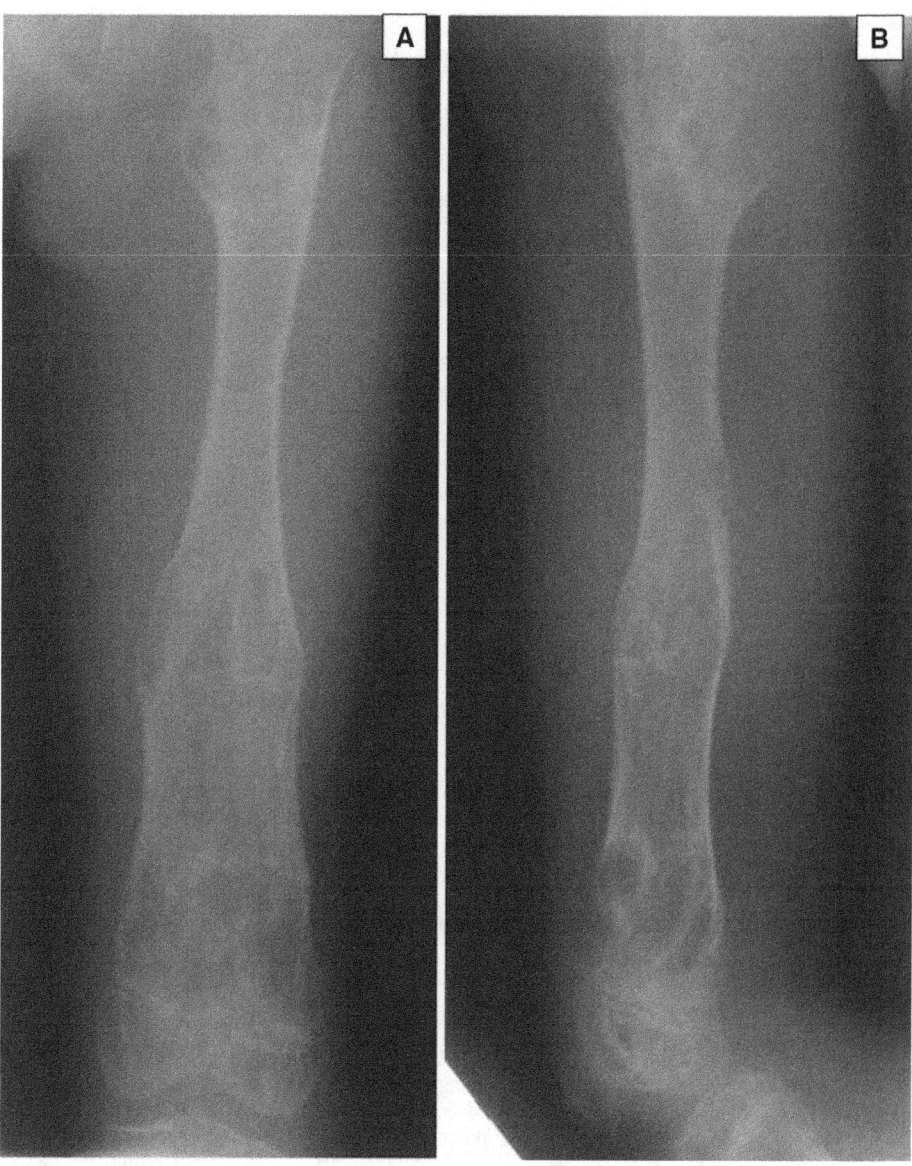

Sakurakichi et al. [17] as the only complications in their series, with the early union requiring repeat osteotomy.

Pandey et al. [18] noted that distraction osteogenesis through predominantly cartilaginous bone converted that into mature corticalized new bone rapidly. This unusual osteogenic capacity and the rapidity of healing was seen in our series also. They reported complications of knee stiffness, which resolved after 2 years. Jesus-Garcia et al. [19] described the results of treatment of 10 patients with Ollier's disease using the Ilizarov technique. The Ilizarov device was used to treat leg length discrepancy and to enhance the conversion of cartilage within the enchondroma into normal mature bone without curettage and bone grafting. The mean duration of treatment was 9.4 months. This led to conversion of the abnormal cartilage into histologically mature bone in all patients. We did not use the Ilizarov device to convert cartilage into new bone on purpose but found that with lengthening or correction there was some conversion of cartilage into new bone. Some caution is needed as enchondromas are actively multiplying lesions with a report of malignant change in fibrous dysplasia with lengthening [20].

One patient fractured the tibia after the fixator was removed in this series. Popkov et al. [21] compared 57 lengthenings in 37 patients with Ollier's disease using external fixation alone with 7 lengthenings using external fixation and elastic stable intramedullary nailing (ESIN). There were three cases of pathologic fractures in the enchondroma region in the external fixation group as well as three cases of bone regenerate deformity and one delayed union. The combined treatment group had no cases of fracture or deformity, and there was no need for plaster immobilization after removal of the external fixator. The BHI was reduced in all the external fixator and ESIN patients, and this was statistically significant for mono-segmental femoral lengthenings.

Conclusion

Patients with Ollier's disease have significant problems with limb length inequality and angular deformities. A need for multiple reconstructive procedures as recurrence of deformities and leg length discrepancy is common. We found ring fixators to be more versatile in managing angular correction, limb lengthening, and soft tissue tension over other types of fixation. There is tendency for premature healing; distraction should start early around 4–5 days and at a faster rate of distraction employed to minimize this complication.

Acknowledgments We thank Dr Simone Swift Ph.D, Orthopaedic Research Assistant and Jonathan Pagdin, B.Sc Nursing, Specialist Nurse, Paediatric limb reconstruction service, Department of Trauma and Orthopaedic Surgery, Sheffield Children's NHS Foundation Trust.

References

1. Ollier L (1900) De la dyschondroplasie. Bull Soc Chir Lyon 3:22–24
2. Herring JA, 2002. Multiple Enchondromatosis. In Skeletal Dysplasias: Tachdjian's Pediatric Orthopaedics, 3rd edn. W B Saunders; Philadelphia, 1927-1929
3. Schwartz HS, Zimmerman NB, Simon MA, Wroble RR, Millar EA, Bonfiglio M (1987) The malignant potential of enchondromatosis. J Bone Joint Surg Am 69:269–274
4. Cannon SR, Sweetnam DR (1985) Multiple chondrosarcomas in dyschondroplasia (Ollier's disease). Cancer 15(55):836–840
5. Liu J, Hudkins PG, Swee RG, Unni KK (1987) Bone sarcomas associated with Ollier's disease. Cancer 1(59):1376–1385
6. Nazzar T, Ilizarov S, Fragomen AT, Rozbruch SR (2008) Humeral lengthening and deformity correction in Ollier's disease: distraction osteogenesis with a multiaxial correction frame. J Pediatr Ortho B 17:127–152
7. Gordon JE, Kelly-Hahn J, Carpenter CJ, Schoenecker PL (2000) Pin site care during external fixation in children: results of a nihilistic approach. J Pediatr Orthop 20:163–165
8. Donnan LT, Saleh M, Rigby AS (2003) Acute correction of lower limb deformity and simultaneous lengthening with a monolateral fixator. J Bone Joint Surg (Br) 85B(2):254–260
9. Shapiro F (1982) Ollier's disease. an assessment of angular deformity, shortening, and pathological fracture in twenty-one patients. J Bone Joint Surg Am 64:95–103
10. Chew DK, Menelaus MB, Richardson MD (1998) Ollier's disease: varus angulation at the lower femur and its management. J Pediatr Orthop 18:202–208
11. Märtson A, Haviko T, Kirjanen K (2005) Extensive limb lengthening in Ollier's disease: 25-year follow-up. Medicina (Kaunas) 41(10):861–866
12. D'Angelo G, Petas N, Donzelli O (1996) Lengthening of the lower limbs in Ollier's disease: problems related to surgery. Chir Organi Mov 81:279–285
13. Baumgart R, Bürklein D, Hinterwimmer S, Thaller P, Mutschler W (2005) The management of leg-length discrepancy in Ollier's disease with a fully implantable lengthening nail. J Bone Joint Surg (Br) 87-B:1000–1004
14. Watanabe K, Tsuchiya H, Sakurakichi K, Yamashiro T, Matsubara H (2007) Treatment of lower limb deformities and limb-length discrepancies with the external fixator in Ollier's disease. J Orthop Sci 12:417–475
15. Curran AR, Kuo KN, Lubicky JP (1999) Simultaneous ipsilateral femoral and tibial lengthening with the Ilizarov method. J Pediatr Orthop 19:386–390
16. Tsuchiya H, Uehara K, Abdel-Wanis ME, Sakurakichi K, Kabata T, Tomita K (2002) Deformity correction followed by lengthening with the Ilizarov method. Clin Orthop Rel Res 402:176–183
17. Sakurakichi K, Tsuchiya H, Kabata T, Yamashiro T, Watanabe K, Tomita K (2005) Correction of juxtaarticular deformities in children using the Ilizarov apparatus. J Orthop Sci 10:360–366
18. Pandey R, White SH, Kenwright J (1995) Callus distraction in Ollier's disease. Acta Orthop Scand 66:479–480
19. Jesus-Garcia R, Bongiovanni JC, Korukian M, Boatto H, Seixas MT, Laredo J (2001) Use of the Ilizarov external fixator in the treatment of patients with Ollier's disease. Clin Orthop 382:82–86
20. Harris NL, Eilert RE, Davino N, Ruyle S, Edwardson M, Wilson V (1994) Osteogenic sarcoma arising from bony regenerate following Ilizarov femoral lengthening through fibrous dysplasia. J Pediatr Orthop 14:123–129
21. Popkov D, Journeau P, Popkov A, Haumont T, Lascombes P (2010) Ollier's disease limb lengthening: should intramedullary nailing be combined with circular external fixator. Orthop Trauma 96:348–353

6

Fibular head transfixion wire and its relationship to common peroneal nerve: cadaveric analysis

Paul Dearden[1] · Kathryn Lowery[1] · Kevin Sherman[1] · Vishy Mahadevan[2] ·
Hemant Sharma[1]

Abstract Proximal tibio-fibular joint is routinely stabilised during leg lengthening, peri-articular fractures and deformity corrections of tibia. Potential injury to the common peroneal nerve at the level of the fibula head/neck junction during wire insertion is a recognised complication. Previous studies have mapped the course of the common peroneal nerve and its branches at the level of the fibular head, and guidelines are published regarding placement of proximal tibial wires. This study aims to relate the course of the common peroneal nerve to the placement of a lateral insertion fibula head transfixion wire. Standard 1.8-mm Ilizarov 'olive' wires were inserted in the fibula head of 10 un-embalmed cadaveric knees. Wires were inserted percutaneously to the fibula head using surface anatomy landmarks and palpation technique. The course of the common peroneal nerve was then dissected. Distances from wire entry point to the course of the common peroneal nerve were measured post-wire insertion. The mean distance of the common peroneal nerve from the anterior aspect of the broadest point of the fibular head was 24.5 mm (range 14.2–37.7 mm). Common peroneal nerve was seen to cross the neck of fibula at a mean distance of 34.8 mm from the tip of fibula (range 21.5–44.3 mm). Wire placement was found to be on average, 52 % of the maximal AP diameter of the fibula head and 64 % of the distance from tip of fibula to the point of nerve crossing fibula neck. When inserting a fibula head transfixion wire, care must be taken not to place wire entry point too distal or posterior on the fibula head. Observing a safe zone in the anterior half of the proximal 20 mm of the fibula head would avoid injury to the nerve. In cases where palpation of fibula is difficult due to patient habitus, we recommend consideration of the use of fluoroscopic guidance during wire transfixion of the proximal tibio-fibular articulation to avoid wire insertion too distally and subsequent potential nerve injury.

Keywords Ilizarov · Peroneal nerve · Anatomy · Frame · Proximal tibial fractures · Limb lengthening

Introduction

Fine wire circular frame fixation for tibial fractures is commonly utilised in the trauma setting, deformity corrections and leg lengthening. In proximal tibial fractures/severe plateau fractures, there is lack of space and fibular head provides not only space and but decent spread of wires, thereby increasing the crossing angle of wires. During leg lengthening and deformity corrections, the fibula has to be transfixed at both ends to prevent any subluxation of either tibio-fibular joint.

Placement of the proximal wires from the lateral side is commonly performed using palpation techniques and observation of Ilizarov 'safe corridors'. The wires are passed percutaneously, without visualisation of the underlying

✉ Kathryn Lowery
Katlowery300@yahoo.com

Paul Dearden
p.dearden@doctors.org.uk

Kevin Sherman
Kevin.Sherman@yh.hee.nhs.uk

Vishy Mahadevan
vmahadev@rcseng.ac.uk

Hemant Sharma
hksorth@yahoo.co.uk

[1] Hull Royal Infirmary, Anlaby Road, Hull, UK

[2] Royal College of Surgeons, England, UK

peroneal nerve. Commonly, wires are passed without radiographic imaging, or with the focus of imaging being on the orientation of wires parallel to the knee articular surface. Injury to the peroneal nerve can have devastating consequences, and its iatrogenic occurrence during external fixation surgery to the proximal tibia has been recognised [1, 2]. The common peroneal nerve supplies motor innervation to the muscles of dorsiflexion of the foot and extension of the toes, and therefore, injury can have a significant effect on the patients' gait. Previous studies have described the anatomy and course of the peroneal nerve and the relationship to the proximal tibia [3–5]. Ruben et al. [6] studied the relationship of the peroneal nerve to Gerdy's tubercle and determined a safe zone for the insertion of proximal tibial wires. Our study aimed to measure the distance of the nerve from a wire inserted into the proximal fibula percutaneously reproducing the clinical environment and to attempt to provide recommendations for the safe placement of wires passed from the lateral aspect into the proximal tibia through the fibula head.

Materials and methods

Ten cadaveric knee specimens were obtained. The specimens were fresh and un-embalmed allowing dissection of the nerve with no concern for the condition of the soft tissues altering the measurements. As the knee specimens had not undergone any form of embalming or tissue 'fixation', the specimens handled in a very similar way to normal healthy tissue with regard to range of movement with no discernible stiffness. The specimens were sectioned knee joints and had been removed from the cadaver at approximately mid-femur and mid-tibia. The details of the specimen in regard to demographics of the donor such as age, sex or height were unknown.

The knees were positioned in slight flexion of approximately 30° and in neutral rotation. Standard 1.8-mm Ilizarov fibula head olive wires were placed to transfix the fibula head to the proximal tibia. The wires were inserted by two orthopaedic registrars, five specimens each, under the supervision of a consultant surgeon experienced with the insertion of such wires in circular frame surgery. This ensured that any bias related to position of wires related to the surgeons experience with wire insertion was reduced. The surface markings of the fibula head were palpated and the wire inserted aiming to be in the centre of the head in both planes. Following insertion, a lateral dissection centred on the fibula was carried out, with the knee remaining slightly flexed. The nerve was identified proximally as it passes posterior to the lateral head of gastrocnemius and gently dissected along its course toward the fibula head,

Fig. 1. Care was taken not to release any soft tissue attachments of the nerve to allow its true anatomical position and course to be as closely maintained as possible during dissection, Fig. 2. Measurements were carefully taken to avoid disturbance of the course of the nerve, if further dissection was required to expose a relevant anatomical point; measurements were taken before further dissection occurred. Measurements were taken using Vernier electronic digital callipers.

Measurements recorded were the point at which the nerve crosses the fibula neck in relation to the distance from the tip of the styloid process of the fibula, the distance from the anterior aspect of the fibula head at its broadest point to the position of the nerve lying posterior to the fibula and the diameter of the fibula at its broadest point. The position of the inserted wire was then analysed in relation to the tip of styloid process of the fibula, the anterior aspect of the fibula and the distance to the nerve as it crosses the fibula neck. These anatomical landmarks were defined following direct visualisation after dissection. From these measurements, ratios were calculated to create guidelines for safe zones of wire insertion to avoid injury to the nerve.

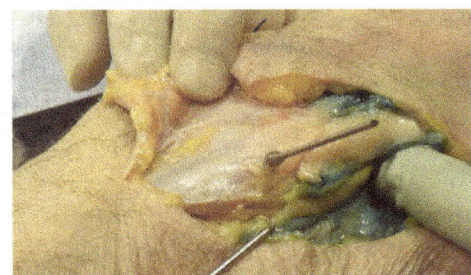

Fig. 1 Demonstrating the lateral approach centred on the fibula. The photograph shows the wire in the fibula and the nerve lying posteriorly to the fibula

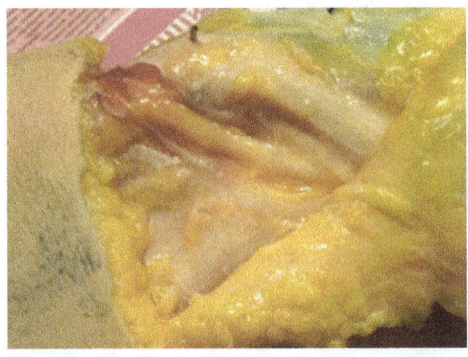

Fig. 2 Demonstration of the nerve released at point which it crosses the fibula neck but the attachments are not released to obtain accurate measurements

Results

The mean diameter of the fibula at its widest point was 22.3 mm (range 18.3–29.9 mm). The wire was inserted on average 11.8 mm from the anterior aspect of the fibula (range 5.5–15.4 mm), Table 1. The mean distance of the common peroneal nerve from the anterior aspect of the broadest point of the fibular head was 24.5 mm (range 14.2–37.7 mm), Table 1. From these measurements, a ratio was determined, thus demonstrating that, on average, the wire was inserted 52 % of the way back from the anterior edge of the fibula (range 24–77 %) in relation to its maximal AP diameter. Wires were on average 49 % of the distance from the anterior aspect of the fibula to the nerve lying posteriorly (range 26–100 %) (Table 1). In one specimen, the wire was inserted in such a way that it was noted to be touching the peroneal nerve in its location at the posterior edge of the fibula. Although the wire was seen to be slightly indenting the nerve, it was not found to be penetrating it, Fig. 3. In this specimen, a comment was recorded during wire insertion that 'anatomical landmark palpation was particularly difficult in this specimen due to the adipose tissue and muscle bulk'.

The distance from the tip of the styloid process of the fibula to the wire insertion point was on average 22.2 mm (range 13.5–32.3 mm) (Table 2). The distance from the tip of styloid process of the fibula to the nerve as it winds around the neck was 34.8 mm (range 21.5–44.3 mm) (Table 2). Calculating these results as a ratio, the wire was on average inserted 64 % of the distance from the fibula styloid to the point of nerve crossing fibula neck (range 43–100 %) (Table 2). The specimen which had the wire touching the nerve posteriorly was also touching the nerve as it crossed the fibula, having been inserted into the fibula

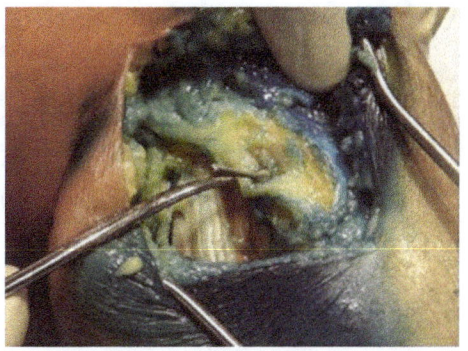

Fig. 3 Demonstration of the specimen in which the wire had been inserted posteriorly and distally near the fibula neck. The wire was touching the peroneal nerve as it was lying at the posterior edge of the fibula; however, although slightly indenting the nerve, it was not penetrating it. *The discolouration* seen in the specimen in this picture is from a previous study which had injected dye into the knee joint and dye had diffused into surrounding tissues. The previous study had no effect on the results of this study (colour figure online)

at a far more distal point, just proximal to the fibula neck. As previously noted, it had not been easy to palpate the fibula head and upon dissection it would appear that the point which had been palpated was not the styloid process of the fibula as this structure is much deeper and posterior. The point palpated is suspected to have been the most prominent subcutaneous superior portion of the anterior border of the fibula.

Discussion

Insertion of a lateral fibular head transfixion wire is often carried out using anatomical landmarks and palpation to plan placement. The surgeon aims to insert the wire in the centre of the fibula head in the sagittal and coronal plane.

Table 1 Average measurements in millimetres of the diameter of the fibula head at its maximum antero-posterior width, distances from the anterior aspect of the fibula to the wire, and to the nerve lying posteriorly

Specimen	AP fib head diameter (mm)	Anterior fibula to wire (mm)	Anterior fibula to nerve (mm)	Wire to nerve ratio (%)	Fib diameter/ wire ratio (%)
1	29.89	15.24	37.77	40	51
2	22.83	5.51	21.33	26	24
3	22.53	6.49	23.69	27	29
4	21.83	11.8	22.71	52	54
5	22.25	10.84	20.89	52	49
6	20.54	7.79	20.44	38	38
7	21.28	14.17	28.16	50	67
8	20.49	12.49	27.35	46	61
9	23.41	15.35	28.56	54	66
10	18.35	14.21	14.21	100	77
Average	22.34	11.389	24.511	48.5	51.6

The last two columns show the ratios in percentages of the distance from the anterior fibula to the wire and to the nerve, and of the wire placement in the fibula head to its AP diameter

Table 2 Average measurements in millimetres of the distance from the tip of the fibula head to the wire and to the nerve as it crosses the fibula neck and the percentage ratio of the distance of the wire from the tip of the fibula to the nerve

Specimen	Tip fibula to wire (mm)	Tip fibula to nerve (mm)	Ratio distance wire to nerve from tip fibula (%)
1	32.87	44.27	74
2	23.50	36.81	64
3	23.78	40.88	58
4	13.50	21.51	63
5	23.52	39.12	60
6	15.21	35.30	43
7	17.21	32.33	53
8	25.14	35.41	71
9	19.64	35.14	56
10	27.23	27.23	100
Average	22.16	34.80	64

Our study examined the proximity of the wire to the common peroneal nerve. We have demonstrated that the distance from the tip of the styloid process of the fibula to the nerve as it winds around the neck was 34.8 mm (range 21.5–44.3 mm). This finding concurs with Rupp et al. [7] who demonstrated the nerve to wraps around the fibular neck at an average of 3.5 cm from the styloid process or tip (range 3–4.4 cm). Stitgen et al. [3] also studied the course and branches of the peroneal nerve at the level of the fibular neck; their study determined that a 'safe zone' from a line drawn between the fibular head and the tibial tuberosity superiorly and extending 2 cm distally minimised the risk of damage to the nerve. Rubel et al. determined an anatomical safe zone for wires inserted into the tibia from the lateral side based on Gerdy's tubercle and mapping out a safe arc. However, these authors recommended that, in the presence of a fibula fracture, these dimensions may be altered and could only be observed reliably in an intact fibula [6]. The nature of the configuration of proximal and intra-articular tibial fractures which require circular frame surgery may often mean that the fibula is not intact. In these circumstances, location of the nerve in relation to fixed fibula landmarks may prove to be more helpful in determining a safe location in which to insert a wire.

The mean diameter of the fibular head at it broadest diameter in the AP plane was found to be 22.3 mm (range 18.3–29.9 mm). The wires in our series were seen to be inserted, on average, 11.8 mm from the anterior aspect of the fibula at its broadest point. From these measurements, a ratio was calculated and demonstrates that the wire was on average inserted in the centre or 52 % of total anterior-to-posterior diameter at its widest point (range 24–77 %)

when using a landmark palpation technique. The distance of the nerve behind the fibula at the widest AP diameter was 24.5 mm (range 14.2–37.7 mm) from the anterior aspect of the fibula. In four of the ten specimens, the course of the nerve traversed the posterior border of the fibula head at its widest AP diameter. This is demonstrated in the discrepancy between the ranges demonstrated in AP diameter of the fibular head when compared to the position of

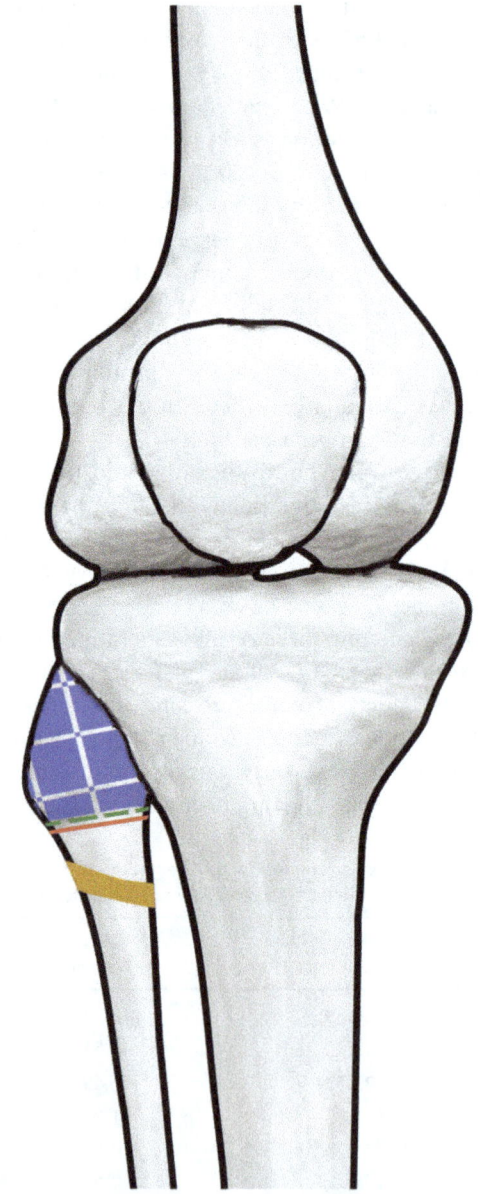

Fig. 4 Illustration demonstrating the area recommended for insertion of the wire in the coronal plane. The *yellow lines* show the range of the nerve crossing the fibula neck measured from the tip of the fibula, range 21.5–44.3 mm. Based on the findings in this study, we recommend that proximal fibula head wires should be inserted no further than 2 cm distal to the tip of the fibular head and aim slightly anterior in the fibula head in sagittal plane at the level of its maximal diameter, (*patchwork area*) (colour figure online)

Fig. 5 Illustration demonstrating the area recommended for insertion of the wire in the sagittal and axial planes

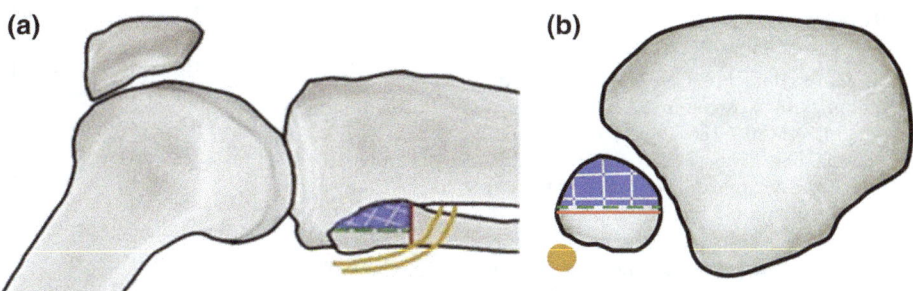

the nerve in relation to the anterior border of the fibula head at its broadest point. As such, if the wire had been inserted too far posterior in the fibular head in these specimens, the nerve was at potentially increased risk of injury.

Calculating a ratio, the wires inserted in this study were 49 % of the distance from the anterior aspect of the fibula to the nerve lying posteriorly (range 26–100 %). However, in one specimen, the nerve lay touching the wire after insertion. In this specimen, the wire had been inserted more posteriorly in the fibula and had been inserted in a more distal position than in the other specimens, where the nerve begins to cross the neck of the fibula. After measurements had been taken, the fibula head was dissected fully in this specimen and was found to extend more proximally than had been felt on palpation. Therefore, using a landmark palpation technique, the wire was inserted too distally and too posterior risking injury to the common peroneal nerve. Following this finding, the authors recommend that, in cases in which the fibula head is easily palpable, surgeons should observe a safe zone located 2 cm from the tip of the styloid process of the fibula and within the anterior half of the fibula Figs. 4 and 5. The surgeon should consider using fluoroscopic guidance to locate this safe point prior to fibula transfixion wire insertion.

The authors recognise the limitations of this study. The cadaveric specimens used were not complete legs, and therefore, measurements of the length of the fibula were not possible. The measurements taken were expressed as ratios in relation to the maximal AP diameter of the fibula head and used to describe proximity of inserted wires to the common peroneal nerve.

In cases of trauma involving either tibial or fibula fracture, the local anatomy may be distorted as described by El-Shazly et al. Similarly, in cases of deformity, the bony anatomy and the course of the nerve around the proximal fibula may be distorted. The observations of this study only describe the anatomical location of the common peroneal nerve in specimens with normal proximal tibiofibula anatomy and without fracture. In such cases, the position of the common peroneal nerve may be displaced during the initial trauma, especially when marked

shortening of the tibia occurs [8], and it may be placed at additional risk during proximal fibula head wire insertion. Special care and consideration of open exposure of the common peroneal nerve may be required in such cases to avoid iatrogenic injury.

It was not possible to obtain information on the origin or demographic details of the specimens used in this study, and therefore, factors such as age or sex were not taken into account. The authors acknowledge that the findings of this study are of limited use in the paediatric population as none of the specimens dissected represented a skeletally immature individual. The anatomy in such cases may vary from that of the adult population and that limited inferences regarding the safe zone of wire insertion can be made from the finding of this paper. The authors appreciate that sample size in this study is small and that further studies allowing for larger numbers of male and female specimens are required to demonstrate any difference between the sexes in the course of the nerve and safe wire insertion zones if one exists.

Based on the findings in this study, we recommend that proximal fibula head wires should be inserted no further than 2 cm distal to the tip of the fibular head and aim slightly anterior in the fibula head in AP plane at the level of its maximal diameter, Fig. 4 and 5. Feeling the anterior edge of the fibula with wire and inserting the wire anteriorly will achieve correct placement of wire in AP plane. This will reduce the risk of placing the wire inadvertently too distal or posterior and injuring the nerve. In cases where the fibular head is not clearly palpable, the use of intraoperative radiographic imaging should be considered to correctly position the wire in both the sagittal and coronal planes.

Research involving Human Participants and/or Animals This article does not contain any studies performed on animals by any of the authors. All procedures performed in studies involving human participants were in accordance with the ethical standards of the institutional and/or national research committee and with the 1964 Helsinki declaration and its later amendments or comparable ethical standards.

Informed consent For this study formal consent was not required.

References

1. Kirgis A, Albrecht S (1992) Palsy of the deep peroneal nerve after proximal tibial osteotomy. An anatomical study. J Bone Joint Surg Am 74(8):1180–1185
2. Slawski DP, Schoenecker PL, Rich MM (1994) Peroneal nerve injury as a complication of pediatric tibial osteotomies: a review of 255 osteotomies. J Pediatr Orthop 14(2):166–172
3. Stitgen SH, Cairns ER, Ebraheim NA, Niemann JM, Jackson WT (1992) Anatomic considerations of pin placement in the proximal tibia and its relationship to the peroneal nerve. Clin Orthop Relat Res 278:134–137
4. Reebye O (2004) Anatomical and clinical study of the common fibular nerve. Part 1: anatomical study. Surg Radiol Anat 26:365–370
5. Moskovich R (1987) Proximal tibial transfixion for skeletal traction. An anatomic study of neurovascular structures. Clin Orthop Relat Res 214:264–268
6. Rubel IF, Schwarzbard I, Leonard A, Cece D (2004) Anatomic location of the peroneal nerve at the level of the proximal aspect of the tibia: Gerdy's safe zone. J Bone Joint Surg Am 86:1625–1628
7. Rupp RE, Podeszwa D, Ebraheim NA (1994) Danger zones associated with fibular osteotomy. J Orthop Trauma 8(1):54–58
8. El-Shazly M, Saleh M (2002) Displacement of the common peroneal nerve associated with upper tibial fracture: implications for fine wire fixation. J Orthop Trauma 16(3):204–207

The effects of tibial fracture and Ilizarov osteosynthesis on the structural reorganization of sciatic and tibial nerves during the bone consolidation phase and after fixator removal

Tatyana N. Varsegova[1] · Natalia A. Shchudlo[1] · Mikhail M. Shchudlo[1] ·
Marat S. Saifutdinov[1] · Mikhail A. Stepanov[1]

Abstract Reactive and adaptive changes in mechanically uninjured nerves during fracture healing have not been studied previously although the status of innervation is important for bone union and functional recovery. This study explores whether subclinical nerve fibre degeneration occurs in mechanically uninjured nerves in an animal fracture model and to quantify its extent and functional significance. Twenty-four dogs were deeply anaesthetized and subjected to experimental tibial shaft fracture and Ilizarov osteosynthesis. Before fracture and during the experiment, electromyography was performed. In 7, 14, 20, 35–37 and 50 days of fixation and 30, 60–90 and 120 days after fixator removal, the dogs were euthanized. Samples from sciatic, peroneal and tibial nerves were processed for semithin section histology and morphometry. On the 37th postoperative day, M-response amplitudes in leg muscles were 70 % lower than preoperative ones. After fixator removal, these increased but were not restored to normal values. There were no signs of nerve injuries from bone fragments or wires from the fixator. The incidence of degenerated myelin fibres (MFs) was less than 12 %. Reorganization of Remak bundles (Group C nerve fibres—principally sensory) led to a temporal increase in numerical nerve fibre densities. Besides axonal atrophy, the peroneal nerve was characterized with demyelination–remyelination, while tibial nerve with hypermyelination. There were changes in endoneural vessel densities. In spite of minor acute MF degeneration, sustained axonal atrophy, dismyelination and retrograde changes did not resolve until 120 days after fracture healing. Correlations of morphometric parameters of degenerated MF with M-response amplitudes from electromyography underlie the subclinical neurologic changes in functional outcomes after tibial fractures even when nerves are mechanically uninjured.

Keywords Shin bone fractures · Nerve fibres degeneration · Dogs

Introduction

The shaft of the tibia is the commonest site of closed and open fractures, but the optimum treatment option remains the subject of debate. The standard treatment for tibial diaphyseal fractures is intramedullary nailing. This treatment option has resulted in a good ability for the patients to return to work, especially after interlocked nailing [1]. In some cohort studies, a high rate of complications from intramedullary nailing has been described [2, 3]. Even in series with a low rate of complications after intramedullary nailing, 60 % of patients experienced limitations in activity and restrictions in quality of life and 44 % reported knee pain [4].

An alternative, external fixation and the Ilizarov fixator, has been labelled "a panacea for the poor" [5] and has found wide use in developing countries [6]. Ilizarov osteosynthesis is considered as a preferred, safe and effective method in open, wedged and complex tibial fractures [7–11], but one disadvantage is the use of wires situated close to nerves [12]. Theoretically, disorders of nerves of the central or peripheral system can have substantial influence on bone health and repair [13], but little is known about reorganization of nerves after fractures in the extremities [14]. The well-known classification of nerve injuries are applied usually to clinical

✉ Natalia A. Shchudlo
nshchudlo@mail.ru

[1] Russian Ilizarov Scientific Center for Restorative Traumatology and Orthopaedics, 6, M.Ulyanova Street, Kurgan, Russian Federation 6640014

evident cases of nerve injury [15], but the role of peripheral nerves in posttraumatic skeletal pain, functional recovery and bone healing is poorly understood [16], although in tissue samples of aseptic delayed union or nonunion of diaphyseal bones the paucity or total lack of peripheral innervation was marked [17].

Aim

The aim of the study was to identify destructive and adaptive histological changes in the sciatic, peroneal and tibial nerves and establish the degree and sequence of recovery after an experimental tibial shaft fracture and Ilizarov osteosynthesis.

Materials and methods

Experimental design

Twenty-nine adult mongrel dogs were used weighing 11–20 kg and 3–5 years of age. Experiments were carried out in accordance with the internationally agreed **Principles of Laboratory Animal Care** (**NIH** Publication **no. 85-23**, revised **1985**) with the experiment protocol approved by the animal care committee at the authors' institution. The control group consisted of five intact and nonoperated dogs, and the experimental group of 24 dogs underwent fracture and osteosynthesis.

Modelling of fracture and surgery

After deep intravenous combined anaesthesia and standard leg positioning, the tibial fracture was created by a standard load of 5 kg falling from the height of 1.5 m. The fracture was reduced and immobilized with a splint in the following 24 h. Ilizarov transosseous osteosynthesis was performed in aseptic conditions of operating room with a repeat of anaesthesia thereafter. Prophylactic Cefazolin was administered postoperatively for 7 days. Wounds and wire channels were monitored daily. After sedation, standard anteroposterior and lateral radiographs (Fig. 1) of the fractured tibia were made at 1-week intervals to assess fracture healing.

Electrophysiological tests

Intramuscular EMG was performed after anaesthesia at four time-points: (1) at 37 and 50 fixation days (F37 and F50); (2) at 30 and 60–90 days postfixator removal (WA30, WA60–90). Stimulus-induced bioelectric activity (M-responses) in gastrocnemius and tibialis anterior muscles was

recorded using a digital EMG-system DISA-1500 (DANTEC, Denmark). Biopotential leads were monopolar with modified needle electrodes. The active recording electrode was inserted transcutaneously in the muscle belly and the reference electrode in its tendon. M-responses were recorded after supramaximal electrical stimulation was applied to the sciatic nerve through paraneural needle electrodes using rectangular wave pulses of 1-ms duration. Muscle action potential amplitudes were measured from the top of the negative peak to the top of maximal positive peak.

Morphological evaluation

The animals were euthanized at eight time-points: 7, 14, 20, 37, 50 fixation days (F7, F14, F20, F37, F50); also at 30, 60–90 and 120 days after the fixator removal (without apparatus WA30, WA60–90, WA120). The nerve samples were processed to obtain epoxy semithin sections at three sites: middle one-third of the thigh for sciatic nerve, middle one-third of the leg for peroneal and tibial nerves. Sections (thickness 0.5–1.0 μm) were made with glass knives using the Nova ultratome LKB (Sweden), mounted on glass slides and then stained with toluidine blue and methylene blue-basic fuchsin. The images were digitized using the photomicroscope "Opton" (Germany) connected to the "DiaMorph" software program (Russia, Moscow). Histomorphometry was performed with the "VT-Master-Morphology" program (VideoTest, Russia, St. Petersburg). In 25 nonoverlapping fields of the endoneural compartment from each nerve, collected in a systematic random order, the numerical densities of endoneural vessels ($N_A$mv), myelinated and unmyelinated nerve fibres ($N_A$mf and $N_A$uf), and per cent of degenerated myelinated nerve fibres (Deg%) were evaluated. About 400 samples of myelinated fibres for each nerve site were made, and morphometric parameters—diameters of myelinated nerve fibres (Dmf), their axons (Dax) and myelin sheath thickness (Lmyel)—were measured.

Statistical evaluation

The data obtained were evaluated for statistical differences using the unpaired Student t test, Mann–Whitney U test and Pearson correlation test (software package Attestat Program, version 9.3.1, developed by I. P. Gaidyshev, Certificate of Rospatent official registration No. 2002611109).

Results

Radiograph assessment

The 24 fractures were classified by the AO/OTA system as: four type 42A3; four type 42B1; two 42B2; nine 42B3;

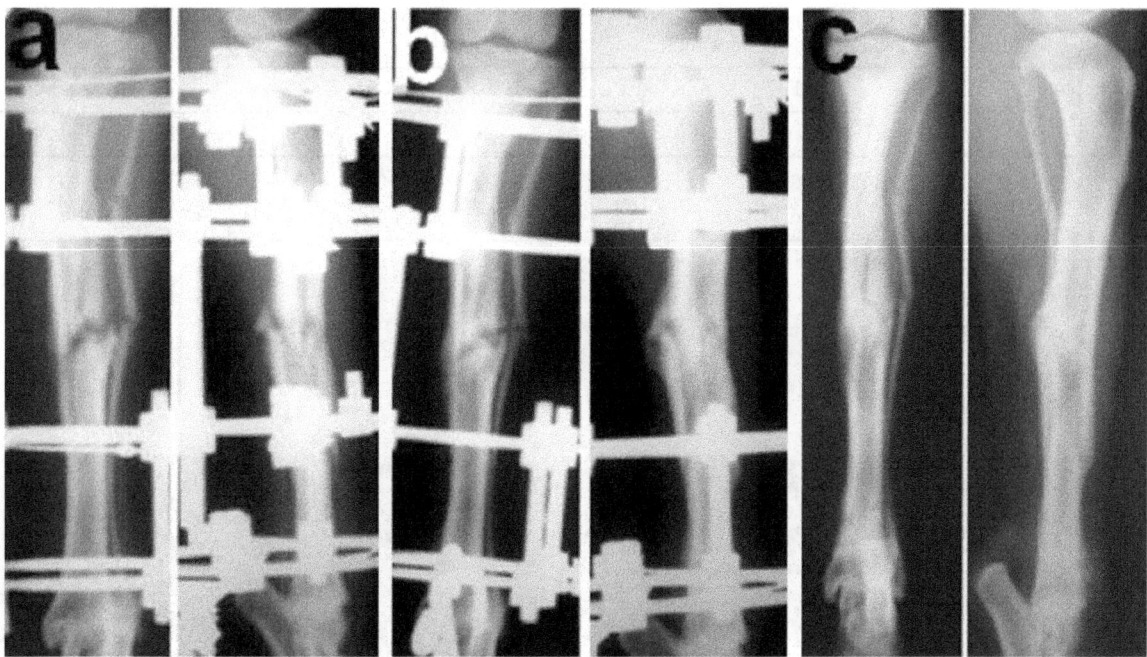

Fig. 1 Tibial fracture in dog on standard X-ray radiographs. **a** Fixation in apparatus 21 days, **b** 50 days—the end of consolidation phase, **c** 30 days after the fixator removal

four 42C1; and one 42C3. Correspondingly, 16.7 % fractures were simple, 62.5 % wedge and 20.8 % complex. Using the Gustilo classification in 22 dogs, the fractures were open and were classed as types II and IIIa. The time for clinical and radiological consolidation from the date of injury to removal of Ilizarov frame varied from 42 to 50 days (46.3 ± 1.5).

Electrophysiological tests

At the end of consolidation phase (F37 and F50), the average recorded M-response amplitudes were substantially decreased in comparison with the initial levels, especially in tibialis anterior muscles (Table 1). After fixator removal, these increased and at WA60–90 days were at 79.5 % of the initial level in gastrocnemius and 62.2 % in tibialis anterior. At the end of experiment, these parameters varied individually and did not reach initial levels.

Microscopic observation

After 7, 14 and 20 fixation days, the peroneal nerve epineurium was oedematous with loci of haemorrhage and paravasal lymphocytic or plasmocytic infiltration. A high content of macrophages, mast cells and plasmocytes was noted in the epineurium until 50–80 days of the experiment. Many of epineural blood vessels possessed thickened walls and widened lumens, with signs of myocyte

dystrophy and death. Large arterioles and capillaries with widened lumens were seen in the endoneural vessels which is unusual for intact nerves. In some fascicles, signs of perineuritis were noted. Axonal and Wallerian degeneration or demyelination occurred more often in thick myelinated fibres at early time-points (F7–F20) in peroneal nerve (Fig. 2a, b), but were very rare in the tibial nerves. Unmyelinated fibre loss was seen in the peroneal nerve (Fig. 2b). At F50 nerve fibre regeneration was the dominant picture. Some sections of regenerated fibres contained elements of paranodal sprouting and were encircled with lemmocytic proliferates; these are signs of repeating de- and remyelination (Fig. 2c). Nerve fibre hypermyelination was typical in the tibial nerve from F20 until the end of experiment (Fig. 3a, b). Most of the unmyelinated nerve fibres contained few axons but many Schwann cell nuclei. An increased number of Remak bundles containing small myelinated axons occurred in tibial nerve, much more than would be seen for an intact nerve. The same remodelling of Remak bundles was noted in sciatic nerve.

Morphometric findings

Table 2 shows that in the leg (tibial and peroneal nerves), maximal degeneration was seen at F7, whereas in the sciatic nerve this occurred at F14.

Figure 4 shows the differences of endoneural vessel densities between nerves of experimental and intact animals. In the peroneal nerve after the first 2 weeks of

Table 1 Mean (±standard deviation) of M-response amplitudes (mV) in gastrocnemius and tibialis anterior muscles before fracture, at consolidation phase (F37 and F50 days) and after the fixator removal (WA30 and WA60–90 days)

Time-points and parameter value/muscle	Ai	F37		F50		WA30		WA60–90	
		Ae	Δ%	Ae	Δ%	Ae	Δ%	Ae	Δ%
Gastrocnemius	26.8 (1.2)	8.9* (0.8)	−66.8 %	11.4* (0.7)	−57.8 %	18.2 (1.5)	−32.1 %	21.3 (2.1)	−20.5 %
Tibialis anterior	23.8 (1.3)	6.1* (1.0)	−74.4 %	6.7* (1.0)	−71.8 %	12.5* (1.3)	−47.5 %	14.8 (1.1)	−37.8 %

Ai initial amplitudes values (before fracture and osteosynthesis), *Ae* experimental values

$\Delta\% = (Ai - Ae)/Ai \times 100\ \%$

* Significant differences (*t* test; $p < 0.05$) between Ai and Ae

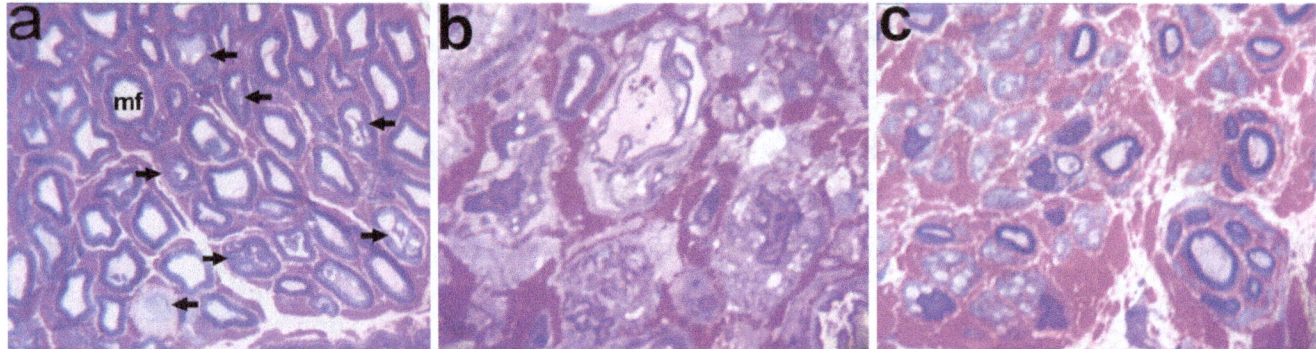

Fig. 2 Fragments of histological transverse semithin sections of the peroneal nerve in dogs with tibial fracture at the consolidation phase. Methylene blue-basic fuchsin staining. **a, b** Endoneurium at 20 days of fixation in Ilizarov apparatus: *mf* normal myelinated fibre, *arrows* degenerated mf, **b** almost all myelinated and unmyelinated fibres are degenerated, **c** regenerated nerve fibres at 50 days of fixation in Ilizarov apparatus. Instrumental magnification 500× (**a**) and 1250× (**b, c**)

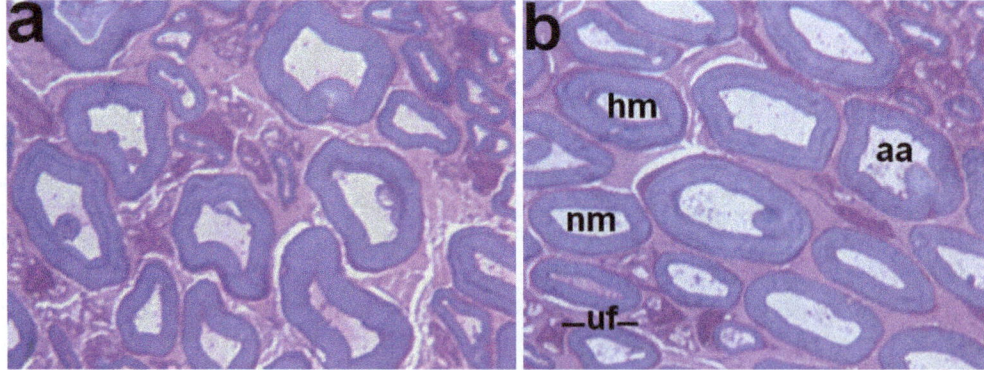

Fig. 3 Fragments of histological transverse semithin sections of the tibial nerve in dogs with tibial fracture at 37 days of the consolidation phase. Methylene blue-basic fuchsin staining. **a** Majority of nerve fibres with myelin decompaction and axonal atrophy, **b** various nerve fibres: *nm* normally myelinated, *hm* hypermyelinated, *aa* severe axonal atrophy, *uf* profiles of unmyelinated nerve fibres containing nuclei. Instrumental magnification 1250×

experiment, endoneural hypovascularity was noted. From F20 until the end of the experiment, the endoneurium of the peroneal nerve of experimental animals was more vascularized than that of intact group. In tibial nerve at F7, $N_A$mv did not change from those in the intact group, but endoneural hypervascularity was recorded with maximums at F14 and WA30 (Fig. 4).

Figure 5 demonstrates the differences of nerve fibre densities between nerves of experimental and intact animals. In the sciatic nerve, the parameters differed significantly from the intact group at all time-points. At F14 the numerical density of unmyelinated fibres was slightly lower but that of myelinated fibres slightly higher than in intact nerves, but both then increased to 26 and 63 %,

Table 2 Per cent rates—mean (±standard deviation)—of degenerated myelin fibres (Deg%) in sciatic, peroneal and tibial nerves of intact and operated animals

Group and time-point/nerve	Intact animals	Operated animals							
		F7	F14	F20	F37	F50	WA30	WA60–90	WA120
Sciatic	1.79 (0.31)	1.85 (0.14)	6.13 (2.34)	5.12 (2.23)	4.25 (1.89)	3.11 (1.68)	3.44 (1.42)	2.89 (1.43)	4.12 (1.09)
Peroneal	1.92 (0.31)	12.51 (2.09)	11.79 (0.30)	8.43 (2.24)	4.64 (0.85)	5.66 (3.52)	5.00 (0.31)	4.74 (0.35)	4.16 (1.00)
Tibial	1.64 (0.20)	10.11 (0.20)	8.65 (3.47)	4.82 (2.32)	5.81 (1.30)	5.44 (0.80)	4.82 (0.37)	5.00 (0.96)	3.77 (0.53)

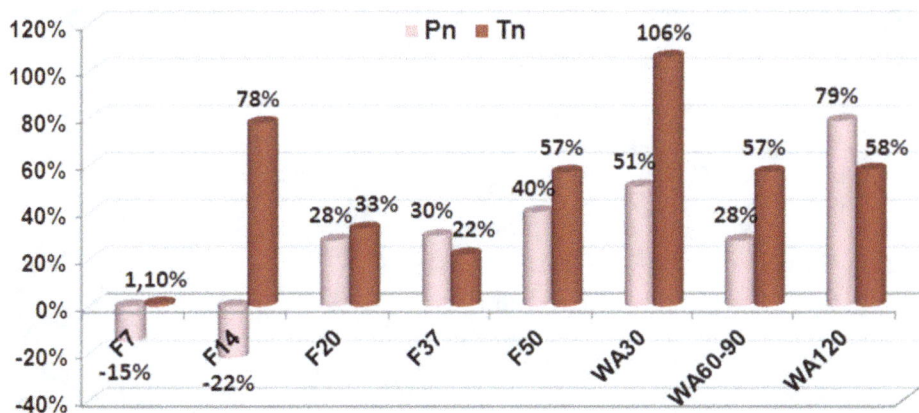

Fig. 4 Endoneural vessel quantification. Per cents of differences of endoneural vessel densities between nerves of intact (i) and experimental (e) animals (N_Amv-i − N_Amv-e/N_Amv-i × 100 %) in peroneal (Pn) and tibial (Tn) nerves at various time-points of experiment (F7–F50—days of consolidation phase; WA30–WA120—days after the fixator removal)

respectively. From F14 to WA30, these decreased and then increased again until the end of the experiment. The oscillation of unmyelinated nerve fibre densities was more marked. In the leg the tibial and peroneal nerves had, at the beginning of experiment, nerve fibre densities lower than in intact nerves especially with the unmyelinated nerve fibre density in the peroneal nerve (Fig. 5). In the peroneal but not in the tibial nerve, oscillations of myelinated and unmyelinated nerve fibre densities were synchronized. At the end of experiment, numerical nerve fibre densities of experimental animals did not differ from nerves in the intact group.

A notable correlation was found between numerical densities of endoneural vessels and unmyelinated nerve fibres in the peroneal nerve ($r = 0.71$) and between numerical densities of endoneural vessels and myelinated nerve fibres in the tibial nerve ($r = 0.66$).

Table 3 shows changes in size of myelinated nerve fibres and their axons in peroneal and tibial nerves of experimental animals in comparison with the intact group. At F7, the average diameters of myelinated nerve fibres and their axons were lower than in intact nerves, but, in the tibial nerves, myelin sheaths were thicker on average than in intact nerves. The greatest decrease in average diameters of myelin fibres and theirs axons was noted at F50 and WA30. Myelin sheaths of nerve fibres in peroneal nerves at F14 and the following time-points of the consolidation phase were significantly thinner on average than in intact nerves especially at F37, but, after fixator removal, the

parameter recovered. For nerve fibres of the tibial nerve, a sustained increase in myelin thickness was seen.

A strong correlation was established between the mid-values of the amplitudes of M-responses in tibialis anterior and the average nerve fibre size of the peroneal nerve: r values for relation between the M-responses and the average myelin nerve fibre diameter, axonal diameter and myelin thickness were 0.84, 0.92 and 0.65, respectively. As for the tibial nerve, a positive correlation between the mid-values of the amplitudes of M-responses in gastrocnemius was established with the average myelin nerve fibre diameter and axonal diameter (r values 0.69 and 0.57, respectively). For an average myelin thickness $r = -0.91$, indicates a negative functional significance of hypermyelination.

Discussion

The recovery of contractile muscle action after tibial fractures is problematic especially for sportsmen [18]. To assess a neurologic impact in such a condition, we have studied histological changes in the peroneal, tibial and sciatic canine nerves after experimental leg fractures. Severe nerve injuries arising from bone fragments were not shown. We used an Ilizarov fixator for fracture stabilization, but nerve injuries from the wires were also not shown. Bone union was achieved earlier than after hybrid fixator use in dogs [19].

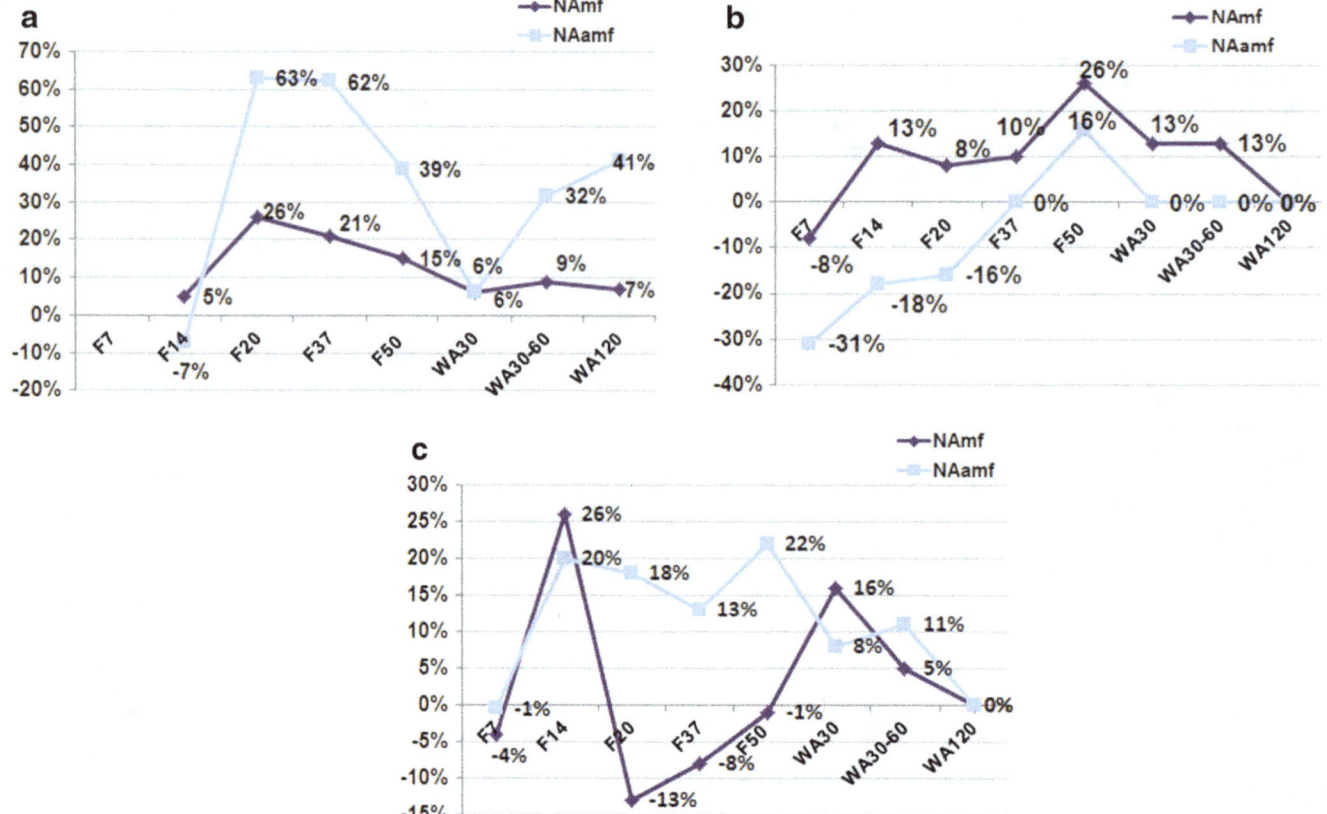

Fig. 5 Numerical densities of myelinated and unmyelinated nerve fibres (N$_A$mf and N$_A$uf). Per cents of differences of nerve fibre densities between nerves of intact and experimental animals at various time-points of experiment (F7–F50—days of consolidation phase; WA30–WA120—days after the fixator removal) **a** sciatic nerve, **b** peroneal nerve, **c** tibial nerve

A greater deficit of bioelectric activity was seen in tibialis anterior muscle than in gastrocnemius. Substantial differences in histological changes within the peroneal and tibial nerves were also recorded. In the peroneal nerve, we observed more destructive changes in the epineurium, endoneural hypovascularity and striking loss of unmyelinated nerve fibres. In spite of active neuroregeneration and remyelination at the end of consolidation phase, even at 120 days after fixator removal, axonal atrophy was sustained and the percentage of degenerated myelinated fibres was higher than in intact nerves. The M-responses amplitudes in tibialis anterior muscle was 40 % lower than initial levels. In tibial nerve, in spite of better preservation of unmyelinated nerve fibres, axonal atrophy was also seen together with degenerative hypermyelination. A probable explanation of differences between peroneal and tibial nerves changes is the diversity of microvascular compression, confirmed by dynamics of endoneural vascularity and consistent with other authors' clinical data about pressure in closed fascial leg compartments after isolated tibial fractures [20]. It is known that in patients with trigeminal

neuralgia, the various types of demyelination correspond to the extent of trigeminal root compression [21].

An unexpected finding in our research was a substantial increase in nerve fibre numerical densities at some time-points of experiment due to remodelling of Remak bundles. The first peak was at 14 days of fixation and the second at the end of consolidation phase. An increase in nerve fibre numerical densities and myelination of unmyelinated axons in Remak bundles was observed in the sciatic nerve of the rat after intraperitoneal injections of GDNF [22]. While the inductive effect of GDNF on osteoblasts proliferation is well known [23], expression of various neurotrophins and their receptors by osteogenic cells has also been shown [24]. It is possible that the fluctuations of numerical nerve fibre densities in the sciatic, peroneal and tibial nerves after tibial fractures reflect a regulatory role of the nervous system in fracture healing.

A limitation of this study is the absence of data on neural growth factor expression. Further research is needed about the relation and influence of the identified destructive and adaptive nerve changes on fracture healing.

Table 3 Mean (±standard deviation) of morphometric parameters (mkm) of myelinated fibres (MF) in peroneal and tibial nerves of intact (I) animals and in nerves of operated animals

Group and time-point/nerve parameter	I	Operated animals							
		F7	F14	F20	F37	F50	WA30	WA60–90	WA120
Peroneal									
MF diameter	6.46 (0.07)	6.29* (0.70)	6.08* (0.08)	5.98* (0.32)	5.78* (0.15)	5.03* (0.56)	5.67* (0.20)	5.89* (0.07)	6.21* (0.39)
Axonal diameter	4.39 (0.08)	4.18* (0.53)	4.17* (0.01)	4.04* (0.35)	3.73* (0.19)	3.40* (0.20)	3.42* (0.06)	3.98* (0.14)	4.15* (0.24)
Myelin thickness	1.04 (0.04)	1.06 (0.11)	0.95* (0.04)	0.97* (0.01)	0.67* (0.48)	0.82* (0.13)	1.00* (0.07)	0.96* (0.05)	1.07 (0.09)
Tibial									
MF diameter	6.75 (0.28)	7.20* (2.91)	6.01* (0.07)	6.44* (0.35)	6.58* (0.35)	6.28* (0.64)	6.31* (0.41)	6.46* (0.36)	6.76 (0.10)
Axonal diameter	4.63 (0.33)	4.18* (1.62)	3.95* (0.44)	4.00* (0.33)	4.14* (0.37)	3.80* (0.21)	3.56* (0.05)	3.97* (0.15)	4.25* (0.16)
Myelin thickness	1.06 (0.05)	1.51* (0.74)	1.03 (0.19)	1.22* (0.17)	1.22* (0.03)	1.24* (0.24)	1.24* (0.23)	1.22* (0.24)	1.25* (0.03)

* Significant differences (Mann–Whitney U test; $p < 0.01$) between experimental and intact groups

Conclusion

In this animal study, we show, for the first time, that even in the absence of nerve injuries either from the fracture or through the application of an Ilizarov fixator, partial degenerative changes, axonal atrophy and demyelination of nerve fibres occur in the peroneal and tibial nerves which influence muscle bioelectric activity negatively during the period of fracture healing and for a long time after fixator removal.

Acknowledgments This work was supported by the Russian Foundation for Basic Research (Project No. 14-44-00010).

Research involving Human Participants and/or Animals Research was conducted in accordance with AVMA Animal Welfare Principles.

Informed consent For this type of study (animal research) formal patient consent is not required.

References

1. Lee Y-S, Lo T-Y, Huang H-L (2008) Intramedullary fixation of tibial shaft fractures: a comparison of the unlocked and interlocked nail. Int Orthop 32(1):69–74
2. Bhandari M, Guyatt G, Tornetta P 3rd et al (2008) Randomized trial of reamed and unreamed intramedullary nailing of tibial shaft fractures. J Bone Joint Surg 90-A:2567–2578
3. Court-Brown CM (2004) Reamed intramedullary tibial nailing, an overview and analysis of 1106 cases. J Orthop Trauma 18:96–101
4. Larsen P, Lund H, Laessoe U, Graven-Nielsen T, Rasmussen S (2014) Restrictions in quality of life after intramedullary nailing of tibial shaft fracture. A retrospective follow-up study of 223 cases. J Orthop Trauma 28(9):507–512. doi:10.1097/BOT.0000000000000031
5. Padhi NR, Padhi P (2007) Use of external fixators for open tibial injuries in the rural third world: Panacea of the poor? Injury 38(2):150–159
6. Ganji SME, Bahrami M, Joukar F (2011) Ilizarov versus AO external fixator for the treatment of tibia open fractures. Iran Red Crescent Med J 13(12):868–872 **(Epub 2011 Dec 1)**
7. Inan M, Tuncel M, Karaoğlu S, Halici M (2002) Treatment of type II and III open tibial fractures with Ilizarov external fixation. Acta Orthop Traumatol Turc 36(5):390–396
8. Hosny G, Fadel M (2003) Ilizarov external fixator for open fractures of the tibial shaft. Int Orthop 27(5):303–306 **(Epub 2003 Jun 17)**
9. Martel II (2011) Chreskostnii osteosintez po Ilizarovu v kompleksnom lechenii bolnih s otkritimi povrejdenijami konechnostei Мартель И.И. [Transosseus Ilizarov osteosynthesis in complex treatment of patients with open extremitas trauma]. Genij Ortopedii 2:44–48
10. Wani N, Baba A, Kangoo K, Mir M (2011) Role of early Ilizarov ring fixator in the definitive management of type II, IIIA and IIIB open tibial shaft fractures. Int Orthop 35(6):915–923
11. Foster PA, Barton SB, Jones SC, Morrison RJ, Britten S (2012) The treatment of complex tibial shaft fractures by the Ilizarov

method. J Bone Joint Surg Br 94(12):1678–1683. doi:10.1302/
0301-620X.94B12.29266

12. Shortt NL, Keenan GF, Muir AY, Simpson AH (2006) The use of
a nerve stimulator to allow safe placement of Ilizarov wires. Oper
Orthop Traumatol 18(4):364–376

13. Sadraie SH, Kaka GhR, Mofid M, Torkaman G, Jalali Monfared
M (2011) Effects of low intensity pulsed ultrasound on healing of
denervated tibial fracture in the rabbit. Iran Red Crescent Med J
13(1):34–41

14. Varsegova TN, Shchudlo NA, Shchudlo MM, Stepanov MA
(2014) Strukturnaja reorganizatsia malobecovogo nerva pri
zajivlenii perelomov kostei goleni v eksperimente [Structural
reorganization of peroneal nerve during the shin bone fracture
healing in the experiment]. Uspehi sovremennogo estestvoznanija
6:13–18

15. Seddon HJ (1943) Three types of nerve injury. Brain
66(4):237–288

16. Mohler LR, Hanel DP (2006) Closed fractures complicated by
peripheral nerve injury. J Am Acad Orthop Surg 14(1):32–37

17. Santavirta S, Konttinen YT, Nordström D, Mäkelä A, Sorsa T,
Hukkanen M, Rokkanen P (1992) Immunologic studies of non-
united fractures. Acta Orthop Scand 63(6):579–586

18. Gaston P, Will E, McQueen MM, Elton RA, Court-Brown CM
(2000) Analysis of muscle function in the lower limb after
fracture of the diaphysis of the tibia in adults. J Bone Joint Surg
Br 82-B(3):326–331

19. Gemmill TJ, Cave TA, Clements DN, Clarke SP, Bennett D,
Carmichael S (2004) Treatment of canine and feline diaphyseal
tibial fractures with low-stiffness external skeletal fixation. J of
Small Anim Pract 45(2):85–91

20. Müller M, Disch AC, Zabel N, Haas NP, Schaser KD (2008)
Initial intramuscular perfusion pressure predicts early skeletal
muscle function following isolated tibial fractures. J Orthop Surg
Res 3:14. doi:10.1186/1749-799X-3-14

21. Devor M, Govrin-Lippmann R, Rappaport ZH (2002) Mechanism
of trigeminal neuralgia: an ultrastructural analysis of trigeminal
root specimens obtained during microvascular decompression
surgery. J Neurosurg 96:532–543

22. Höke A, Ho T, Crawford TO, LeBel C, Hilt D, Griffin JW (2003)
Glial cell line-derived neurotrophic factor alters axon schwann
cell units and promotes myelination in unmyelinated nerve fibers.
J Neurosci 23(2):561–567

23. Gale Z, Cooper PR, Scheven BA (2012) Glial cell line-derived
neurotrophic factor influences proliferation of osteoblastic cells.
Cytokine 57(2):276–281

24. Asaumi K, Nakanishi T, Asahara H, Inoue H, Takigawa M (2000)
Expression of neurotrophins and their receptors (TRK) during
fracture healing. Bone 26(6):625–633

8

Hook plate fixation for acute acromioclavicular dislocations without coracoclavicular ligament reconstruction: a functional outcome study in military personnel

Narinder Kumar[1] · Vyom Sharma[1]

Abstract The aim of our study was to evaluate the shoulder function after clavicular hook plate fixation of acute acromioclavicular dislocations (Rockwood type III) in a population group consisting exclusively of high-demand military personnel. This prospective study was carried out at a tertiary care military orthopaedic centre during 2012–2013 using clavicular hook plate for management of acromioclavicular injuries without coracoclavicular ligament reconstruction in 33 patients. All patients underwent routine implant removal after 16 weeks. The functional outcome was assessed at 3, 6 and 12 months after hook plate removal and 2 years from the initial surgery using the Constant Murley and UCLA Scores. All the patients were male serving soldiers and had sustained acromioclavicular joint dislocation (Rockwood type III). Mean age of the patient group was 34.24 years (21–55 years). The mean follow-up period in this study was 23.5 months (20–26 months) after hook plate fixation and an average of 19.9 months (17–22 months) after hook plate removal. The average Constant Score at 3 months after hook plate removal was 60.3 as compared to 83.7 and 90.3 at 6 months and 1 year, respectively, and an average of 91.8 at the last follow-up that was approximately 2 years after initial surgery which was statistically significant (p value <0.05). The UCLA Score was an average of 15.27, 25.9 and 30.1 at 3, 6 months and 1 year, respectively, after removal of hook plate which improved further an average of 32.3 at the last follow-up, which was also statistically significant (p value <0.05). Clavicular hook plate fixation without coracoclavicular ligament reconstruction is a good option for acute acromioclavicular dislocations producing excellent medium-term functional results in high-demand soldiers.

Keywords Acromioclavicular dislocation · Hook plate · Military personnel

Introduction

Acromioclavicular joint injuries are a common entity with an ever-evolving approach towards management of these injuries from the days of Hippocrates [1] and Galen [2]. The quantum of these injuries is on the rise constituting approximately 9–12 % of all shoulder injuries following fall on an outstretched hand [3–6]. The commonly used and validated classification proposed by Rockwood divides these injuries into six types [7]. Though there is general consensus about conservative management for Rockwood type I and II injuries and surgical treatment for Rockwood type IV, V and VI injuries, the most suitable treatment for Rockwood type III injuries remains controversial [8–11].

Different approaches have been described for management of these injuries ranging from conservative management with bandages and slings to multiple surgical options including fixation of the acromioclavicular joint with pins, tension band wiring, the modified Weaver–Dunn procedure, fixation with washer and screw, suspensory fixation devices and clavicular hook plate. All of these options have their own specific advantages and disadvantages, but no clearly superior option has been established as yet [12].

The clavicular hook plates are pre-contoured plates with varying sizes and depths as well as side to fit different

✉ Narinder Kumar
kumarnarinder1969@gmail.com

Vyom Sharma
vyom120.sharma@gmail.com

[1] Military Hospital, Kirkee, Pune, Maharashtra 411020, India

anatomy. After reduction in the acromioclavicular joint, the hook is placed under the acromion process posteriorly and the screws are used to fix the plate to lateral clavicle maintaining the reduction. The manufacturers of the plate recommend routine removal of the plate after 3 months to avert the complications of subacromial impingement and acromial osteolysis. Clavicular hook plates have been demonstrated to be an effective implant option for surgical treatment of Rockwood type III acromioclavicular dislocation but concerns have been raised about acromial osteolysis, subacromial impingement and even possibly rotator cuff injuries [13–15].

In view of absence of any concrete evidence for an ideal implant for fixation of a Rockwood type III acromioclavicular joint dislocation and necessity of coracoclavicular ligament reconstruction, we undertook this prospective study to establish the efficacy of clavicular hook plate for fixation of acute type III injuries without coracoclavicular/acromioclavicular ligament reconstruction in soldiers involved in high-demand activities and athletics.

Materials and methods

The study design was a prospective study at a tertiary care military orthopaedic centre during 2012–2013 for management of acromioclavicular injuries. All patients with Rockwood type III acromioclavicular injuries were included in the study after approval of the institutional ethical committee. Exclusion criteria included Rockwood type I, II, IV, V, VI injuries, open injuries, polytrauma, neurovascular injury and concomitant shoulder or upper limb trauma. No other management modalities, including conservative management, were employed.

All the patients were subjected to radiographic analysis of an anteroposterior view of the shoulder and stress views which were accordingly classified by the attending surgeon

[16] The radiographs were also assessed for coracoclavicular distance comparing in the injured versus noninjured shoulder (Fig. 1). Type III acromioclavicular injuries were treated surgically within 48 h of arrival at the centre with open reduction and fixation with clavicular hook plate (DePuy Synthes) in beach chair position under general anaesthesia. Surgery was delayed in some cases due to concomitant injuries or delay in referral of the patient to our centre. The surgical approach was a transverse incision over lateral third of clavicle. The acromioclavicular joint was exposed after assessing the torn acromioclavicular ligaments. The fixation of the acromioclavicular separation was done with titanium clavicular hook plate (4, 5 or 6 hole) in templated hook offset (12, 15 or 18 mm) without any supplemental ligamentous repair or reconstruction of coracoclavicular or acromioclavicular ligaments. Post-operatively, arm sling was used for 10 days to 2 weeks. Passive- and active-assisted shoulder range of motion (ROM) was commenced on second post-operative day as per pain tolerance. Active shoulder movements including abduction up to 90° were initiated 2 weeks post-operatively onwards.

All patients were taken up for removal of the hook plate after a mean period of 16 weeks (14–22 weeks) and subsequently enrolled in an institutional shoulder rehabilitation programme to regain shoulder range of motion including cuff-strengthening exercises. The patients were followed up for a minimum period of 24 months after hook plate fixation. The patients were subjected to radiographic assessment at 12 weeks, 6 months, 1 and 2 years which included the congruency of acromioclavicular joint and restoration of the coracoclavicular distance or any increase in the same at later follow-up examinations. The functional outcome was assessed using the Constant and Murley Score and UCLA Score with assessment at all follow-ups. The Constant Score and UCLA Score prior to and following hook plate removal were subjected to paired t test for statistical significance.

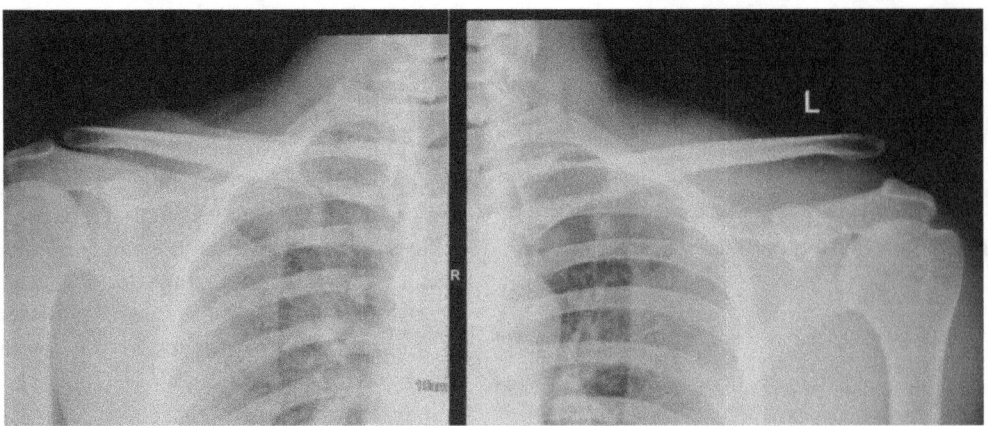

Fig. 1 Pre-operative radiograph showing grade III acromioclavicular dislocation and an increased coracoclavicular distance

Results

A total of 45 patients with acromioclavicular dislocations were managed at a tertiary military orthopaedic centre from Dec 2011 to Apr 2013. The study population comprised of soldiers who were diagnosed with Rockwood type III acromioclavicular dislocation. The sample size was eventually thirty-three soldiers after excluding Rockwood type I, II, IV, V, VI injuries, open injuries, polytrauma, neurovascular injury and concomitant shoulder or upper limb trauma (12 cases excluded). All the included patients were male. The mean age of the patients was 34.24 years (21–55 years) with 40 % in their thirties and 32 % in twenties. The common mechanism of injury was fall on shoulder or outstretched hand following sports injuries (60 %) and road traffic accident (28 %). All the patients had acute injuries (less than 2 weeks). Twenty-three patients (69 %) had injury in the nondominant arm. The average duration of surgical intervention from the day of injury was 9.06 days (4–15 days). All the patients in this study had Rockwood's type III acromioclavicular dislocation. The operating surgeons varied from residents to consultants with experience ranging from 2 to 15 years. The mean duration of the procedure was 43 min (35–55 min). The average length of the incision was 84.2 mm (70–100 mm). The most commonly used hook plate was 5 holes in twenty-four (72 %) patients with 18 mm hook offset. There was no incidence of surgical site infection or any post-operative complications. The average hospital stay was 7.6 days after surgery (5–10 days) as all soldiers undergo supervised rehabilitation. The hospital stay was longer than usual due to peculiar nature of

clientele (soldiers) which hails from all parts of the country. The hospital caters for extra beds required for convalescence till suitable arrangements can be made for convalescing soldier to travel home. The hospital stay includes stay in convalescence beds which would normally be at home in other facilities.

The patients were taken up for removal of the hook plate after an average period of 16 weeks (14–22 weeks) from the day of surgery with 48 % patients in 14- to 16-week period. There were three patients (9 %) who reported after the stipulated period of implant removal (12–14 weeks) at 20–22 weeks.

The mean follow-up period in this study was 23.5 months (20–26 months) after hook plate fixation and an average of 19.9 months (17–22 months) from the day of hook plate removal.

The functional outcome was assessed after hook plate removal at all follow-ups. The average Constant Score at 3 months after hook plate removal was 60.3 (95 % Confidence Interval between 58.7 and 61.9) as compared to 83.7 and 90.3 at 6 months and 1 year, respectively, and an average of 91.8 (95 % Confidence Interval between 88.5 and 93.05) at the last follow-up which was approximately 2 years after initial surgery. This was statistically significant (*p* value <0.05) as shown in Fig. 2. The UCLA Score was an average of 15.27 (95 % Confidence Interval between 14.6 and 15.8), 25.9 and 30.1 at 3, 6 months and 1 year, respectively, after removal of hook plate which was further an average of 32.3 (95 % Confidence Interval between 31.9 and 32.6) at the last follow-up, which was also statistically significant (*p* value <0.05) as shown in Fig. 3.

Fig. 2 Constant Score at 3, 6 months and 1 year after hook plate removal and 2 years post hook plate fixation

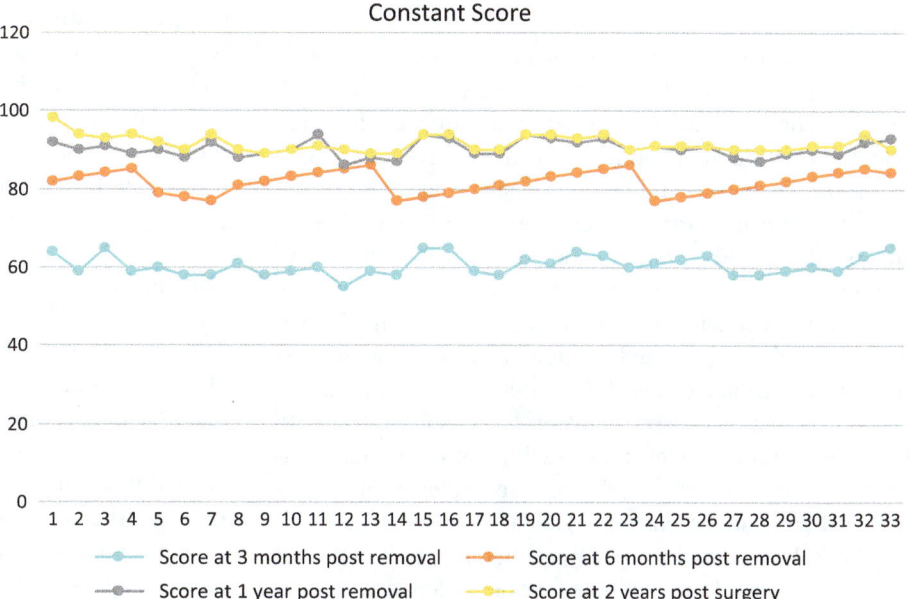

Fig. 3 UCLA Score at 3, 6 months and 1 year after hook plate removal and 2 years post hook plate fixation

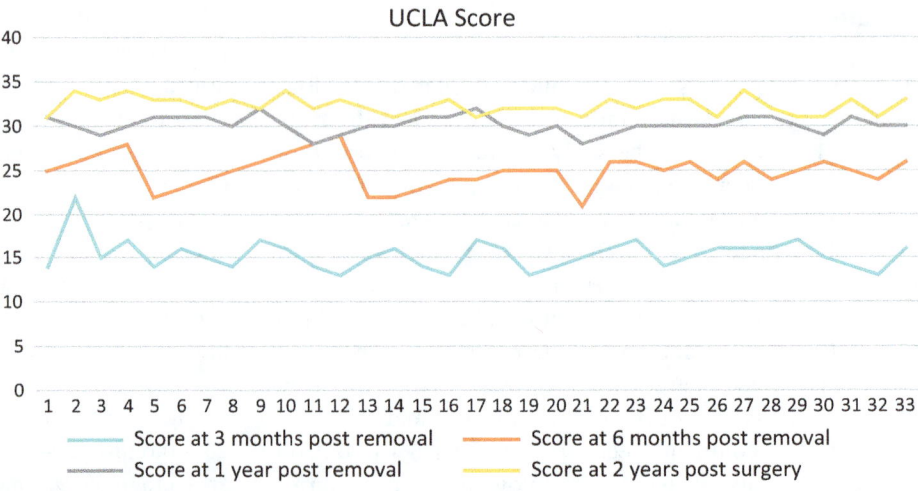

UCLA Score

Legend: Score at 3 months post removal · Score at 6 months post removal · Score at 1 year post removal · Score at 2 years post surgery

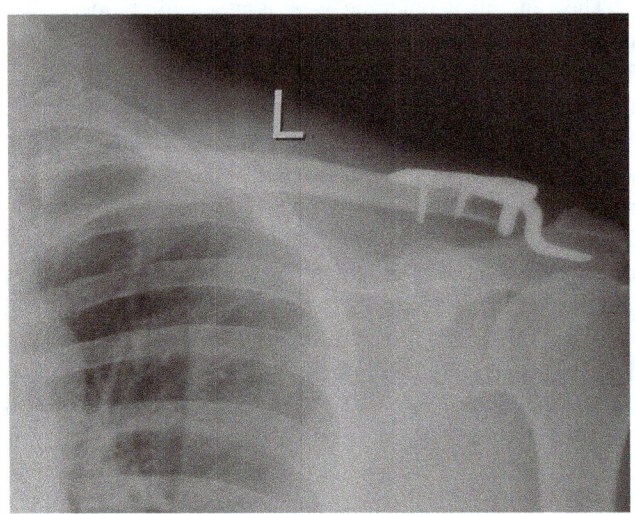

Fig. 4 Post-operative radiograph at 12 weeks showing a congruent acromioclavicular joint and hook plate in situ

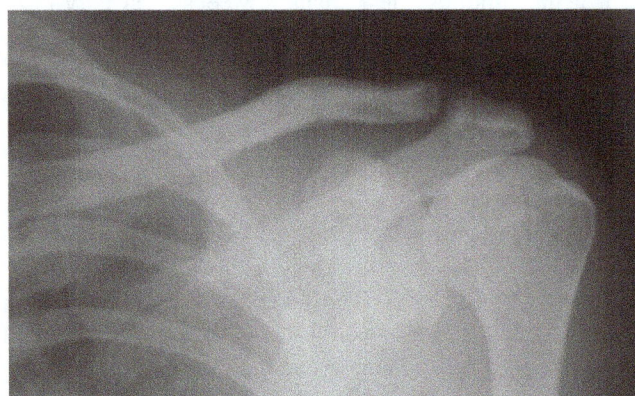

Fig. 5 Stress radiograph at 2 years post hook plate fixation: Congruent acromioclavicular articulation and normal coracoclavicular distance with mild sclerosis

The significant functional limitations in the period prior to hook plate removal were mild-to-moderate pain in 15 (45 %) patients, restricted overhead abduction and terminal internal rotation in majority of patients. The functional evaluation at the last follow-up revealed that none of the patients had pain in the affected shoulder and had achieved full overhead abduction. All the patients had returned to pre-injury activity level including sports except one patient who felt moderate impairment in this regard though he had achieved full range of painless motion. None of the patients had any recurrence of instability after hook plate removal.

The radiological assessment at 12–14 weeks (prior to hook plate removal) by plain radiographs revealed congruent acromioclavicular joint and no evidence of osteolysis and comparable coracoclavicular distance (Fig. 4).

The follow-up radiographs immediately after hook plate removal revealed no subluxation or dislocation and a comparable coracoclavicular distance to the unaffected shoulder on stress radiograph. There was no evidence of osteolysis at the last follow-up post hook plate removal, and screw tracks had healed adequately. There was evidence of sclerosis in acromion and distal end clavicle in three cases, though the patients were completely asymptomatic with full functional recovery (Fig. 5).

Discussion

There has been a shift in the management of acromioclavicular injuries with an ever-increasing consensus towards nonoperative treatment for Rockwood type I–II and surgical treatment for type IV–VI [17]. However, despite more than 150 surgical techniques being described for type III acromioclavicular joint dislocation, there is still no consensus on the ideal fixation method/device for fixation of a type III dislocated acromioclavicular joint [18].

The debate of nonoperative versus operative treatment for type III injuries remains undecided as studies have found advantages and disadvantages of both in young athletic population [19].

The probability of any surgical procedure and fixation device to maintain a congruent acromioclavicular joint and a good shoulder function is dependent on the fixation device which mimics the biomechanics of native acromioclavicular joint. The role of Kirschner wires and pins for fixation of acromioclavicular dislocation has definitely gone into disrepute due to complications like pin breakage and pin migration [20]. The results of coracoclavicular screw with or without ligament reconstruction has also shown variable results in small sample of patients [21]. The basis of using an anatomically contoured clavicular hook plate is the proximity of this device to mimic the amphiarthrotic nature of the acromioclavicular articulation. In view of this, we preferred to use the hook plate in our subset of patients who were primarily athletic and involved in strenuous physical activities as soldiers. Recent literature has reported excellent results using tightrope (arthrex), but these results were not available at the time of our study to consider as an option [17].

The demographic pattern of acromioclavicular injuries has depicted a steep trend towards males sustaining these injuries with 50 % or more in the age group of 20–39 years [22]. Our study population reflected the same with 72 % of the patients belonging to this age group. The role of sport-induced factors in these injuries has been well established, and a large number of patients (60 %) in our study sustained injury during basketball, wrestling, cycling or even fall from a vertical rope in our study population [23].

The most significant disadvantages of conservative management of an acromioclavicular injury are an impaired shoulder function, pain, cosmetic deformity and effect on performance of athletes involved in upper limb activities. All the earlier fixation methods led to an extremely rigid fixation which impaired the rotational movement between clavicle and scapula [24]. This aspect is taken care of by an implant-like clavicular hook plate which forms leverage between proximal ends of plate fixed to distal clavicle; hook penetrates the undersurface of acromion and maintains the amphiarthrotic acromioclavicular articulation [25].

The functional outcome of shoulder following removal of the hook plate improved significantly during subsequent follow-ups. The Constant Score after 12 weeks post hook plate removal hook was on an average 60, primarily due to improving but painful shoulder motion and moderate pain. In this study, we did not allow the patients to attempt overhead abduction beyond 90 degrees, while hook plate was in situ to avoid inadvertent damage to acromion and subsequent acromial osteolysis and subacromial bursitis

which has been reported in the earlier studies on hook plate fixation [26, 27]. There was a significant improvement in the Constant Score at 18 months post hook plate removal in all the patients. There were 19 patients (57 %) with Constant Score above 90 at the last follow-up. All the patients had significant improvement in overhead abduction (beyond 120°) and returned to active sports such as basketball, handball and kabaddi. The functional outcome was similarly excellent as seen in UCLA Scores at the last follow-up at around 2 years post-surgery. The ultimate goal of surgical intervention in this set of injuries was to facilitate return to their pre-injury level of active sports which was achieved in all the patients which is comparable to the results of earlier studies where hook plate has been used [26]. The major disadvantages of hook plate cited in earlier series have been repeat surgery, persistent shoulder pain, incomplete shoulder function, acromial osteolysis and acromioclavicular subluxation [27]. In our study, we had no surgical site infection, and in the early and midterm follow-up, there was no incidence of osteolysis, subluxation of acromioclavicular joint after hook plate removal. There was no requirement of any repeat surgical intervention other than the removal of hook plate itself. The concern of subacromial impingement was pertinent till the hook plate was in situ. However, after plate removal, there was no clinicoradiological evidence of the same. The radiological assessment of a sound acromioclavicular joint can be done with stress radiographs and measurement of the coracoclavicular distance comparing with the contralateral side or an absolute value which should be 11–13 mm generally [28].

The hook plate in our experience is an excellent device to obtain a congruent acromioclavicular joint due to its unique biomechanical characteristics and stiffness which are most similar to a physiologic acromioclavicular articulation [25].

The debate on surgery versus conservative treatment in type III injuries is not applicable to young athletic individuals, like soldiers in our study, in view of their high functional requirements which are met better with surgical stabilisation. An extension of the same debate is whether surgery restores the strength of ligaments. This has been proven by the excellent functional outcome in all the patients in our study with all the patients returning to their pre-injury athletic performance [29, 30]. The hook plate works quite well as an "internal splint" that keeps the acromioclavicular joint reduced during the time necessary for biological healing of the ligaments. In addition, the accuracy of joint reduction can be clearly visualised peroperatively. Though quite a few arthroscopic procedures have been described recently using suspensory fixation devices, an extremely high level of accuracy is required in terms of placement of tunnels. Faulty placement of tunnels may lead to fractures of coracoid or clavicle [31, 32]. Though these techniques are appealing in view of cosmesis and ability to treat concomitant shoulder injuries, the technique remains restricted to experienced shoulder arthroscopists. Good to excellent results have also been reported with open techniques using suspensory devices, e.g. tightrope [17]. In comparison, the results of hook plate fixation have been consistent in our study despite variable experience of the operating surgeons as the surgical technique is simple and easily reproducible.

The major drawback of using a hook plate is requirement of another surgery for removal of implant. Though there were no complications in our study, the hook plates can cause disturbances over the subacromial bursa, supraspinatus tendinitis, disturbances over the plate end and acromial osteolysis, if retained for long time. We were able to avoid these complications by timely removal of the implant. The limitation of our study is a relatively small sample size (thirty-three) and absence of a control group. A major advantage of our study was that the entire population group of soldiers was homogenous with similar functional requirements.

Conclusion

It can be concluded that precontoured clavicular hook plate is a good implant option to be considered for fixation of type III acromioclavicular dislocations without requiring any additional ligamentous procedures. The recommendation to apply this conclusion across all types of acromioclavicular dislocations would not be absolutely pertinent as this study primarily dealt with type III injuries. Young active athletic patients like soldiers with such injuries would definitely benefit with an early reduction and fixation with hook plate followed by its timely removal.

Informed consent Informed consent was obtained from all individual participants included in the study.

References

1. Adams FL (1986) The Genuine Works of Hippocrates vols. 1 and 2. William Wood, New York
2. Arenas AJ, Pampliega T, Iglesias J (1993) Surgical management of bipolar clavicular dislocation. Acta Orthop Belg 59:202–205
3. Trainer G, Arciero RA, Mazzocca AD (2008) Practical management of grade III acromioclavicular separations. Clin J Sport Med 18(2):162–166
4. Motta P, Bruno L, Maderni A et al (2012) Acromioclavicular motion after surgical reconstruction. Knee Surg Sports Traumatol Arthrosc 20(6):1012–1018
5. Mazzocca AD, Arciero RA, Bicos J (2007) Evaluation and treatment of acromioclavicular joint injuries. Am J Sports Med 35(2):316–329
6. Fraser-Moodie JA, Shortt NL, Robinson CM (2008) Injuries to the acromioclavicular joint. J Bone Joint Surg Br 90(6):697–707
7. Rockwood CA (1984) Injuries to the acromioclavicular Joint. In: Rockwood CA, Green DP (eds) Fractures in adults vols. 1, 2. JB Lippincott, Philadelphia
8. Rolf O, Hann von Weyhern A, Ewers A, Boehm TD, Gohlke F (2008) Acromioclavicular dislocation Rockwood III–V: results of early versus delayed surgical treatment. Arch Orthop Trauma Surg 128(10):1153–1157
9. Hootman JM (2004) Acromioclavicular dislocation: conservative or surgical therapy. J Athl Train 39(1):10–11
10. Tauber M (2013) Management of acute acromioclavicular joint dislocations: current concepts. Arch Orthop Trauma Surg 133(7):985–995
11. Rockwood C, Green D, Bucholz R, Heckman J (1996) Fractures in adults, vol 1, 4th edn. Lippincott-Raven, Philadelphia, pp 1341–1413
12. Smith TO, Chester R, Pearse EO, Hing CB (2011) Operative versus non-operative management following Rockwood grade III acromioclavicular separation: a meta-analysis of the current evidence base. J Orthop Traumatol 12:19–27
13. Steinbacher G, Sallent A, Seijas R, Boffa JM, Espinosa W, Cugat R (2014) Clavicular hook plate for grade-III acromioclavicular dislocation. J Orthop Surg (Hong Kong) 22(3):329–332
14. Kashii M, Inui H, Yamamoto K (2006) Surgical treatment of distal clavicle fractures using the clavicular hook plate. Clin Orthop Relat Res 447:158–164
15. Yoon JP, Lee BJ, Nam SJ, Chung SW, Jeong WJ, Min WK, Oh JH (2015) Comparison of results between hook plate fixation and ligament reconstruction for acute unstable acromioclavicular joint dislocation. Clin Orthop Surg 7(1):97–103
16. Schneider MM, Balke M, Koenen P, Fröhlich M, Wafaisade A, Bouillon B, Banerjee M (2014). Inter- and intraobserver reliability of the Rockwood classification in acute acromioclavicular joint dislocations. Knee Surg Sports Traumatol Arthrosc [Epub ahead of print]
17. Balke M, Schneider MM, Akoto R, Bäthis H, Bouillon B, Banerjee M (2014). Acute acromioclavicular joint injuries: changes in diagnosis and therapy over the last 10 years. Unfallchirurg [Epub ahead of print]
18. Beitzel K, Cote MP, Apostolakos J, Solovyova O, Judson CH, Ziegler CG et al (2013) Current concepts in the treatment of acromioclavicular joint dislocations. Arthroscopy 29(2):387–397
19. Korsten Koos, Gunning Amy C, Leenen Luke P H (2014) Operative or conservative treatment in patients with Rockwood type III acromioclavicular dislocation: a systematic review and update of current literature. Int Orthop 38(4):831–838
20. Franssen BB, Schuurman AH, Van der Molen AM, Kon M (2010) One century of Kirschner wires and Kirschner wire insertion techniques: a historical review. Acta Orthop Belg 76(1):1–6
21. EL-Menawy M (2014) Acute acromioclavicular dislocations: results of coracoclavicular screw fixation. Egypt Orthop J 49:38–42
22. Claudio C, Vincenzo F, Luca DG, et al (2013) Epidemiology of isolated acromioclavicular joint dislocation. Emerg Med Int. Article ID 171609, 5 pp. doi:10.1155/2013/171609
23. Rios CG, Mazzocca AD (2008) Acromioclavicular joint problems in athletes and new methods of management. Clin Sports Med 27(4):763–788
24. Fung M, Kato S, Barrance PJ, Elias JJ, McFarland EG, Nobuhara K et al (2001) Scapular and clavicular kinematics during humeral

elevation: a study with cadavers. J Shoulder Elbow Surg 10:278–285

25. McConnell AJ, Yoo DJ, Zdero R, Schemitsch EH, McKee MD (2007) Methods of operative fixation of the acromioclavicular joint: a biomechanical comparison. J Orthop Trauma 21:248–253

26. Ejam Samir, Lind Thomas, Falkenberg Boe (2008) Surgical treatment of acute and chronic acromioclavicular dislocation Tossy type III and V using the Hook Plate. Acta Orthop Belg 74:441–445

27. Charity RM, Haidar SG, Ghosh S, Tillu AB (2006) Fixation failure of the clavicular hook plate: a report of three cases. J Orthop Surg 14(3):333–335

28. Harris J, Harris W (2000) Radiology of emergency medicine, 4th edn. Lippincott Williams & Wilkins, Philadelphia

29. Bahk MS, Kuhn JE, Galatz LM, Connor PM, Williams GR Jr (2010) Acromioclavicular and sternoclavicular injuries and clavicular, glenoid, and scapular fractures. Instr Course Lect 59:209–226

30. Gstettner C, Tauber M, Hitzl W, Resch H (2008) Rockwood type III acromioclavicular dislocation: surgical versus conservative treatment. J Shoulder Elbow Surg 17(2):220–225

31. Salzmann GM, Walz L, Buchmann S, Glabgly P, Venjakob A, Imhoff AB (2010) Arthroscopically assisted 2-bundle anatomical reduction of acute acromioclavicular joint separations. Am J Sports Med 38(6):1179–1187

32. Gerhardt DC, VanDerWerf JD, Rylander LS, McCarty EC (2011) Postoperative coracoid fracture after transcoracoid acromioclavicular joint reconstruction. J Shoulder Elbow Surg 20(5):e6–e10

9

Predicting translational deformity following opening-wedge osteotomy for lower limb realignment

Richard C. Barksfield[1] · Fergal P. Monsell[1]

Abstract An opening-wedge osteotomy is well recognised for the management of limb deformity and requires an understanding of the principles of geometry. Translation at the osteotomy is needed when the osteotomy is performed away from the centre of rotation of angulation (CORA), but the amount of translation varies with the distance from the CORA. This translation enables proximal and distal axes on either side of the proposed osteotomy to realign. We have developed two experimental models to establish whether the amount of translation required (based on the translation deformity created) can be predicted based upon simple trigonometry. A predictive algorithm was derived where translational deformity was predicted as $2(\tan \alpha \times d)$, where α represents 50 % of the desired angular correction, and d is the distance of the desired osteotomy site from the CORA. A simulated model was developed using TraumaCad online digital software suite (Brainlab AG, Germany). Osteotomies were simulated in the distal femur, proximal tibia and distal tibia for nine sets of lower limb scanograms at incremental distances from the CORA and the resulting translational deformity recorded. There was strong correlation between the distance of the osteotomy from the CORA and simulated translation deformity for distal femoral deformities (correlation coefficient 0.99, $p < 0.0001$), proximal tibial deformities (correlation coefficient 0.93–0.99, $p < 0.0001$) and distal tibial deformities (correlation coefficient 0.99, $p < 0.0001$). There was excellent agreement between the predictive algorithm and simulated translational deformity for all nine simulations (correlation coefficient 0.93–0.99, $p < 0.0001$). Translational deformity following corrective osteotomy for lower limb deformity can be anticipated and predicted based upon the angular correction and the distance between the planned osteotomy site and the CORA.

Keywords Opening-wedge osteotomy · Deformity analysis · Osteotomy rules · Translational deformity · Limb realignment · Obligatory translation

Introduction

The management of lower limb deformity by corrective osteotomy is complex and requires a thorough understanding of the deformity analysis. The advent of computerised imaging systems and the availability of digital templating software have simplified the pre-operative planning process but still require an appreciation of the limitations imposed by simple mathematical principles.

Paley et al. [1] stressed the importance of the centre of rotation of angulation (CORA) in planning corrective osteotomies and highlighted that where a corrective osteotomy was performed at an alternative position to the CORA, translation at the osteotomy would be needed if the limb axis was to be correctly realigned. This phenomenon, described as obligatory translation, follows the principles of mechanics in deformity correction [2].

It is not always possible to perform a corrective osteotomy at the CORA due to a number of factors: severe juxta-articular deformities or previous instrumentation may render bone stock insufficient to provide adequate fixation, and soft tissue scarring or tenuous skin

✉ Richard C. Barksfield
rcbarksfield@hotmail.com

Fergal P. Monsell
Fergal.Monsell@UHBristol.nhs.uk

[1] Bristol Royal Hospital for Children, Paul O'Gorman Building, Upper Maudlin Street, Bristol BS2 8BJ, UK

coverage may prevent access to the osteotomy site altogether [3].

Whilst the need for obligatory translation in an osteotomy away from the CORA has been appreciated, the amount required for a size of angular correction plus distance from the CORA has yet to be calculated. We designed a study to establish the relationship between translational malalignment occurring following osteotomy using a digital image model. Our null hypothesis was that there was no correlation between the site of corrective osteotomy and the resultant translational deformity based on our suggested trigonometric method.

Materials and methods

The study looked at a single uniplanar corrective osteotomy to restore the anatomical alignment of the affected bone in the coronal plane. We assumed obligatory translation would apply equally to osteotomies at any level within the lower limb but sought to confirm this by analysis of osteotomies at three different levels: the distal femoral metaphysis, the proximal tibial metaphysis and the distal tibial metaphysis.

Derivation of predictive algorithm

The predictive algorithm was developed using a simplified model comprising of a CORA at the intersection of a proximal anatomical axis and a distal anatomical axis. The angle subtended at the intersection of these axes was the angular correction needed. The predicted translation was calculated by resolving the model into two identical right-angled triangles. In this way, the anticipated translation would be $2(\tan \alpha \times d)$, where α represents 50 % of the desired angular correction, and d is the distance of the desired osteotomy site from the CORA (Figs. 1, 2).

Fig. 1 Derivation of predictive algorithm. The anatomical axis of the proximal and distal fragments intersects at the centre of rotation of angulation (CORA). Where the osteotomy is performed away from the CORA, the translation encountered is $2(\tan \alpha \times d)$

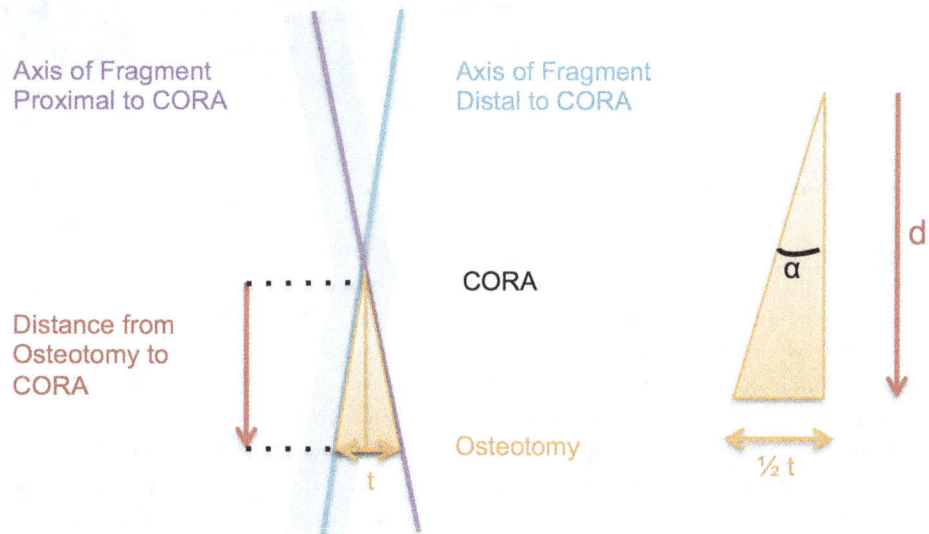

Fig. 2 Demonstration of where an opening-wedge osteotomy is performed at the CORA, no translation is necessary in order to correct the axis of deformity (**a**). Where the osteotomy is at in an alternative position to the CORA, translation is obligatory if the axis of deformity is to be realigned (**b**)

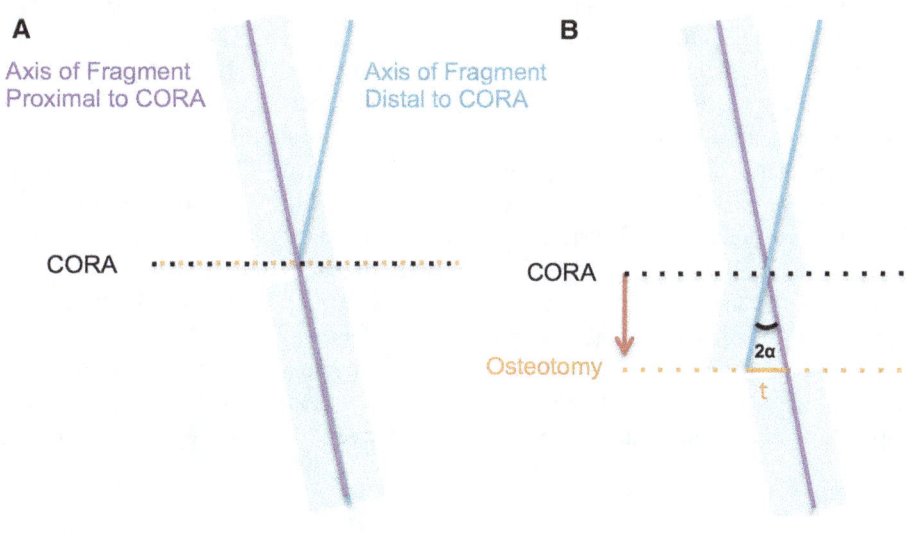

Fig. 3 Demonstration of the use of the deformity templating software for a typical distal femoral deformity simulation. Note the translation that occurs where the osteotomy is performed proximal to the CORA

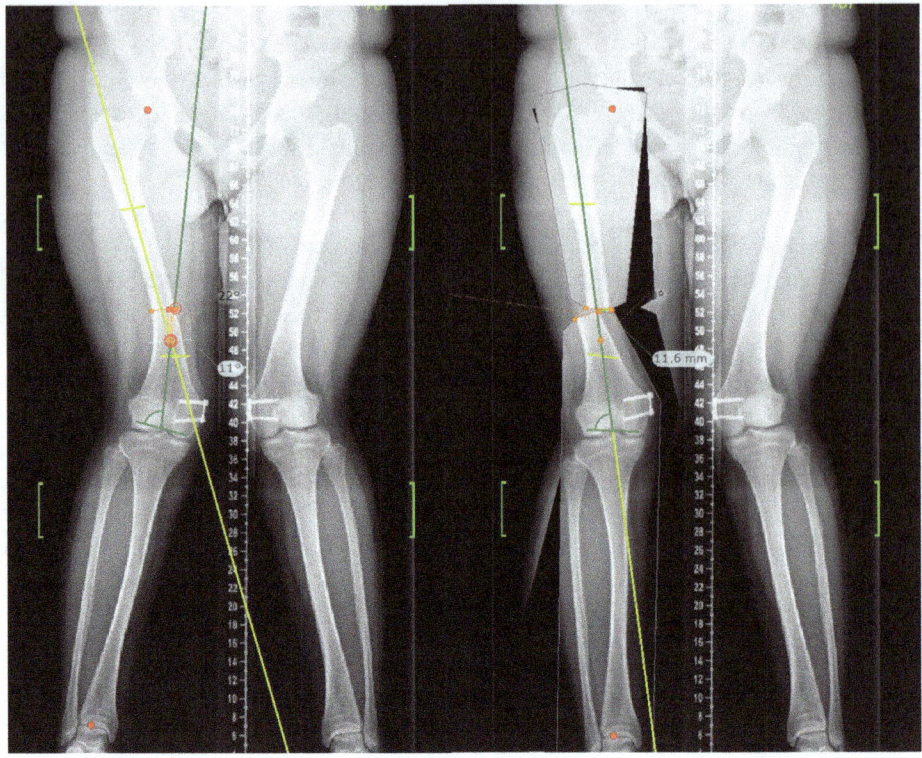

Digital image simulation

Experimental data were simulated using the TraumaCad online digital software suite (Brainlab AG, Germany). Anonymised lower limb scanograms were uploaded and calibrated using the inbuilt "Deformity Correction model". A lower limb deformity analysis was performed for each scanogram, and a CORA derived for correcting each deformity. A corrective osteotomy and limb realignment were then simulated at the level of the CORA; this was repeated at intervals of 5 mm proceeding proximally from the distal femoral and distal tibial metaphyses, and proceeding distally from the proximal tibial metaphysis (Fig. 3). For each simulation, a series of measurements was performed that included the angular correction, the distance to CORA, the measured translation and the percentage translation.

The predicted values for each angular deformity were calculated for each level of osteotomy and correlated with the data generated from the simulated radiological data. Data were analysed using GraphPad Online Statistics Calculator [4] and STATA (StataCorp LP, TX, USA). Agreement between simulated and predicted models was then assessed using Bland and Altman limits of agreement and Lin's concordance correlation coefficient. This was an important step in determining true agreement between the experimental models rather than a linear association that may be affected by systematic bias.

Results

Digital simulation

Simulated data were collected for nine experimental models that comprised of three distal femoral, three proximal tibial and three distal tibial deformities. The mean angular correction simulated was 23.0° and this ranged from 9.8° to 40.4°.

Distal femur

Data for the distal femoral deformities are presented in Fig. 4. The correlation coefficient between distance of the osteotomy from the CORA and translational deformities produced was 0.99 ($p < 0.0001$) for all femurs studied.

Proximal tibia

Data for proximal tibial simulations are presented in Fig. 5. The correlation coefficient for the distance of the osteotomy to the CORA and the measured translation was 0.99

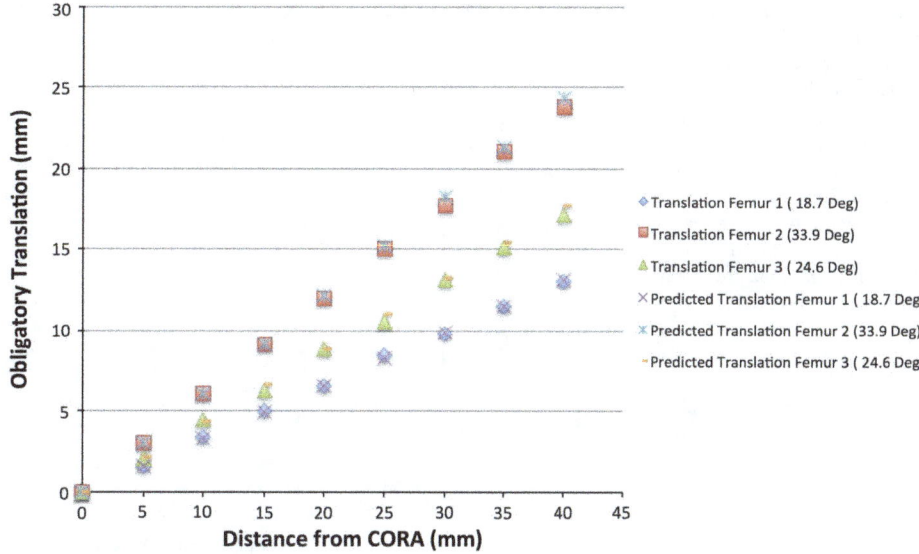

Fig. 4 Simulated and predicted data for correction of distal femoral deformities. There was strong correlation between translational deformity and increasing distance of the osteotomy from the CORA in the simulated model. In addition, there was strong correlation between predicted translation and the translation measured during simulation

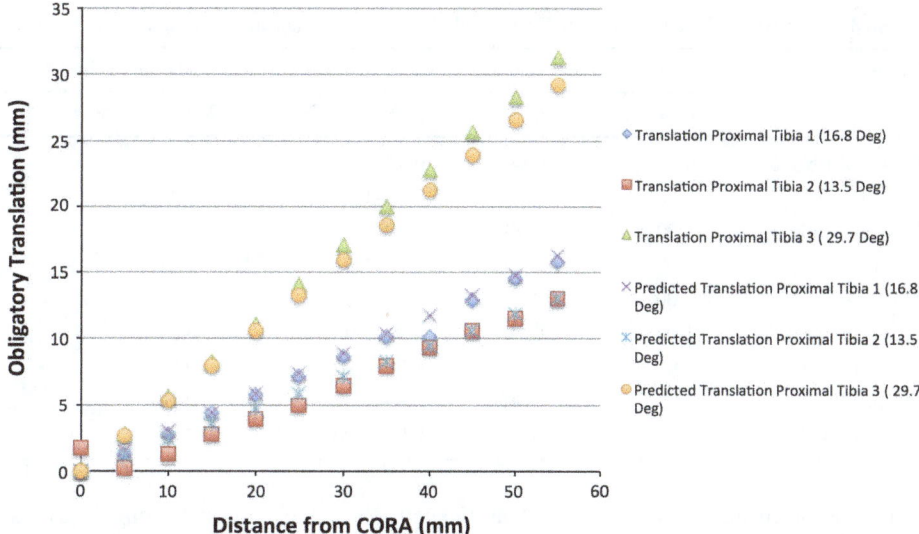

Fig. 5 Simulated and predicted data for correction of proximal tibial deformities. There was strong correlation between translational deformity and increasing distance of the osteotomy from the CORA in the simulated model. Note that translation for tibia 2 decreased initially as distance from the CORA increased, but then followed the predictive model

for tibia 1 ($p < 0.0001$), 0.93 for tibia 2 ($p < 0.0001$) and 0.99 for tibia 3 ($p < 0.0001$).

Distal tibia

Simulated modelling data for distal tibial deformity corrections are presented in Fig. 6. In keeping with data from both distal femoral and proximal tibial simulations, there was a clear correlation between distance of the osteotomy to the CORA and resulting translation [correlation coefficient 0.99 ($p < 0.0001$) for all simulations].

Agreement between experimental models

The analysis of agreement between predicted and simulated models is presented in Table 1. Substantial agreement

(Lin's concordance coefficient >0.99) was seen in eight of the nine models and even better (Lin's concordance coefficient 0.95–0.99) in the remaining model. The Bland and Altman limits of agreement were low and include zero for all models, indicating that there was no clinically significant difference between experimental models and that no systematic bias was apparent.

Discussion

Translation following corrective osteotomy for lower limb deformity can be anticipated and predicted based upon the angular correction and the relationship between the planned osteotomy site and the CORA. In most cases, significant translational deformity can be avoided by an

Fig. 6 Simulated and predicted data for correction of distal tibial deformities. There was strong correlation between translational deformity and increasing distance of the osteotomy from the CORA in the simulated model. There was also a clear correlation between the predicted translational deformity and that produced by the simulated model

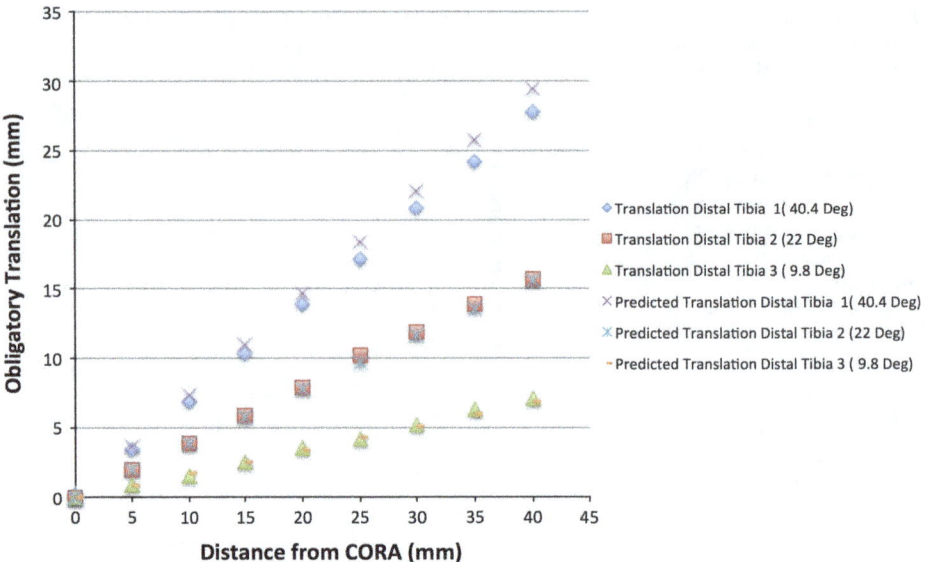

Table 1 Lin's concordance coefficient (LCC) and Bland and Altman limits of agreement between simulated and predicted models

Variable	Lin's concordance coefficient			Bland and Altman agreement		
	PPMCC	LCC	95 % CI LCC	Mean difference	SD	Limits of agreement (95 %)
Proximal tibia 1	0.99	0.99	0.97–1.00	−0.31	0.497	−1.28 to 0.67
Proximal tibia 2	0.96	0.95	0.89–1.00	−0.45	0.865	−2.14 to 1.25
Proximal tibia 3	1.00	0.99	0.99–1.00	0.71	0.551	−0.37 to 1.78
Distal femur 1	1.00	1.00	0.99–1.00	0.01	0.124	−0.23 to 0.26
Distal femur 2	1.00	0.99	0.99–1.00	−0.22	0.234	−0.68 to 0.24
Distal femur 3	1.00	0.99	0.99–1.00	−0.21	0.220	−0.64 to 0.22
Distal tibia 1	1.00	0.99	0.99–1.00	−0.86	0.613	−2.06 to 0.34
Distal tibia 2	1.00	0.99	0.99–1.00	0.16	0.156	−0.15 to 0.46
Distal tibia 3	0.99	0.99	0.99–1.00	0.04	0.160	−0.28 to 0.35

appreciation of the site of the CORA and execution of the osteotomy at this level. There are, however, occasions where optimal placement of the osteotomy site is not possible either due to soft tissue considerations and previous instrumentation, or periarticular deformity in which fixation may become tenuous in the resulting bone fragments [5]. Under these circumstances, it is useful to have an appreciation of the obligatory translation that will result, and we have therefore developed a predictive model to estimate this in most cases (Fig. 7; Table 1).

We have demonstrated a strong correlation between translational deformity and osteotomy site, and excellent agreement between predictive and simulated models. This is not surprising when considering that the predictive model was derived from a simplified mathematical model and these are the laws upon which the deformity correction software is based. We recognise that both models may be an oversimplification, particularly when considering the

constraints of the soft tissue envelope on the angle of correction achievable and the actual translation observed at the osteotomy site (Table 2).

The next logical step in this process would be to compare the translation predicted by our model with the actual translation produced across a range of angular corrections "in vivo". The practicalities of doing this are complicated. Many of our corrections are performed using circular fixators which make early radiographs difficult to interpret, and we found follow-up films after fixator removal difficult to analyse due to the overlying callus formation, poor distinction of osteotomy edges and loss of the true site of the CORA. Whilst an "in vivo" model would be preferable, we did not find early pilot data to be reliable and hence this was not included in the analysis.

With the advent of digital imaging software, a number of studies have examined the reliability of computer-assisted measurements in assessment of lower limb

Fig. 7 Chart demonstrating the predicted translational deformity for opening-wedge osteotomy for a range of angular corrections and distances from the CORA

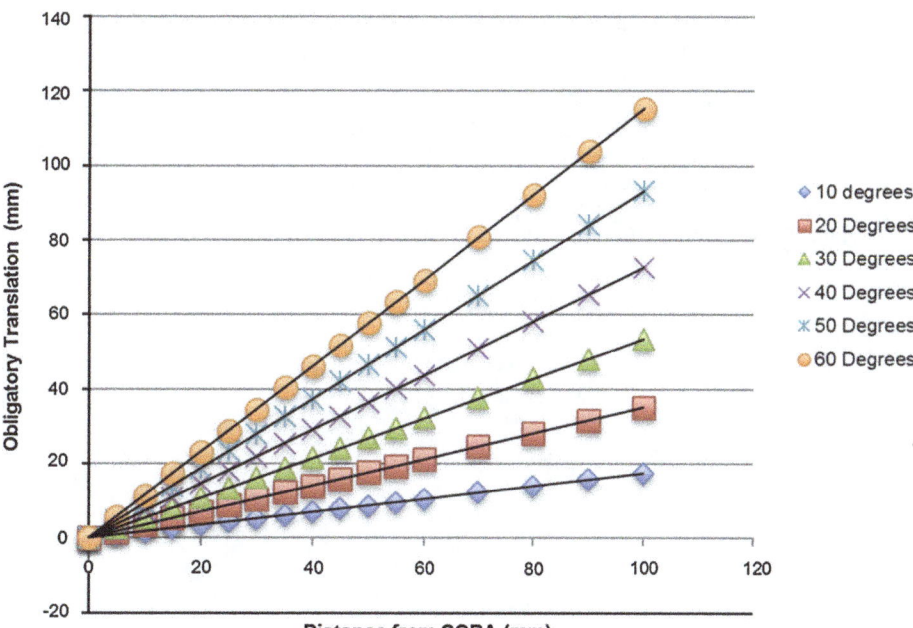

Table 2 Maximum distance osteotomy can be performed from CORA before 10-mm obligatory translation ensues

Angular correction (°)	Maximum distance of osteotomy to CORA (mm)
10	57
20	28
30	19
40	14
50	11
60	9

alignment and deformity measurement [6–8]. In the present study, the simulated modelling was performed using the TraumaCad online software suite and a single observer (RB). We have not evaluated the intra-observer and inter-observer reliability of measurements using this technique, but are aware of a previous study that has specifically examined the reliability of measurements performed using the TraumaCad software suite and found them to be reliable [9]. We therefore believe the results presented to be both relevant and reproducible.

Our null hypotheses were that there would be no relationship between the position of osteotomy with regard to the CORA and the resultant obligatory translation produced. On the basis of our results, we have rejected this hypothesis and have demonstrated not only a clear correlation between position of osteotomy and resultant translation, but also that this can be predicted by an appreciation of the geometric equation.

Acknowledgments Online access to TraumaCad Quentry was provided by Brainlab AG, Germany. We would like to acknowledge the work of Mr. Daniel C. Perry, Senior Lecturer, University of Liverpool, Honorary Consultant Orthopaedic Surgeon and NIHR Clinical Scientist, who kindly assisted with the statistical analysis.

Research involving Human Participants and/or Animals This article does not contain any studies with human participants or animals performed by any of the authors.

Informed consent Informed consent was not required for this work.

References

1. Paley D, Herzenberg JE, Tetsworth K, McKie J, Bhave A (1994) Deformity planning for frontal and sagittal plane corrective osteotomies. Orthop Clin N Am 25(3):425–465
2. Monsell FP, Barnes JR, Kirubanandan R, McBride AM (2011) Distal tibial physeal arrest after meningococcal septicaemia: management and outcome in seven ankles. J Bone Joint Surg Br 93(6):839–843. doi:10.1302/0301-620X.93B6.26276
3. Fabricant PD, Camara JM, Rozbruch SR (2013) Femoral deformity planning: intentional placement of the apex of deformity. Orthopedics 36(5):e533–e537. doi:10.3928/01477447-20130426-11
4. GraphPad Software (2015) QuickCalcs Online Software Suite. http://www.graphpad.com/quickcalcs/. Accessed 18 Sept 2015
5. Kulkarni GS (2004) Principles and practice of deformity correction. Indian J Orthop 38:191–198
6. Rozzanigo U, Pizzoli A, Minari C, Caudana R (2005) Alignment and articular orientation of lower limbs: manual vs computer-aided measurements on digital radiograms. Radiol Med 109(3):234–238
7. Nowicki PD, Vanderhave KL, Farley FA, Kuhns LR, Dahl W, Caird MS (2012) Reliability of digital radiographs for pediatric lower extremity alignment. J Pediatr Orthop 32(6):631–635. doi:10.1097/BPO.0b013e3182694e07

8. Sailer J, Scharitzer M, Peloschek P, Giurea A, Imhof H, Grampp S (2005) Quantification of axial alignment of the lower extremity on conventional and digital total leg radiographs. Eur Radiol 15(1):170–173 **(Epub 5 Aug 2004)**

9. Segev E, Hemo Y, Wientroub S, Ovadia D, Fishkin M, Steinberg DM, Hayek S (2010) Intra- and inter-observer reliability analysis of digital radiographic measurements for pediatric orthopedic parameters using a novel PACS integrated computer software program. J Child Orthop 4(4):331–341. doi:10.1007/s11832-010-0259-5

10

Combined use of the Ilizarov method, concentrated bone marrow aspirate (cBMA), and platelet-rich plasma (PRP) to expedite healing of bimalleolar fractures

Edgardo R. Rodriguez-Collazo[1] · Maria L. Urso[2]

Abstract Distal tibial and fibular fractures, particularly in patients with comorbidities, heal slowly and have a high incidence of postoperative nonunion and infection. Autologous concentrated bone marrow aspirate (cBMA) and platelet-rich plasma (PRP) increase osteogenic potential of demineralized bone matrix (DBM). The purpose of this case series was to evaluate the efficacy of cBMA, PRP, DBM in conjunction with the Ilizarov fixator as compared to DBM and the Ilizarov fixator alone in expediting fracture healing. Ten patients (mean age 52.9 years) were in the cBMA Group, and 10 patients (mean age 54 years) were in the Control Group. Comorbidities included diabetes, obesity, smoking, and renal disease. Radiographs showed a significant difference in the rate of complete healing in the cBMA Group at 16 ± 1.6 weeks post-surgery as compared to 24 ± 1.3 weeks in the Control Group ($P < 0.001$). No differences were observed between groups in infection rate or nonunions. We conclude that the Ilizarov fixator combined with DBM, cBMA, and PRP expedites fracture healing of the distal tibia and fibula in patients with significant comorbidities.

Keywords Mesenchymal stem cell · Tibia · Fracture Fibula · Nonunion · Comorbidities

✉ Maria L. Urso
urso.maria@gmail.com

Edgardo R. Rodriguez-Collazo
erodriguez@cfaas.com

[1] Department of Surgery, Presence Saint Joseph Hospital, 2900 N Lake Shore Dr., Chicago, IL 60657, USA

[2] Arteriocyte Medical Systems, 45 South St., Suite 3, Hopkinton, MA 01748, USA

Introduction

Distal tibial and fibula fractures can be treated successfully with the Ilizarov fixator [1]. However, complications include contractures, pin track infections, loss of range of motion, and articular damage. Patients who are experiencing soft-tissue loss, comorbidities, and chronic infection increase the complexity of these cases. Patients who are smokers and of advanced age with a high rate of systemic illness are the most difficult to treat because these factors negatively impact the rate of healing and incidence of infection [2, 3]. The challenge surgeons face with these patients is to achieve a stable, well-aligned, mobile and pain-free joint while minimizing the risk of infection and post-traumatic osteoarthritis. The classic Ilizarov technique has several advantages when treating patients with various comorbidities [4]. With this technique, the reduction and fixation of the fracture is performed with minimal soft-tissue exposure and blood loss and the fixation stable enough to allow weight-bearing soon after surgery. The external fixator gives the surgeon the opportunity to adjust the alignment and compress or distract during or after surgery. These factors improve the success rate of the Ilizarov method in fracture repair and contribute a positive effect on patient quality of life [5].

In the treatment for complicated fractures, surgeons may use autologous iliac bone graft (ICBG) to augment healing. Unfortunately, in patients with multiple comorbidities, autologous bone grafting may introduce new complications. These include bleeding, infection, and chronic pain at the donor site. There can be limited bone graft material available for treatment [6]. Since the success of a bone graft is determined by the ability of the grafted tissue to recruit progenitor cells to the injured area to form osteoblasts for healing, alternative methods are needed in compromised patients.

Safe and effective alternative graft materials have become popular for use in patients with significant comorbidities. Demineralized bone matrix (DBM) is donor tissue that has been processed to remove inorganic mineral content resulting in an organic collagen matrix [7]. This leaves DBM with minimal osteoinductive properties. Additional material which improves the osteogenic environment can be obtained from bone marrow aspirate which is concentrated for osteoprogenitor cells. The benefit of bone marrow separation is twofold: Red blood cells are removed since they can interfere with bone formation and healing [6], and concentrated osteoprogenitor cells increase the osteogenic stimulus. This use of concentrated bone marrow aspirate (cBMA) combined with an osteoinductive bone graft substitute (DBM) insures that two of the main properties for bone growth and healing, osteogenesis and osteoinduction, are present with minimal risk and morbidity to the patient. Concentrated BMA provides osteogenic mesenchymal stem cells (MSCs) and hematopoietic stem cells (HSCs). Mesenchymal stem cells secrete various bioactive factors, have inherent differentiation potential, and modulate angiogenic and growth factors in the local microenvironment [8–10]. In addition, MSCs exert anti-inflammatory and immunosuppressive signaling which protect against tissue destruction while facilitating regeneration. Pluripotent hematopoietic stem cells (HSCs) derived from autologous bone marrow may also provide pro- and anti-inflammatory signaling while stimulating the production of angiogenic growth factors via paracrine effects in the treated area [11]. Together, cBMA combined with DBM may expedite healing rates.

The use of platelet-rich plasma (PRP) can augment the healing process of soft tissues following surgical interventions. PRP is a biological intervention prepared as a platelet concentrate after centrifugation of the patient's whole blood. Through centrifugation, the majority of the red blood cell components and the plasma volume are removed resulting in a post-processed concentration of therapeutic factors (i.e., platelets and white blood cells). Production of PRP also concentrates endogenous growth factors in circulating blood. These factors include platelet-derived growth factor (PDGF), vascular endothelial growth factor (VEGF), transforming growth factor-beta (TGF-β1), epidermal-derived growth factor (EGF), and fibroblast growth factor (FGF) [12–15]. Collectively, PRP stimulates hemostasis, reduces infection, and enhances skin regeneration [16].

The aim of this retrospective case series was to compare the outcome of cBMA and PRP in expediting healing of distal tibial and fibula fractures when used with DBM and the Ilizarov fixator as compared to DBM and the Ilizarov fixator alone.

Patients and methods

Study population

Twenty patients ($n = 20$) were included in this retrospective study. Ten patients ($n = 10$, mean age 52.9 years) were in the cBMA Group, and 10 patients ($n = 10$, mean age 54 years) were in the Control Group. Comorbidities included diabetes, obesity, smoking, and renal disease. Ten patients in the cBMA Group had abnormal bone metabolism indicated by vitamin D and calcium deficiency as to seven patients in the Control Group. All patients had closed distal tibial and fibula fractures with a poor soft-tissue envelope.

The study protocol, medical record review procedures, and data analysis were approved by the Presence[SM] Saint Joseph Hospital Institutional Review Board. Patients were treated between January 2010 and December 2012 with a mean follow-up time of 18 months. Patients were identified by a retrospective review of the electronic medical records. The two cohorts (treatment and control) were identified through the case note review. All identifying data (name, DOB (only age included), demographics) were removed from electronic medical records prior to data analysis.

Intervention

Bone marrow aspiration and concentration

For the 10 patients in the cBMA Group, 26 ml of bone marrow was harvested from the medial aspect of the proximal tibia (Fig. 1a). First, the 30-ml syringe was primed with 4 ml of anticoagulant citrate dextrose solution (ACD-A) (Arteriocyte Medical Systems, Hopkinton, MA). A mallet was then used to advance the 15-gauge Jamshidi needle (Arteriocyte Medical Systems, Hopkinton, MA) until a decrease in resistance was met. The decreased resistance was used to indicate that the needle had entered the marrow cavity. Bone marrow was then drawn back gently (to prevent lysing of the cells) into the 30-ml syringe that was primed with 4 ml of ACD-A. During the marrow draw, if significant resistance was met, the needle was repositioned until the marrow flowed easily. This prevented clotting and unnecessary physical disruption of the aspirate and avoid cell lysis and a reduction in growth factor content of the platelets. The needle was repositioned until a total volume of 30 ml, including the ACD-A, was harvested.

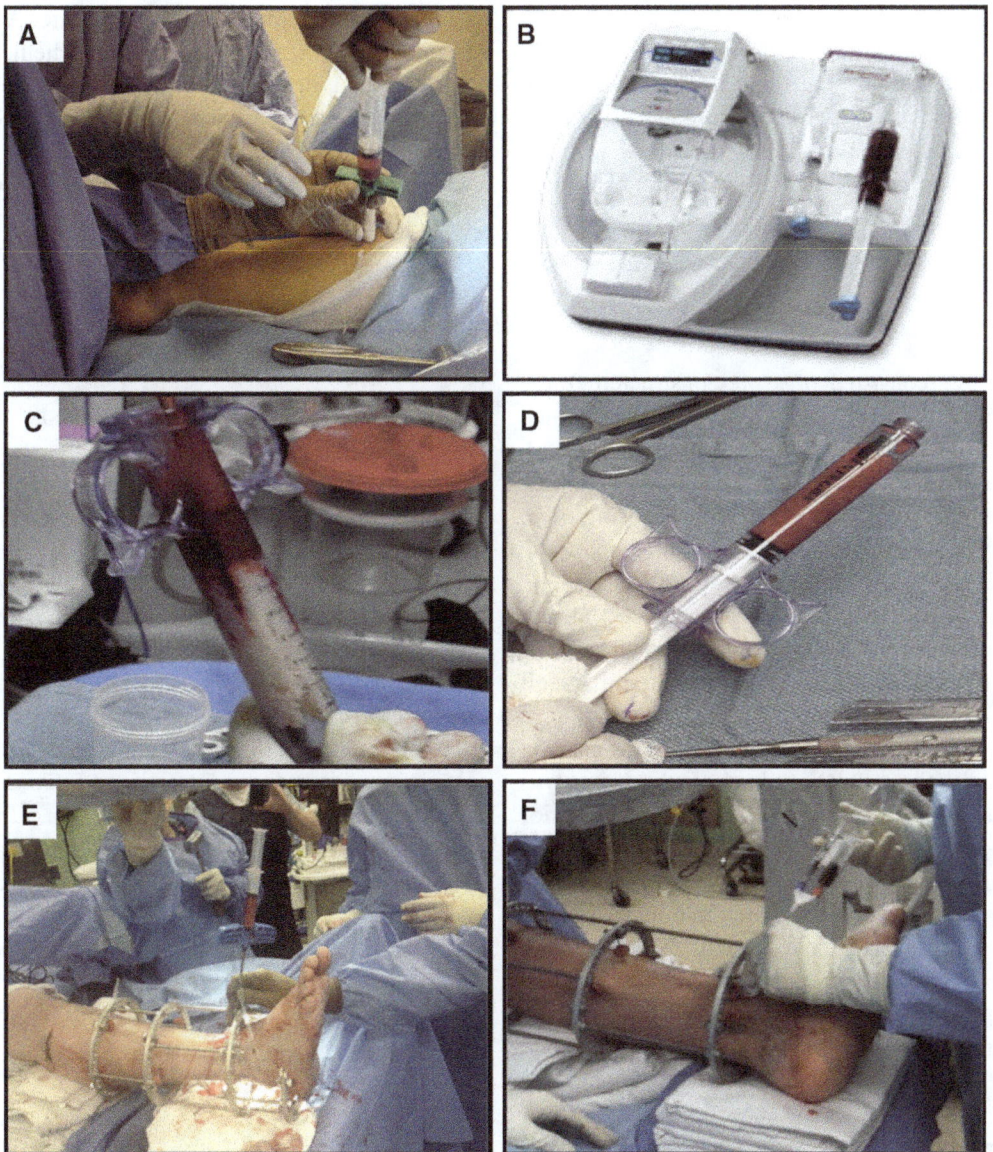

Fig. 1 Tissue harvesting and application. **a** Bone marrow aspiration method. **b** Magellan platelet separator. **c** Syringe containing initial mixture of cBMA and DBM. **d** Final implantable mixture of cBMA and DBM. **e** Application of cBMA and graft material to fracture site. **f** Application of PRP using a spray tip cannula

The harvested marrow was then filtered and processed in the Arteriocyte Magellan® system (Arteriocyte Medical Systems, Inc., Hopkinton, MA) (Fig. 1b). The Magellan® is an automatic, dual spin, closed system allowing for safe and rapid bedside concentration of whole blood and bone marrow aspirate. For each case, the Magellan® was customized to obtain a final volume of cBMA of approximately 3 ml from 30 ml of bone marrow aspirate.

Phlebotomy and concentration of PRP

For each patient in the cBMA Group, 30 ml of whole blood was drawn from an antecubital vein. The 30-ml syringe was primed with 4 ml of ACD-A before 26 ml of whole blood was obtained from each patient using standard phlebotomy procedures. On reaching the final volume of 30 ml, the syringe was loaded into the Magellan System. The Magellan® was programmed to produce 3 ml of PRP from the 30 ml volume (Fig. 1b).

DBM

Integra Accell EVO, which is a DBM and poloxamer Reverse-Phase Medium produced by Integra (Irvine, CA), was used in all patients (cBMA Group and Control Group). This form of DBM provides a high surface area which facilitates binding access for natural bone proteins and a scaffold and signal for new bone formation. The Accell EVO DBM is moldable putty at room temperature which becomes more viscous at body temperature.

Prior to use, the Accell EVO DBM was mixed with the cBMA (cBMA Group only) to achieve desired consistency (Fig. 1c, d). Five cc. of the Accell EVO DBM was injected into fracture sites in both groups (Fig. 1e).

Ilizarov technique

The circular fixator consisted of a pre-constructed frame that consisted of four rings (Fig. 2). A proximal reference wire was fixed and tensioned to the most proximal ring. A distal reference wire was fixed directly proximal to the ankle. After the bone ends were fixed with opposing olive wires, radiology was used to ascertain alignment of the bone. In cases where the fracture was close to the ankle, the foot was incorporated into the frame to enhance stability and prevent equinus or varus contracture. With the bones were aligned, the cBMA (cBMA Group only) and Accell EVO DBM mixture (cBMA and Control Groups) were injected percutaneously using the 15-gauge bone marrow aspiration needle (Fig. 1e). Viability of the foot was assessed via palpation of the dorsalis pedis and posterior tibial pulses and measurement of oxygen saturation of the hallux. If circulation appeared to be disrupted, the length was adjusted as necessary to return circulation to normal. PRP combined with calcium chloride and thrombin solution was applied using a spray tip cannula at all surgical wound sites in the cBMA Group (Fig. 1f).

Patients were assessed every 2 weeks via X-ray to determine whether the fracture was completely healed and whether frame removal was appropriate. A single observer evaluated the X-rays to determine whether cortices were fully ossified, determined by a sharp outline of the cortical bone. In addition, each patient needed to be able to bear weight on the limb for the frame to be removed. If patients were not healed by week 12, a CT scan was performed. Patients then returned every 2–4 weeks for X-ray or CT scan, respectively, until complete healing was determined. Once the frame was removed, patients were fitted with a patellar tendon brace and instructed to wear the brace for 6 months after frame removal.

Data collection and statistical analysis

A sample size estimation was performed to identify the number of subjects needed to detect a significant difference in rate of healing between treatment conditions (control vs. cBMA). Sample size estimate ranges were generated using effect sizes and standard deviations at a power of 0.8 and alpha of 0.05 (SigmaPlot v 10.0, Systat Software Inc., Germany). The outcome measures were assessed by physical examination, radiographic examination, and chart review. The mean ± standard deviation was calculated for all measurements reported. To describe the outcomes of the surgical intervention, frequencies and percentages were used for the categorical variables. A one-way analysis of variance (ANOVA) between groups was performed to determine whether there was a significant difference between the rate of healing in the cBMA Group and the Control Group. The critical alpha level was set at 0.05.

Results

Figure 3 illustrates outcome measures for the cBMA and Control Groups. The mean fixator time was 24 ± 1.3 weeks in the Control Group and 16 ± 1.6 weeks in the cBMA Group ($P < 0.001$). In the Control Group, postoperative radiographs for seven of 10 patients showed complete bone healing at the time of external fixator removal. In the cBMA Group, eight of 10 patients showed complete bone healing when the external fixator was removed at approximately 16 weeks post-surgery (Fig. 4). There were no significant differences between groups in the number of patients with complete bone healing ($P = 0.6$) at the time of fixator removal. Of the two patients in the cBMA Group who experienced delayed union, only one revision was required due to consistent pain. Four weeks post-revision, the patients' pain had subsided. The second patient did not require a revision, but a percutaneous injection of cBMA was used to augment healing. Both patients healed within approximately

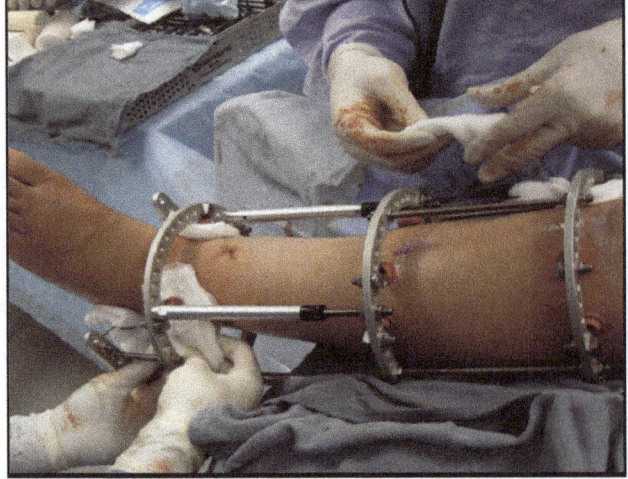

Fig. 2 Ilizarov method of fixation. The circular fixator consisted of a pre-constructed frame that consisted of four rings. A proximal reference wire was fixed and tensioned to the most proximal ring. A distal reference wire was fixed directly proximal to the ankle

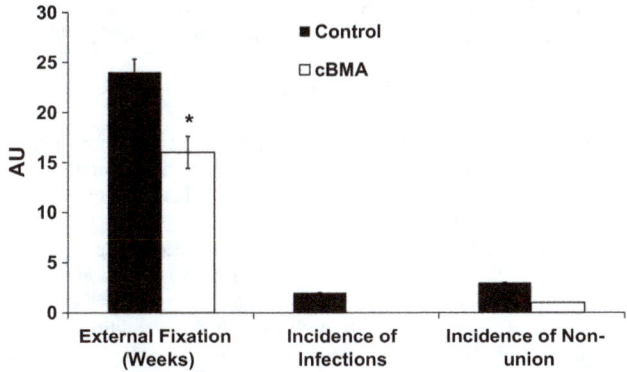

Fig. 3 Postoperative outcome measures. There was a significant reduction in the time of external fixation in the cBMA Group. No differences were reported in incidence of infection or nonunion between groups. Data are mean ± SD. *$P < 0.001$

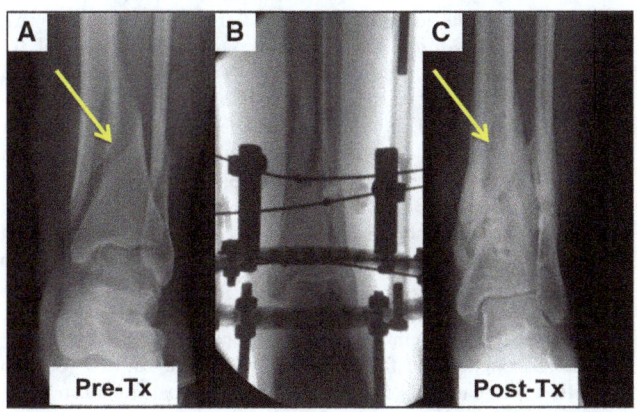

Fig. 4 Serial radiographs. **a** Pre-treatment radiograph of a female patient in the cBMA Group with a bimalleolar fracture (*yellow arrow*). **B** Fluoroscopy image of olive wire stabilization of the fracture. **c** Post-treatment radiographs of same female patient at 16 weeks post-procedure. Fracture is healed (*yellow arrow*) (color figure online)

4 months without residual deformity or morbidity. In the Control Group, three patients developed a stiff nonunion without deformity. These patients were braced and were followed for 18 months until complete healing was observed. No surgical revisions were necessary.

Two patients in the cBMA Group experienced superficial irritation as a result of the wires. Antibiotics were not needed in these patients. In the Control Group, two patients developed an infection that required treatment with oral antibiotics. The incidence of infection was not different between groups ($P = 0.2$). No limbs were amputated in this series.

Discussion

The aim of the author's strategy in combining cBMA and PRP with the Ilizarov technique and DBM was to decrease the period of external fixation, expedite fracture healing,

and diminish the rate of complications, specifically infections. In agreement with our hypothesis, patients treated with cBMA and PRP healed significantly faster than patients in the Control Group. Complications experienced by patients in the cBMA Group were minor, and only one required additional surgery. In the Control Group, three patients experienced nonunion complications, and two experienced skin infections requiring treatment with oral antibiotics. These were not statistically significant, but the trend of fewer skin infections may have arisen from use of PRP at the incision sites in the cBMA Group [17]. Previous reports have evaluated the potent antimicrobial effects of PRP and suggested the combined actions of concentrated levels of leukocytes, platelets, and their derived growth factors have strong bacterial inhibitory effects.

Nonunion is a major challenge to surgeons when treating complex fractures in a patient with multiple comorbidities. Open bone grafting techniques for the treatment for complex fractures have remained unchanged since the early work of Phemister and colleagues [18]. Complications of this technique range from infection, hematoma, and to donor site morbidity. As bone growth is optimal when osteogenic cells are present, techniques that induce osteogenesis while not inducing donor site morbidity in an already-compromised patient are still needed.

This retrospective cohort comparison highlights the benefits of using an autologous source of cells derived from a patient's bone marrow aspirate to provide an osteogenic milieu. Specifically, mesenchymal cells concentrated from the patient's bone marrow are multipotent and are able to differentiate into osteoprogenitor cells and osteocytes [19]. Both groups of cells have critical roles in bone remodeling. It is suggested that when osteogenic cells were combined with the inductive properties of the DBM and the stable environment of Ilizarov fixation in this series, healing outcomes were improved and time to union reduced as compared to the Control Group without osteoprogenitor cells. This strategy is of importance in this patient sample as patients here had multiple comorbidities that are associated with poor fracture healing.

There are few reports in the literature evaluating the efficacy of cBMA in conjunction with DBM to promote fracture healing. To our knowledge, this is the first cohort comparison to evaluate the combined use of PRP, cBMA, DBM, and the Ilizarov method in patients with various comorbidities; there was a significant reduction in external fixator time and time to healing. Several reports in the literature suggest the use of PRP on chronic wounds or at postoperative incisions promotes antimicrobial activity, and reduces infection [20]. There was a trend suggested here as no patients in the cBMA Group required oral antibiotics for superficial skin infections.

The limitations of this study include the retrospective nature, the limited number of patients, and the time points at which data were collected. Another factor, currently under investigation in our research group, is the potential variability in the number of progenitor cells (MSCs and HSCs) in a sample of cBMA from each patient. In the population studied, the presence of multiple comorbidities introduces the possibility that patients in the cBMA Group with delayed healing had suboptimal numbers of progenitor cells in their cBMA sample; a larger sample size will be required as well as prior progenitor cell analysis so that patients can be randomized according to progenitor cell number.

In conclusion, the use of DBM saturated with cBMA in combination with the Ilizarov technique results in an 85 % healing rate in approximately 4 months. We conclude this strategy is safe, reliable, and effective with good clinical outcomes for the treatment for complex fractures in patients with significant comorbidities.

Acknowledgments This work was supported in part by Arteriocyte Medical Systems.

References

1. Krappinger D, Irenberger A, Zegg M, Huber B (2013) Treatment of large posttraumatic tibial bone defects using the Ilizarov method: a subjective outcome assessment. Arch Orthop Trauma Surg 133(6):789–795. doi:10.1007/s00402-013-1712-y

2. Blum AL, BongioVanni JC, Morgan SJ, Flierl MA, dos Reis FB (2010) Complications associated with distraction osteogenesis for infected nonunion of the femoral shaft in the presence of a bone defect: a retrospective series. J Bone Joint Surg Br 92(4):565–570. doi:10.1302/0301-620X.92B4.23475

3. Sella EJ (2008) Prevention and management of complications of the Ilizarov treatment method. Foot Ankle Spec 1(2):105–107. doi:10.1177/1938640008315349

4. Ramos T, Karlsson J, Eriksson BI, Nistor L (2013) Treatment of distal tibial fractures with the Ilizarov external fixator—a prospective observational study in 39 consecutive patients. BMC Musculoskelet Disord 14:30. doi:10.1186/1471-2474-14-30

5. Brinker MR, O'Connor DP (2007) Outcomes of tibial nonunion in older adults following treatment using the Ilizarov method. J Orthop Trauma 21(9):634–642. doi:10.1097/BOT.0b013 e318156c2a2

6. Pieske O, Wittmann A, Zaspel J, Loffler T, Rubenbauer B, Trentzsch H, Piltz S (2009) Autologous bone graft versus demineralized bone matrix in internal fixation of ununited long bones. J Trauma Manag Outcomes 3:11. doi:10.1186/1752-2897-3-11

7. Gruskin E, Doll BA, Futrell FW, Schmitz JP, Hollinger JO (2012) Demineralized bone matrix in bone repair: history and use. Adv Drug Deliv Rev 64(12):1063–1077. doi:10.1016/j.addr.2012.06.008

8. Barry FP (2003) Mesenchymal stem cell therapy in joint disease. Novartis Found Symp 249:86–96 (**discussion 96–102, 170–104, 239–141**)

9. Gobbi A, Bathan L (2009) Biological approaches for cartilage repair. J Knee Surg 22(1):36–44

10. Hauser RA, Orlofsky A (2013) Regenerative injection therapy with whole bone marrow aspirate for degenerative joint disease: a case series. Clin Med Insights Arthritis Musculoskelet Disord 6:65–72. doi:10.4137/CMAMD.S10951

11. Turajane T, Chaweewannakorn U, Larbpaiboonpong V, Aojanepong J, Thitiset T, Honsawek S, Fongsarun J, Papadopoulos KI (2013) Combination of intra-articular autologous activated peripheral blood stem cells with growth factor addition/preservation and hyaluronic acid in conjunction with arthroscopic microdrilling mesenchymal cell stimulation Improves quality of life and regenerates articular cartilage in early osteoarthritic knee disease. J Med Assoc Thail Chotmaihet Thangphaet 96(5): 580–588

12. Mehta S, Watson JT (2008) Platelet rich concentrate: basic science and current clinical applications. J Orthop Trauma 22(6):432–438. doi:10.1097/BOT.0b013e31817e793f

13. Crovetti G, Martinelli G, Issi M, Barone M, Guizzardi M, Campanati B, Moroni M, Carabelli A (2004) Platelet gel for healing cutaneous chronic wounds. Transfus Apheresis Sci 30(2):145–151. doi:10.1016/j.transci.2004.01.004

14. Lubkowska A, Dolegowska B, Banfi G (2012) Growth factor content in PRP and their applicability in medicine. J Biol Regul Homeost Agents 26(2 Suppl. 1):3S–22S

15. Yang HS, Shin J, Bhang SH, Shin JY, Park J, Im GI, Kim CS, Kim BS (2011) Enhanced skin wound healing by a sustained release of growth factors contained in platelet-rich plasma. Exp Mol Med 43(11):622–629. doi:10.3858/emm.2011.43.11.070

16. Guo Y, Qiu J, Zhang C (2008) Follow-up study on platelet-rich plasma in repairing chronic wound nonunion of lower limbs in 47 cases. Zhongguo xiu fu chong jian wai ke za zhi = Zhongguo xiufu chongjian waike zazhi = Chin J Repar Reconstr Surg 22(11):1301–1305

17. Anitua E, Alonso R, Girbau C, Aguirre JJ, Muruzabal F, Orive G (2012) Antibacterial effect of plasma rich in growth factors (PRGF(R)-Endoret(R)) against Staphylococcus aureus and Staphylococcus epidermidis strains. Clin Exp Dermatol 37(6):652–657. doi:10.1111/j.1365-2230.2011.04303.x

18. Phemister DB (1947) Treatment of ununited fractures by onlay bone grafts without screw or tie fixation and without breaking down of the fibrous union. J Bone Joint SurgAm 29(4):946–960

19. Kasemkijwattana C, Hongeng S, Kesprayura S, Rungsinaporn V, Chaipinyo K, Chansiri K (2011) Autologous bone marrow mesenchymal stem cells implantation for cartilage defects: two cases report. J Med Assoc Thail Chotmaihet Thangphaet 94(3):395–400

20. Khalafi RS, Bradford DW, Wilson MG (2008) Topical application of autologous blood products during surgical closure following a coronary artery bypass graft. Eur J Cardio Thorac Surg 34(2):360–364. doi:10.1016/j.ejcts.2008.04.026

11

A prospective observational study of 56 patients treated with ring fixator after a complex tibial fracture

Rasmus Elsoe[1] · Søren Kold[1] · Peter Larsen[2] · Juozas Petruskevicius[1]

Abstract The objective of this prospective study was to evaluate the patient-reported outcomes for patients with complex tibial fractures treated with a ring fixator. The secondary aim was to analyse the variables affecting patient-reported outcomes and time to union. Fifty-six patients participated in the study. The mean age at the time of fracture was 56.5 years (range 30–86). All fractures united during the study period. The ring fixator was removed at an average of 25.3 weeks (range 9–53). During treatment, the function and QOL increased with time. Compared with an established reference population, the study population showed a significantly worse EQ5D-5L index both throughout the treatment period and 8 weeks after frame removal. 18% of patients reported mild to severe depression 8 weeks after frame removal.

Keywords Ilizarov · Ring fixator · Complex fracture tibial bone · Plateau fracture · Pilon fracture · Short-term outcome

✉ Rasmus Elsoe
  rae@rn.dk

1   Department of Orthopaedic Surgery, Aalborg University
    Hospital, Aalborg University, 18-22 Hobrovej, 9000 Aalborg,
    Denmark

2   Department of Occupational Therapy and Physiotherapy,
    Aalborg University Hospital, Aalborg University, 18-22
    Hobrovej, 9000 Aalborg, Denmark

Introduction

Complex fractures of the tibial bone involving the joint surfaces and multi-fragmented tibia shaft fractures with soft tissue damage are challenging [1–3]. Conservative management is often not feasible and, consequently, most fractures are treated operatively [4, 5].

Surgical management methods include open reduction and internal fixation [6], angle-stable locking plates [7], ring fixators [8] and percutaneous screw fixation [9]. The literature does not favour a single surgical method from objective measures or patient-reported outcomes. There are ongoing discussions concerning the patient-reported QOL throughout the treatment period between the different surgical methods.

The authors prefer the use of ring fixation for the treatment of complex fractures of the tibial bone. The period from surgery to union and removal of the frame is considerable and can vary from 8 to 87 weeks [10–12]. To the authors' knowledge, no studies have evaluated the patient-reported outcomes during the treatment period. Moreover, no studies have undertaken an analysis of the variables affecting short-term patient-reported outcome and with one study only reporting factors affecting time to union [13].

The primary aim of this study was to report the patient-reported quality of life (HRQOL) from surgery to eight weeks after frame removal in patients with a complex tibial fracture. The secondary aim was to analyse variables affecting patient reported outcomes and time to union.

The hypothesis was that patients would report worse outcome compared with the Danish reference population on EQ5D-5L index score from time of surgery to eight weeks after frame removal following a complex tibial fracture.

Patients and methods

Study design

The study design was a prospective follow-up study including all patients treated with a ring fixator after a complex fracture of the tibial bone. The Danish Data Protection Agency (J. nr. 2008-58-0028) approved the study. The main outcome measurement was the EQ5D-5L index [14].

The Trauma Ilizarov Database (TID)

All patients treated with a ring fixator following a complex fracture of the tibial bone between December 2012 and May 2014 at Aalborg University Hospital, Denmark, were included in the Trauma Ilizarov Database. Patients with complex tibial fractures treated without a ring fixator were excluded. Patients who were unable to fill out the questionnaires due to physical or mental disabilities were excluded. A detailed overview is shown in Fig. 1.

Patient baseline characteristics were obtained at the time of admission to hospital. All patients were systematically examined at the outpatient clinic after 2, 6 weeks, 3 and 6 months. A final examination was conducted 8 weeks after removal of the fixator.

Data on age, gender, trauma mechanism, type of trauma, fracture classification, type of surgery, comorbidities and complications were registered. Fracture classification was performed using the AO classification [15] and based on a CT scan pre-operatively.

Surgical treatment

Bicondylar fractures of the tibial bone, complex fractures with soft tissue damage of the tibial shaft and distal fractures of the tibial bone not treatable by intramedullary nailing were all treated by an external ring fixator. The authors preferred to manage proximal and distal tibial fractures with initial screw fixation of joint bearing bone fragments and, if necessary, with exposure of the joint surface. Both autogenous and allogeneous bone grafting were used. The metaphyseal–diaphyseal fractures were bridged by one or more rings. The frame was connected to the bone by hydroxyapatite-coated half-pins and k-wires with olives as needed. After applying the ring fixator alignment was assessed and corrected if needed. Amendments such as footplates and proximal fixation of the femur were used where deemed appropriate.

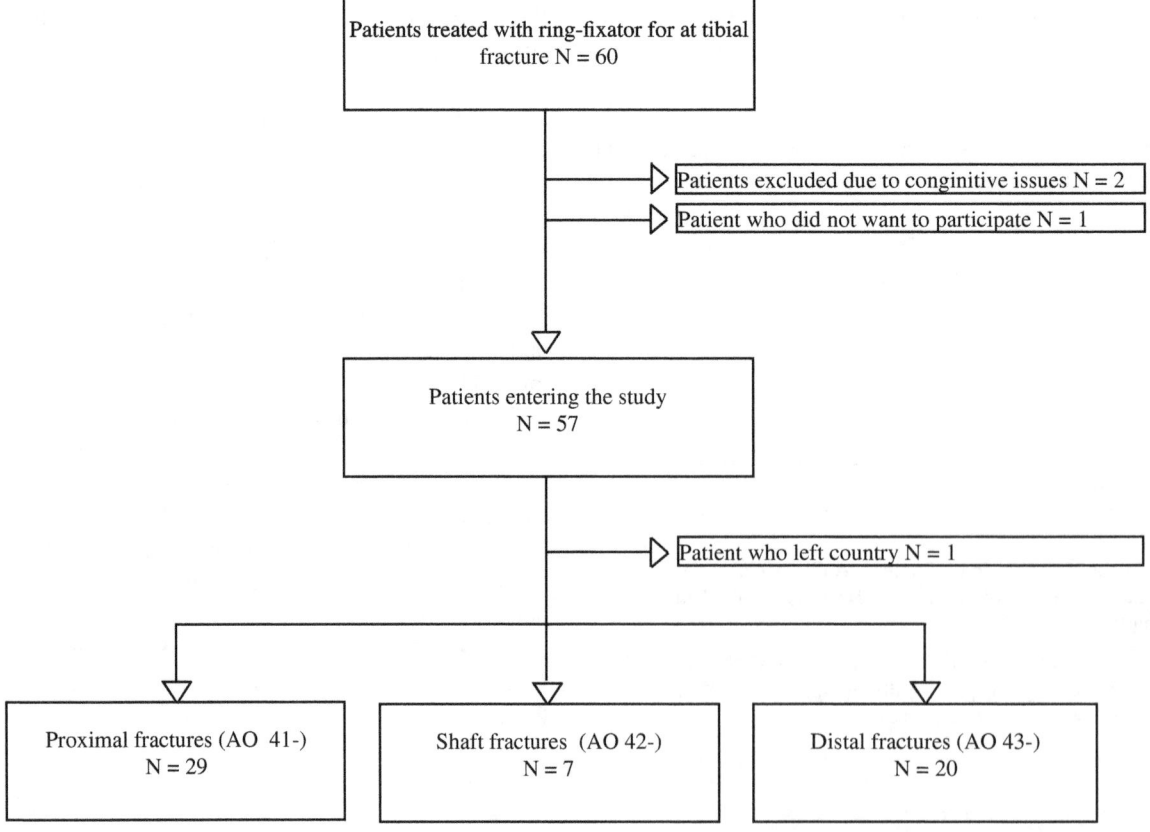

Fig. 1 Patient recruitment flow

All patients were systematically examined at the outpatient clinic every 6 weeks until fracture union. In general, patients with fractures of the joint surfaces were kept non-weight bearing for 6 weeks. The decision of fracture union and the removal of the frame was as described by Ramos et al. [8]; the fracture was regarded as united when 3 of 4 cortices on antero-posterior and lateral X-rays showed bridging callus; the fracture was stable under manual stress and the patients were able to walk without pain after the connection rods had been removed.

All patients had a standardized physiotherapy programme from the first day following surgery and daily until discharge. After discharge, the patients were managed in the outpatient clinic. The rehabilitation programme has special focus on knee and ankle range of motion, muscle function and the ability to maintain these functions in conjunction with management of activities of daily living. In general, patients were seen in the outpatient clinic 1–3 times a week for 3–5 months.

Outcome measurements

Patient reported measurements

EQ5D-5L is a standardized and validated instrument to assess health outcome [14]. It consists of 5 dimensions: mobility, self-care, usual activities, pain/discomfort and anxiety/depression and a self-rated health scale on a 20 cm vertical, visual analogue scale with endpoints labelled 'the best health you can imagine' and 'the worst health you can imagine'. Each dimension has 5 levels: no problems, slight problems, moderate problems, severe problems and extreme problems. A Danish data set was used to calculate the EQ5D-5L index [16]. An EQ5D-5L index at 1.0 indicates full health and 0.0 denotes death. Reference population from Denmark is available [17].

Knee Injury and Osteoarthritis Outcome Score (KOOS) [18] is a standardized and validated instrument used to evaluate knees and associated problems. The questionnaire includes 42 items, and each item obtains a score from 0 to 4; a total score from 0 to 100 is calculated for each subscale. A total score of 100 indicates no symptoms and 0 indicates major symptoms. KOOS reference data [19] from a general population-based sample in southern Sweden is available.

The Olerud–Molander Ankle Score (OMAS) [20] is a standardized and validated instrument used to evaluate ankle and associated problems. The OMAS is a patient-reported questionnaire developed to evaluate function after ankle fracture. The scale is a functional rating scale from 0 (totally impaired) to 100 (completely unimpaired) and is based on nine different items: pain, stiffness, swelling, stair climbing, running, jumping, squatting, supports and activities of daily living.

The Major Depression Inventory (MDI) score [21] is a validated system designed to measure depression symptoms in accordance with the symptom guidelines defined by the WHO classification for unipolar depression (ICD-10) and the American Psychiatric Association classification for major depression (DSM-IV). The instrument consists of 12 questions. On a 6-point Likert scale, the individual items measure how much of the time the symptoms have been present during the last 14 days. The MDI was scored according to specific guidelines. A score of 0 indicates no depression and 50 severe depression. The categories, no depression, less than 20, mild, 20–24, moderate, 25–29 and severe depression, 30 or more, were used [21, 22].

Radiological outcome measurements

Radiographic examination included X-rays and pre-operative CT scans for all patients. Postoperatively, X-rays of the entire lower leg were obtained and used to evaluate the quality of reduction. Radiological examination was performed at 6 weeks, 3 months and every 6 weeks until union. At the final examination 8 weeks after fixator removal, the radiological assessments were made on AP and lateral X-rays. Proximal tibial fractures were evaluated by alignment and depression of the articular surface and condylar widening as described by Rasmussen et al. [23]. Shaft fractures were evaluated by alignment. Distal fractures were evaluated with regard to alignment, talar subluxation, central depression and mortise widening as described by Ramos et al. [2] Furthermore, an assessment of the postoperative reduction for distal fractures was performed as described by March and co-workers [24], modified by Burwell and Charnley [25]. Two authors carried out radiological evaluations separately (RE & JP). In case of disagreement, consensus was obtained.

Objective outcome measurements

Range of motion (ROM) Knee range of motion was assessed by active extension and flexion of the knee with the patient supine on the examination table. The patient was asked to perform maximal flexion and extension, and the angle was measured by a goniometer. Ankle range of motion was assessed by active dorsal and plantar flexion of the talocrural joint with the patient supine on the examination table. The patient was asked to perform maximal dorsal and plantar flexion, and the angle was measured by a goniometer.

Pain was assessed with a visual analogue scale (VAS) ranging from 0 to 100 mm. Patients were asked to classify pain while resting.

Statistics

Continuous data were expressed with mean and standard deviation (SD). Categorical data were expressed as frequencies. The assumption of normal distribution variables was checked visually by Q–Q plots. Linear or logistic regression was used to analyse variables affecting time to union and patient-reported outcome. The Chi-squared test was used to compare patients' reported outcome between categorical variables. A P value of <0.05 was considered significant.

The statistical analysis was performed by Stata (version 13).

Results

A total of 60 patients were treated for a tibial facture with ring fixator during the study period. Four patients met one or more of the exclusion criteria, and 56 patients participated in the study (Fig. 1).

There were 32 females and 24 males in the study population. The mean age at the time of fracture was 56.5 years, range 30–86. The baseline variables for all patients concerning trauma mechanism, type of trauma, fracture classification, open or closed fracture, comorbidities and complications are presented in Table 1. Thirty-two patients (57%) patients had antibiotics during the treatment period due to pin or wire infections. One patient was

Table 1 Baseline characteristics

Age at time of fracture, mean (range)	56.5 (30–82)
Gender male/female	24/32
Smoker yes/no	37/19
Side of injury, right/left/bilateral	27/27/2
High-/low-energy trauma	19/37
Comorbidities	
ASA score, mean(SD)	1.8 (0.7)
Charlson comobidity score, mean(SD)	2.9 (1.9)
Diabetes mellitus	8
Fracture classification	
AO-41	29
AO-42	7
AO-43	20
Open/closed fracture	9/47
Complications	
Pin site infection, number of patients	33
Pin or wire infection treated in hospital	1
Pin or wire infection treated with peros antibiotics	32
Pin or wire exchange during treatment period	12

readmitted to hospital for antibiotics intravenously. Twelve (21%) patients had one or more wires exchanged due to infection. No instances of compartment syndrome or osteomyelitis were observed, and all patients united during the study period.

Twenty-nine patients presented with a proximal tibia fracture AO 41- (A2 = 1, A3 = 1, C1 = 4, C2 = 1, C3 = 22). Seven patients presented with a complex shaft fracture AO 42- (A1 = 1, A2 = 3, C1 = 2, C3 = 1). Twenty patients presented with a distal fracture AO 43- (A2 = 1, A3 = 4, B1 = 3, B2 = 1, B3 = 3, C1 = 1, C2 = 1, C3 = 6).

Patient-reported outcome

MDI

Overall, 18% of patients reported mild to severe depression 8 weeks after frame removal. Five patients reported MDI scores between 20 and 30 indicating mild to moderate depression, and 5 patients had a score of >30 indicating severe depression. No significant difference in MDI scores was observed throughout the treatment period (Fig. 3).

Six patients with proximal fractures, 2 patients with shaft fractures and 2 patients with distal fractures reported mild to severe depression.

Proximal fractures (AO 41-)

The mean EQ5D-5L index from surgery to union is presented in Fig. 2. Eight weeks after frame removal, the mean EQ5D-5L index was 0.695 (CI 0.63–0.76). The mean EQ5D-5L VAS was 74.5 (CI 65.2–83.9). Compared with the established reference population from Denmark [17], the study population showed a significantly worse EQ5D-5L index at the time of union (Table 2).

Eight weeks after frame removal, the mean KOOS score was pain 65.6 (CI 56.1–75.2), symptoms 54.5 (CI 44.3–64.6), ADL 69.8 (CI 58.6–81.0), sport 28.6 (CI 17.3–39.8) and QOL 48.0 (CI 38.1–57.8). Compared with the established reference population [19], the study population showed a significantly worse KOOS outcome for all the five subgroups (Table 2).

Shaft fractures (AO 42-)

The mean EQ5D-5L index from surgery to union is presented in Fig. 2. Eight weeks after frame removal, the mean EQ5D-5L index was 0.58 (CI 0.43–0.73). The mean EQ5D-5L VAS was 57.9 (CI 29.6–86.1). Compared with the established reference population from Denmark [17], the study population showed a significantly worse EQ5D-5L index at the time of union (Table 2).

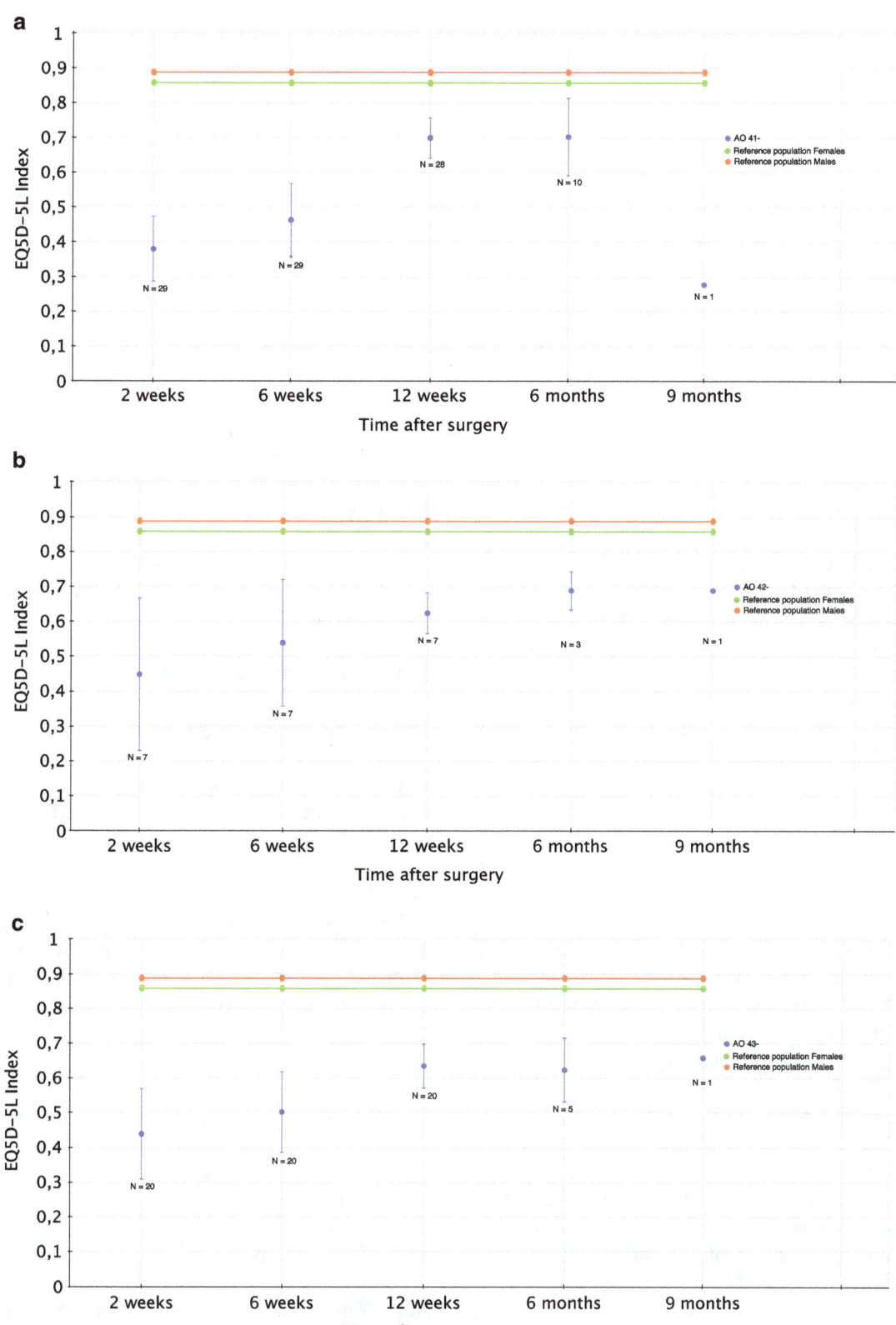

Fig. 2 a Patient reported outcome, proximal tibial fractures (AO 41-), patient-reported outcome from surgery to frame removal, proximal tibial fractures. **b** Patient reported outcome, tibial shaft fractures (AO 42-), patient-reported outcome from surgery to frame removal, tibial shaft fractures. **c** Patient reported outcome, distal tibial fractures (AO 43-), patient-reported outcome from surgery to frame removal, distal tibial fractures

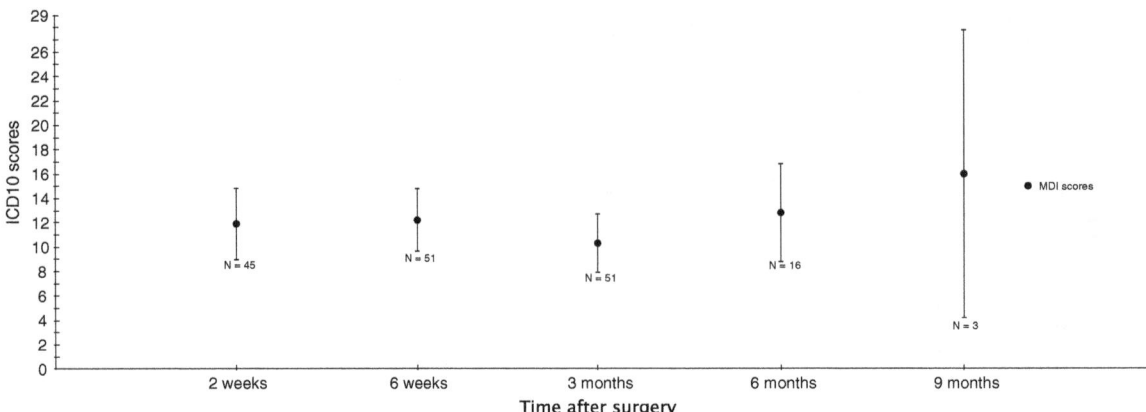

Fig. 3 Patient-reported MDI scores from surgery to frame removal

Distal fractures (AO 43-)

The mean EQ5D-5L index from surgery to union is presented in Fig. 2. Eight weeks after frame removal, the mean EQ5D-5L index was 0.65 (CI 0.57–0.72). The mean EQ5D-5L VAS was 66.0 (CI 55.4–76.5). Compared with the established reference population from Denmark [17], the study population showed a significantly worse EQ5D-5L index (Table 2).

The mean Olerud–Molander Ankle Score 8 weeks after frame removal was 40.3 (CI 29.6–50.9). No reference population was available for the Olerud–Molander Ankle Score.

Radiological outcome measurements

Proximal fractures (AO 41-)

All fractures united during the study period. The ring fixator was removed at an average of 23.5 weeks, range 9.1–45.4. At the final examination 8 weeks after frame removal, 9 patients were out of alignment or had an articular depression of more than 3 mm (Table 3).

Shaft fractures (AO 42-)

All fractures united during the study period. The ring fixator was removed at an average of 27.4 weeks, range 16.1–42.0. At the final examination 8 weeks after frame removal, one patient was out of alignment, representing a varus deformity of 5° (Table 3).

Distal fractures (AO 43-)

All fractures united during the study period. The ring fixator was removed at an average of 24.9 weeks, range 13.4–51.3. At the final examination 8 weeks after frame

removal, three patients were out of alignment and three patients had a central depression of more than 3 mm. No talar subluxation of more than 0.5 mm or mortise widening of more than 0.5 mm was present. The Burwell and Charnley classification shows 12 patients with good reduction, six patients with fair reduction and one with poor reduction (Table 3).

Objective outcome measurements

Proximal fractures (AO 41-)

At the final examination 8 weeks after frame removal, the mean knee flexion was 116.9° (CI 112.1–121.7). Twelve patients experienced a knee extension limitation of 5° or less, and 2 patients had a knee extension limitation exceeding 10°.

The VAS score for rest pain 8 weeks after frame removal was reported with a range from 0 to 6. Twenty-two patients reported no pain, five patients reported VAS between 1 and 5 and two patients reported VAS 6.

Shaft fractures (AO 42-)

The VAS score for rest pain 8 weeks after frame removal was reported with a range from 0 to 7. Two patients reported no pain, 4 patients reported VAS between 1 and 5 and 1 patient reported VAS 7.

Distal fractures (AO 43-)

At the final examination 8 weeks after frame removal, the mean dorsal flexion of the ankle was 9.5° (CI 5.2–13.7). The mean plantar flexion of the ankle was 22.5° (CI 18.3–26.8).

The VAS score for rest pain 8 weeks after frame removal was reported with a range from 0 to 8. Twelve

Table 2 Patient-reported outcome 8 weeks after frame removal compared with reference populations

| | KOOS | | | | | | | | | |
| | PAIN | | ADL | | SYMP | | QOL | | SPORT | |
	Mean	95% CI	Mean	95% CI	Mean	95% CI	Mean	95% CI	Mean	95% CI
Proximal fracture (AO 41-)										
Study population	65.6	56.1–75.2*	69.8	58.6–81.0*	54.5	44.3–64.6*	48	38.1–57.8*	8.6	17.3–39.8*
Reference population**,***		86.7–88.2		86.5–88.1		85.4–86.9		77.4–79.6		72.5–75.1

| | EQ5D-5L | | | VAS | |
| | Index | | | | |
	Mean		95% CI	Mean	95% CI
Study population	0.695		0.627–0.763*	74.5	65.2–83.9
Reference population**** (male/female 50–59 years)	0.888/0.858		0.880–0.896/0.850–0.866		
Shaft fracture (AO 42-)					
Study population	0.579		0.429–0.728*	57.9	29.6–86.1
Reference population**** (male/female 50–59 years)	0.888/0.858		0.880–0.896/0.850–0.866		
Distal fracture (AO 43-)					
Study population	0.646		0.570–0.7*	66	55.4–76.5
Reference population**** (male/female 50–59 years)	0.888/0.858		0.880–0.896/0.850–0.866		

* Significantly different compared with reference population
** Paradowski PT et al. BMC Musculoskeletal Disord, 2006[18]
*** Unpublished data. Ewa Roos 'Personal communication' Nov 13, 2 01 2. Paradowski et al. 2006
**** Sorensen J et al. Scand. J. Public Health, 2009[16]

patients reported no pain, five patients reported VAS between 1 and 5 and two patients reported VAS between 7 and 8.

Analysis of variables affecting time to union

The analysis of variables affecting time to union shows a significant association between time to union and smoking ($P = 0.04$). No significant association between age, BMI, Charlson comorbidity score, pin or wire infection and high-/low-energy trauma was observed ($P \geq 0.05$, Table 4).

Analysis of variables affecting patient-reported outcome

Eight weeks after frame removal, baseline variables (age, BMI, Smoking, Charlson comorbidity score, infection and high-/low-energy trauma) show no significant influence on patient-reported outcome (EQ5D-5L; $P \geq 0.26$, Table 4).

Eight weeks after frame removal, a comparison of patients with a fracture out of alignment or with an articular depression and patients with fractures in alignment or without articular depression shows no significantly worse EQ5D-5L index ($P = 0.50$).

Discussion

This study shows that ring fixation of complex fractures of the tibial bone has a high rate of union and a low rate of complications. These findings are supported by a number of recent studies [2, 12, 26–28]. Moreover, the fracture and subsequent treatment was associated with significant persisting disability and depression until 8 weeks after removal of the frame.

This is the first study to prospectively evaluate the patient-reported QOL and function throughout the treatment period in patients treated with a ring fixator after a complex tibial bone fracture. Throughout the treatment period, patients with complex fractures of the tibial bone treated with a ring fixator experience worse function and QOL compared with the established reference populations. Unfortunately the study has no information regarding pre-injury health status, and it could be argued that the pre-injury health status of the study population is not comparable to the established national reference population. Skoog et al. [29] have reported comparable pre-injury QOL values in a population of tibial fractures compared to reference populations. The second limitation was the study could not distinguish whether poor QOL was influenced by injury or by the treatment with circular frame.

Table 3 Observed deformities, depressions and condylar widening

	Varus deformity measured in °	Valgus deformity measured in °	Flexion deformity measured in °	Extension deformity measured in °	Depression AP mm	Depression lateral mm	Condylar widening mm
Proximal							
Patient ID							
2		5			3		
11			10		2	3	
3			8		1	1	
17					6	3	10
34					6	2	8
39			3		5	3	0
46						4	
52			3		4		
55	4				1		

	Varus deformity measured in °	Valgus deformity measured in °	Flexion deformity measured in °	Extension deformity measured in °
Shaft				
Patient ID				
8				4
13	5			

	Varus deformity measured in °	Valgus deformity measured in °	Flexion deformity measured in °	Extension deformity measured in °	Central depression > 3 mm
Distal					
Patient ID					
5					3
25	3				
26					4
33		3			
45	8				
51					7
53					5

Eight weeks after frame removal, the radiological assessments were made on AP and side X-rays. Proximal tibial fractures were evaluated concerning alignment and depression of the articular surface and condylar widening as described by Rasmussen et al. [22]. Shaft fractures were evaluated concerning alignment. Distal fractures were evaluated with regard to alignment, talar subluxation, central depression and mortise widening as described by Ramos et al. [2] Furthermore, an assessment of the postoperative reduction for distal fractures was performed as described by March and co-workers [23], modified by Burwell & Charnley [24]

During the treatment period, function and QOL increased with time. No studies evaluating other surgical treatment methods have prospectively reported the patient-reported QOL from the time of fracture to union. In summary, more research is needed regarding patient-reported function and QOL throughout the treatment period between different surgical methods.

A number of studies have reported the outcome after complex fractures of the tibia bone. Ramos et al. [2, 8] have, in two recent studies, evaluated the patient-reported functional outcome after complex fractures to the distal and proximal end of the tibial bone treated with ring fixator. These studies do not compare the results to an established reference population but still show that, even after successful treatment, patients reported a low score on the KOOS/FAOS subscales for sports and QOL. A retrospective study by Ahearn et al. [28] support these findings and reported poor outcome scores after complex tibial plateau fractures evaluated on WOMAC and SF-36, despite satisfactory reduction and alignment. Furthermore,

Table 4 Variables affecting time to union and patient-reported outcome

	Time to union	EQ5D-5L
Age	$b = 0.51, P = 0.06$	$b = 0.02, P = 0.70$
BMI	$b = 0.24, P = 0.63$	$b = 0.06, P = 0.56$
Smoking	$\mathbf{b = 0.09, P = 0.04^*}$	$b = 0.27, P = 0.88$
Charlson comorbidity	$b = 0.07, P = 0.05$	$b = 0.007, P = 0.32$
Pin/wire infection	$b = 0.07, P = 0.11$	$b = 2.13, P = 0.26$
High-/low-energy trauma	$b = 0.05, P = 0.23$	$b = 0.93, P = 0.61$

b = regression coefficient

Bold represents statistically significant difference

a large-scale retrospective study by O'Toole et al. [30] reported that the most important drivers in patients' satisfaction following major lower limb trauma seem to be physical function, less pain, the absence of depression and the ability to return to work. Moreover, O'Toole et al. [30] reported that patients' satisfaction was not related to details of the injury, patient demographics or psychological profile of the patient. These findings indicate that complex fractures of the tibial bone are severe in nature and may result in some disability. It is the authors' intention to report the objective and patient-reported outcome 1 and 3 years after frame removal in order to evaluate the development in patient-reported QOL and function.

This study shows an unexpected high rate of mild to severe depression 8 weeks after frame removal. These findings are new and, to the authors' knowledge, no earlier studies have reported mental disability for the present study population. The severe nature of the fractures and the long treatment period in combination with a high degree of socioeconomic consequences and a significantly worse QOL may be contributory factors leading to mental vulnerability. Krappinger et al. [3] support these findings in a recent study of patients treated with the Ilizarov technique after large post-traumatic tibial bone defects. The study reported a major burden of mental and physical stress for both patients and their relatives. In contrast, Baschera et al. [11] reported no significantly worse SF-12 mental component score compared to a normal population in patients treated with ring fixator after 1–9 years' follow-up. The overall mental health for patients with complex fractures of the tibial bone may be a point of further interest in clinical evaluation, treatment and research in the future.

This study shows a significant negative effect between smoking and time to union. A recent systematic review by Patel et al. 2013 [31] evaluated the effect of smoking on bone healing after tibial fractures and support the findings from the present study. Patel et al. [31] reported a significant longer time to fracture healing for smokers and concluded an overall negative effect of smoking on bone healing after tibial fractures. In contrast, Alemdaroglu

et al. [13] reported no significant difference in the time to union for smokers for patients treated with ring fixator of the tibial bone. This study shows no significant correlation between any of the other baseline characteristics and time to union. The rate of complications in this patient population was low thus larger studies should be conducted to reveal the influence of variables such as high-energy trauma, open fractures, soft tissue injuries, diabetes, age and malnutrition that affect fracture union [13, 32–35].

Conclusion

This study shows a major morbidity related to the treatment of complex tibial fractures until 8 weeks after frame removal. Treatment of complex tibial fractures involving joint surfaces is challenging, and this study shows a significant burden on QOL, mental and physical disabilities for the patients throughout the prolonged treatment period. Even eight weeks after union and removal of the frame, patients experienced a significantly worse patient-reported outcome compared with an established reference population. At the time of frame removal, no significant difference in EQ5D-5L index between AO type 41-, 42- and 43-was found. Eight weeks after frame removal, 18% of the patients reported mild to severe depression.

Acknowledgements The Department of Orthopaedic Surgery and the Department of Occupational and Physiotherapy, Aalborg University Hospital, Denmark are acknowledged for proving unrestricted grants.

Informed consent Proper informed consent was taken and patients explained about the procedure before entering the study.

References

1. Joveniaux P, Ohl X, Harisboure A et al (2010) Distal tibia fractures: management and complications of 101 cases. Int Orthop 34:583–588

2. Ramos T, Karlsson J, Eriksson BI, BINistor L (2013) Treatment of distal tibial fractures with the Ilizarov external fixator–a prospective observational study in 39 consecutive patients. BMC Musculoskelet Disord 14:30

3. Krappinger D, Irenberger A, Zegg MHuber B (2013) Treatment of large posttraumatic tibial bone defects using the Ilizarov method: a subjective outcome assessment. Arch Orthop Trauma Surg 133:789–795

4. Jansen H, Frey SP, Doht S et al (2013) Medium-term results after complex intra-articular fractures of the tibial plateau. J Orthop Sci 18:569–577

5. Ali AM (2013) Outcomes of open bicondylar tibial plateau fractures treated with Ilizarov external fixator with or without minimal internal fixation. Eur J Orthop Surg Traumatol 23:349–355

6. Manidakis N, Dosani A, Dimitriou R et al (2010) Tibial plateau fractures: functional outcome and incidence of osteoarthritis in 125 cases. Int Orthop 34:565–570

7. Lee JA, Papadakis SA, Moon C, Zalavras CG (2007) Tibial plateau fractures treated with the less invasive stabilisation system. Int Orthop 31:415–418

8. Ramos T, Ekholm C, Eriksson BI et al (2013) The Ilizarov external fixator–a useful alternative for the treatment of proximal tibial fractures. A prospective observational study of 30 consecutive patients. BMC Musculoskelet Disord 14:11

9. Sament R, Mayanger JC, Tripathy SKSen RK (2012) Closed reduction and percutaneous screw fixation for tibial plateau fractures. J Orthop Surg (Hong Kong) 20:37–41

10. Subasi M, Kapukaya A, Arslan H et al (2007) Outcome of open comminuted tibial plateau fractures treated using an external fixator. J Orthop Sci 12:347–353

11. Baschera D, Kingwell D, Wren MZellweger R (2014) A holistic perspective of patients' lives post-Ilizarov external fixation. ANZ J Surg 84:776–780

12. Kapoor SK, Kataria H, Patra SR, Boruah T (2010) Capsuloligamentotaxis and definitive fixation by an ankle-spanning Ilizarov fixator in high-energy pilon fractures. J Bone Joint Surg Br 92:1100–1106

13. Alemdaroglu KB, Tiftikci U, Iltar S et al (2009) Factors affecting the fracture healing in treatment of tibial shaft fractures with circular external fixator. Injury 40:1151–1156

14. Eq-5d questionnary (2012). http://www.euroqol.org/about-eq-5d/publications/user-guide.html

15. Marsh JL, Slongo TF, Agel J, et al., (2007) Fracture and dislocation classification compendium—2007: orthopedic trauma association classification, database and outcome committee. J Orthop Trauma 21:1–133

16. Wittrup-Jensen KU, Lauridsen J, Gudex C, Pedersen KM (2009) Generation of a Danish TTO value set for EQ-5D health states. Scand J Public Health 37:459–466

17. Sorensen J, Davidsen M, Gudex C et al (2009) Danish EQ-5D population norms. Scand J Public Health 37:467–474

18. KOOS questionnary [KOOS web site]. http://www.koos.nu. Accessed 12 June 2011

19. Paradowski PT, Bergman S, Sunden-Lundius A et al (2006) Knee complaints vary with age and gender in the adult population. Population-based reference data for the Knee injury and Osteoarthritis Outcome Score (KOOS). BMC Musculoskelet Disord 7:38

20. Olerud C, Molander H (1984) A scoring scale for symptom evaluation after ankle fracture. Arch Orthop Trauma Surg 103:190–194

21. Olsen LR, Jensen DV, Noerholm V et al (2003) The internal and external validity of the Major Depression Inventory in measuring severity of depressive states. Psychol Med 33:351–356

22. Bech P, Rasmussen NA, Olsen LR et al (2001) The sensitivity and specificity of the Major Depression Inventory, using the Present State Examination as the index of diagnostic validity. J Affect Disord 66:159–164

23. Rasmussen PS (1973) Tibial condylar fractures. Impairment of knee joint stability as an indication for surgical treatment. J Bone Joint Surg Am 55:1331–1350

24. Marsh JL, Buckwalter J, Gelberman R et al (2002) Articular fractures: does an anatomic reduction really change the result? J Bone Joint Surg Am 84-A:1259–1271

25. Burwell HN, Charnley AD (1965) The treatment of displaced fractures at the ankle by rigid internal fixation and early joint movement. J Bone Joint Surg Br 47:634–660

26. Ramos T, Ekholm C, Eriksson BI et al (2013) The Ilizarov external fixator–a useful alternative for the treatment of proximal tibial fractures. A prospective observational study of 30 consecutive patients. BMC Musculoskelet Disord 14:11

27. Korkmaz A, Ciftdemir M, Ozcan M et al (2013) The analysis of the variables, affecting outcome in surgically treated tibia pilon fractured patients. Injury 44:1270–1274

28. Ahearn N, Oppy A, Halliday R et al (2014) The outcome following fixation of bicondylar tibial plateau fractures. Bone Joint J 96-B:956–962

29. Skoog A, Soderqvist A, Tornkvist H, Ponzer S (2001) One-year outcome after tibial shaft fractures: results of a prospective fracture registry. J Orthop Trauma 15:210–215

30. O'Toole RV, Castillo RC, Pollak AN et al (2008) Determinants of patient satisfaction after severe lower-extremity injuries. J Bone Joint Surg Am 90:1206–1211

31. Patel RA, Wilson RF, Patel PAPalmer RM (2013) The effect of smoking on bone healing: a systematic review. Bone Joint Res 2:102–111

32. Adams CI, Keating JF, Court-Brown CM (2001) Cigarette smoking and open tibial fractures. Injury 32:61–65

33. Demiralp B, Atesalp AS, Bozkurt M et al (2007) Spiral and oblique fractures of distal one-third of tibia-fibula: treatment results with circular external fixator. Ann Acad Med Singapore 36:267–271

34. Smith TK, Reed JB, Sanders KM (1987) Interaction of two electrical pacemakers in muscularis of canine proximal colon. Am J Physiol 252:C290–C299

35. Gaston P, Will E, McQueen MM et al (2000) Analysis of muscle function in the lower limb after fracture of the diaphysis of the tibia in adults. J Bone Joint Surg Br 82:326–331

12

Lengthening of the humerus with intramedullary lengthening nails

Julian Fürmetz[1] · Søren Kold[2] · Nikola Schuster[1] · Florian Wolf[1] ·
Peter H. Thaller[1]

Abstract Distraction osteogenesis of the humerus with fully implantable lengthening is now possible since the diameter of the available nails was reduced to 10 mm and below. We report on the first intramedullary lengthening cases of the humerus with two different lengthening devices (FITBONE and PRECICE). Two different approaches and implantation techniques were used. We retrospectively reviewed clinical and radiographic data and pointed out results, pitfalls and complications of the procedure. Four adult patients with relevant length discrepancy of the humerus were treated with fully implantable systems in two centers between 2012 and 2015. Three patients were treated with FITBONE by an antegrade approach; one patient had lengthening with a PRECICE and a retrograde approach. Average nail lengthening was 55 mm (40–65 mm), and the average duration of lengthening was 70 days (52–95 days). The average distraction index was 0.72 mm/day (range 0.4–1.0 mm/day) or 12.5 days/cm (range 8.0–16.2 days/cm). The average consolidation index was 33.6 days/cm (range 25–45 days/cm). There was an implant failure (arrest) with the PRECICE. After consolidation and exchange with a technically improved implant, the course of treatment was uneventful. In patients with antegrade lengthening shoulder abduction decreased, and in the patient with the retrograde approach it improved but elbow extension decreased marginally. Reduced motion of the adjacent joints can be a major problem in intramedullary lengthening of the humerus. This first case series in the field of a rare indication suggests that lengthening of the humerus by fully implantable lengthening nails might be a valuable alternative to lengthening with external fixation. Main advantage of the PRECICE technology is the possible shortening in-between of lengthening.

Keywords Humerus lengthening · Intramedullary lengthening · Distraction osteogenesis · Lengthening nail · FITBONE · PRECICE

Introduction

Today, distraction osteogenesis has become a crucial tool in limb lengthening and deformity correction. Regarding leg lengthening, it has already been described at the beginning of the last century and since the work of Ilizarov it has been more and more understood and brought into clinical use [1].

Compared to leg length discrepancies, arm length discrepancies are less frequent and subsequent secondary damage is lower [2]. But, functional impairment, cosmetic reasons and muscular problems may be an indication for a correction. Lengthening of the humerus was first reported by Dick and Tietjen in 1978 using a Wagner fixator, plating and bone grafting [3]. Since then, different ways of external fixation have been described for lengthening of the humerus [4–9]. Currently, circular frames like the Ilizarov frame and monolateral fixators are the most common fixation techniques and lead to similar results [8, 9]. The results indicate a significant improvement of function, and therefore, lengthening of the humerus is not just a cosmetic procedure.

✉ Julian Fürmetz
Julian.Fuermetz@med.uni-muenchen.de

[1] 3D-Surgery, Department of General, Trauma and Reconstructive Surgery, Munich University Hospital LMU, Germany, Nußbaumstraße 20, 80336 Munich, Germany

[2] Department of Orthopaedics, Aarhus University Hospital, Århus, Denmark

Regarding the lower limb, lengthening by intramedullary devices gained popularity over the past decades. In the first decades of intramedullary lengthening, the diameter of the available lengthening devices was too large for smaller bones and thus for the upper limb. To this date, there is only one other report in the literature about lengthening of the humerus by an intramedullary device, but lacking to provide any results or details [10].

Lengthening nails have many advantages such as no pin site infections, lesser soft-tissue damage and pain, better joint movement and more patient comfort compared to external devices [10–16]. In the past years, technological progress made smaller diameters, as low as 8.5 mm possible [10].

Presently, the most frequently implanted systems are the FITBONE nail, (WITTENSTEIN Intens GmbH, Igersheim, Germany) and the PRECICE nail (Ellipse Technologies Inc., CA, USA) after the ISKD was withdrawn from the market 2009 and the last PHENIX nail was implanted in 2013 [17]. The diameters range from 11 to 13 mm (FITBONE) and 8.5 to 12.5 mm (PRECICE). The FITBONE nail is a motorized (electromotive) system which was developed in 1990 [11]. The PRECICE nail is a magnetically actuated, mechanical system and was introduced to the market in 2011 [10].

In the following, we present two different approaches and implantation techniques regarding intramedullary lengthening of the humerus with two different systems (FITBONE and PRECICE).

Patients and methods

Study patients

We reviewed four patients who underwent five intramedullary lengthening procedures between 2012 and 2015. Three patients underwent three lengthenings with FITBONE, and one patient underwent two lengthenings with PRECICE. All patients were fully informed about the nature of the procedure and the technology involved. All patients explicitly wanted an internal lengthening procedure and declined an external lengthening procedure. Details regarding patient age, sex, etiology, length discrepancy, surgery, lengthening details and complications were tabulated (see Table 1). Calibrated humerus AP radiographs were performed to obtain the humerus length discrepancy before the procedure.

Two patients suffered from a posttraumatic shortening of the humerus, one in childhood (patient Y.G.; FITBONE) and one adult patient (G.K. PRECICE). The other two patients (FITBONE) had unilateral humeral shortening caused by Erb–Duchenne-type obstetric palsy. All FITBONE patients had a minimum follow-up of 6 months after nail removal.

The PRECICE patient (G.K.) has still the nail in situ, and follow-up is 18 months after nail implantation. The case of M.J. has been published previously [18].

Treatment strategy

The first three patients received lengthening with the FITBONE nail using an antegrade approach. The PRECICE lengthening nail (second generation) was used twice for lengthening of the humerus of patient G.K. using a retrograde approach. The second PRECICE nail was the technical improved version P2.1 which has no 'thru-slots' or tack welds at the end of the proximal nail [10]. To protect the radial nerve from damage during osteotomy, a careful soft-tissue dissection is performed to the bone, and a drill guide and soft-tissue protectors are placed to perform safe drilling and chiseling.

Antegrade approach

For antegrade humeral nailing, an anterolateral transdeltoid approach provided access to the humeral canal, and the supraspinatus tendon was split in the direction of its fibers. A protective steel sleeve was passed through the split supraspinatus tendon prior to reaming. Reaming was performed with straight reamers. In two patients (M.J. and Y.G.) the osteotomy was completed with a chisel after careful dissection and predrilling through a small lateral incision. In patient T.K. a previously inserted humeral plate had to be removed prior to nail insertion (see Fig. 1), and the drill and chisel osteotomy was completed through this larger approach. The motor unit inside the nail was connected to a subcutaneously placed receiver by a cord passing through the split in the supraspinatus tendon.

During distraction procedure, the patient had to hold a transmitter over the receiver to activate the motor unit inside the lengthening nail. Lengthening was started at the eighth postoperative day at a maximum rate of 1/3 mm three times per day.

Retrograde approach

Patient G.K. had a posttraumatic decreased shoulder function. A retrograde approach was chosen to protect the rotator cuff and to avoid proximal migration of the humeral head (see Figs. 2, 3).

For retrograde technique in supine position, the supinated patient's elbow has to be fully flexed (up to 140°). Through a small triceps split, the guide wire enters the cortex of the olecranon fossa roof. A steel sleeve was passed through the triceps tendon, and the reaming was performed with straight reamers. Two 3-mm K-wires were placed in the proximal and distal part of the humerus for torsion control. Through a

Table 1 Patients and methods

Patient	M.J.	T.K.	Y.G.	G.K.
Sex	Male	Female	Male	Male
Age	19	19	27	51
History	Erb–Duchenne-type obstetric palsy	Erb–Duchenne-type obstetric palsy	Traumatic growth arrest in childhood	Posttraumatic shortening after complex fracture and nonunion
Disorders	Neck pain, back pain, functional deficit	Neck pain, functional deficit	Functional deficit	Posttraumatic stress disorder, functional deficit
Side	Left	Right	Left	Left
Preoperative humerus shortening (mm)	50	65	65	40
Type of nail	TAA 1160 Tibia FITBONE	TAA 1160 Custom straight FITBONE	TAA 1160 Custom straight FITBONE	PRECICE retrograde femur, 2nd generation P2 and P2.1
	Diameter 11 mm	Diameter 11 mm	Diameter 11 mm	Diameter 8.5 mm
	Length 225 mm	Length 205 mm	Length	Length 215
	Stroke 60 mm	Stroke 60 mm	205 mm	Stroke 50 mm
			Stroke 60 mm	
Osteotomy height from tip of greater tuberculum (mm)	120	130	90	200; 190
Distraction index (mm/day)	0.8	0.6	0.8	0.45 and 1.0
Consolidation index (days/cm)	27.5	25	45	40.0 and 30.3
Problems/obstacles	Proximal humeral head migration, stop of lengthening and remaining shortage of 10 mm	Z-plastic of biceps tendon due to flexion contracture of the elbow	Removal of receiver and chord penetrating rotator cuff to gain better ROM	Early consolidation after "crown breakage" (PRECICE P2)

minimally invasive lateral approach below, the insertion of the deltoid muscle a drill bit osteotomy was performed and completed with a small chisel. Lengthening with the PRE-CICE nail was started at the fifth postoperative day at rate of 1/3 mm, three times per day. After detailed instruction we provided the patient an external magnet controller for his personal use. For the lengthening procedure, the controller was placed on a table hooked into its transport box in an upright position (see Fig. 3).

Postoperative care and follow-up

Before starting the lengthening procedure, a two-plane radiograph of the humerus and a calibrated AP radiograph from the osteotomy site were taken. During lengthening, the distraction was weekly controlled clinically and radiologically by calibrated radiographs of the osteotomy site and adjusted according to radiological signs of bone formation in the regenerate. To preserve the range of motion of the

adjacent joints, physiotherapy was carried out on a regular basis. After the desired length was achieved, radiographs were taken every 2 weeks until full consolidation.

Outcome

After finishing lengthening, the humeral length and the length of the regenerate were obtained on calibrated radiographs or CT Scouts. Consolidation was classified as three out of four cortices being present on the AP and lateral radiographs. Measurement of pre- and postoperative range of motion of the shoulder and elbow joints was performed by a senior surgeon. Subjective functional deficits in daily living, e.g., personal hygiene, clothing or type writing, were noted before and after the treatment. Additional procedures during the lengthening or consolidation period were noted. Complications which led to additional procedures during treatment were divided into implant- and non-implant-related complications.

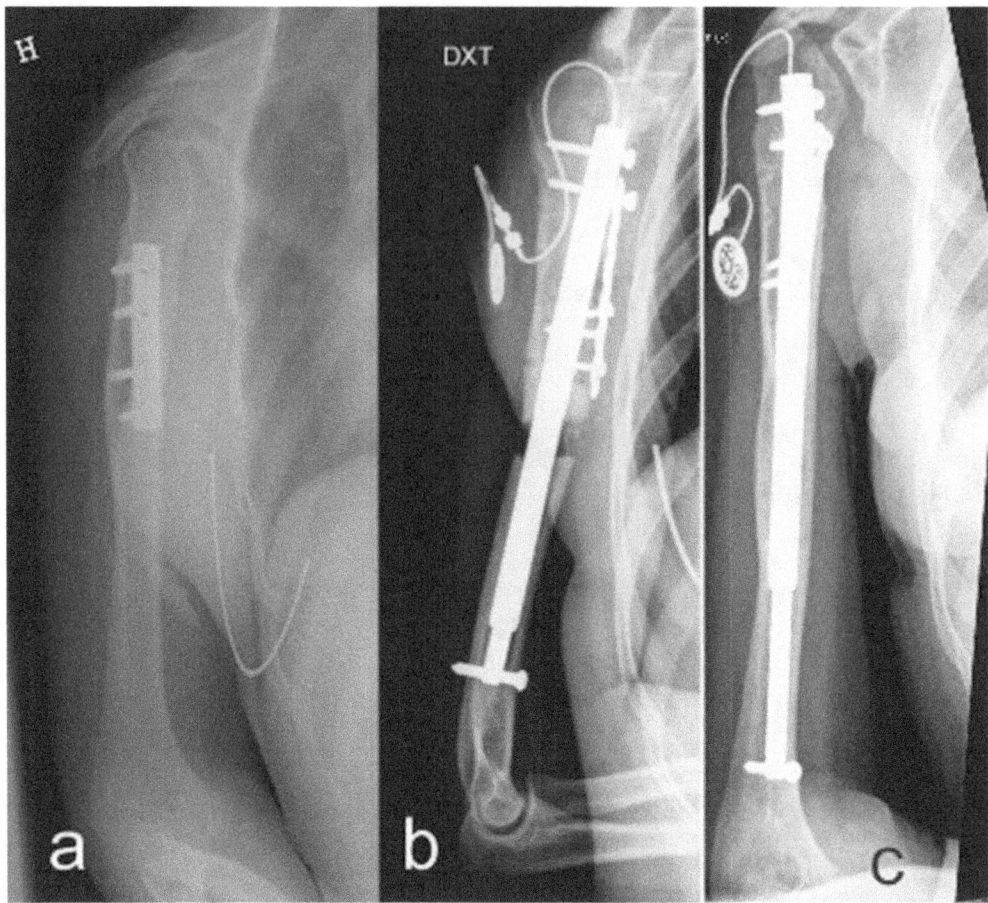

Fig. 1 a Preoperative radiograph of 19-year-old patient T.K. with 65 mm shortening of the right humerus after Erb–Duchenne-type obstetric palsy. The patient had at the age of 12 years an external rotation osteotomy fixed with a plate. **b** Follow-up radiograph after lengthening has been initiated by the inserted FITBONE. After the previously inserted plate was removed at the time of FITBONE insertion a cortical defect existed. In order to securely lock the proximal part of the nail, a new plate was fixed in good cortical bone distally and one of the proximal locking screws were inserted through a plate hole. **c** Radiograph after consolidation of 6-cm lengthened humerus

IRB approval

The study was carried out according to the Declaration of Helsinki. The Ethic Committee of the University of Munich approved this study with the ID number 8-16.

Results

Lengthening

Full lengthening was achieved in one patient (patient G.K.). Two patients (Y.G. and T.K.) had a residual discrepancy of 5 mm, and due to reduced shoulder motion (Y.G.) and elbow motion (T.K.) a minor difference was tolerated. In patient M.J. lengthening was terminated leaving the left humerus 1 cm short compared with the right side. After 4 cm of intramedullary nail lengthening (and a total of 9 cm lengthening due to prior 5 cm extramedullary lengthening with an Ilizarov fixator in childhood), the humeral head migrated proximal and the shoulder abduction declined, so lengthening was terminated.

Average nail lengthening was 55 mm (range 40–65 mm), and the average duration of lengthening was 70 days (range 52–95). The average distraction index was 0.72 mm/day (range 0.4–1.0 mm/day) or 12.5 days/cm (range 8.0–16.2 days/cm). Mean time to reach consolidation was 165 days after the distraction, and the average consolidation index was 33.6 days/cm (range 25–45 days/cm).

Range of motion

Patient Y.G. showed no change in elbow motion. Shoulder abduction decreased 20°.

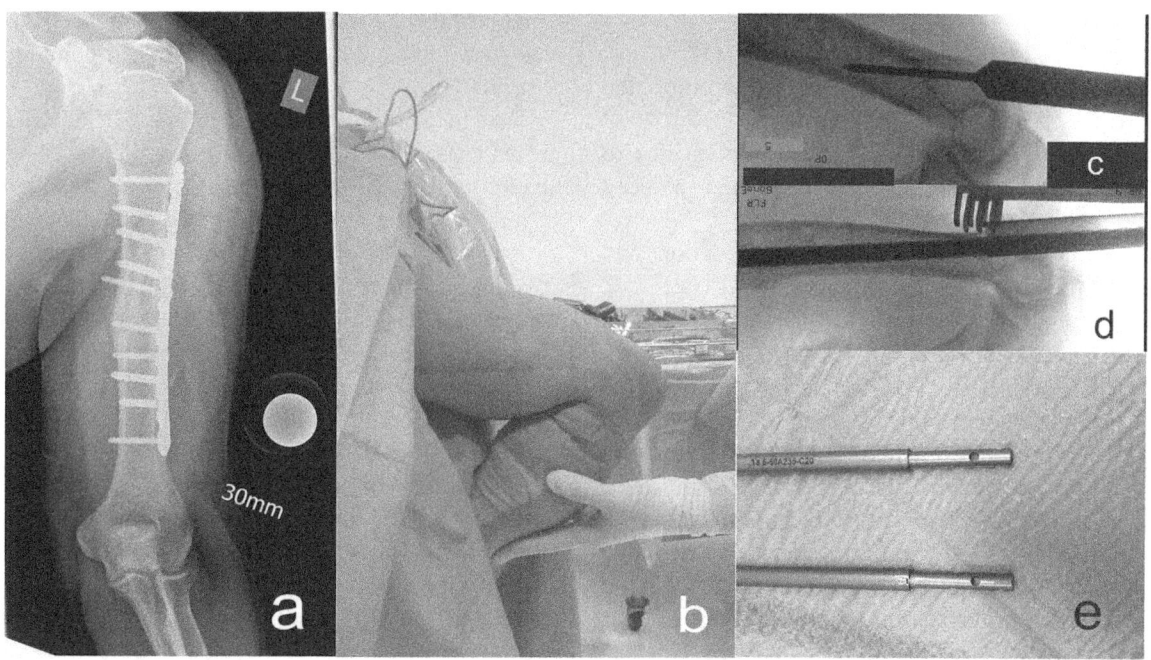

Fig. 2 a Preoperative radiograph of patient G.K. with 40 mm shortening of the left humerus after a successfully treated nonunion; **b** intraoperative supine positioning of the patient for retrograde approach; **c** and **d** steel sleeves and rigid reamers for preparing the intramedullary canal; **e** crown breakage of the first PRECICE (P 2) below, predistracted nail above (P 2.1)

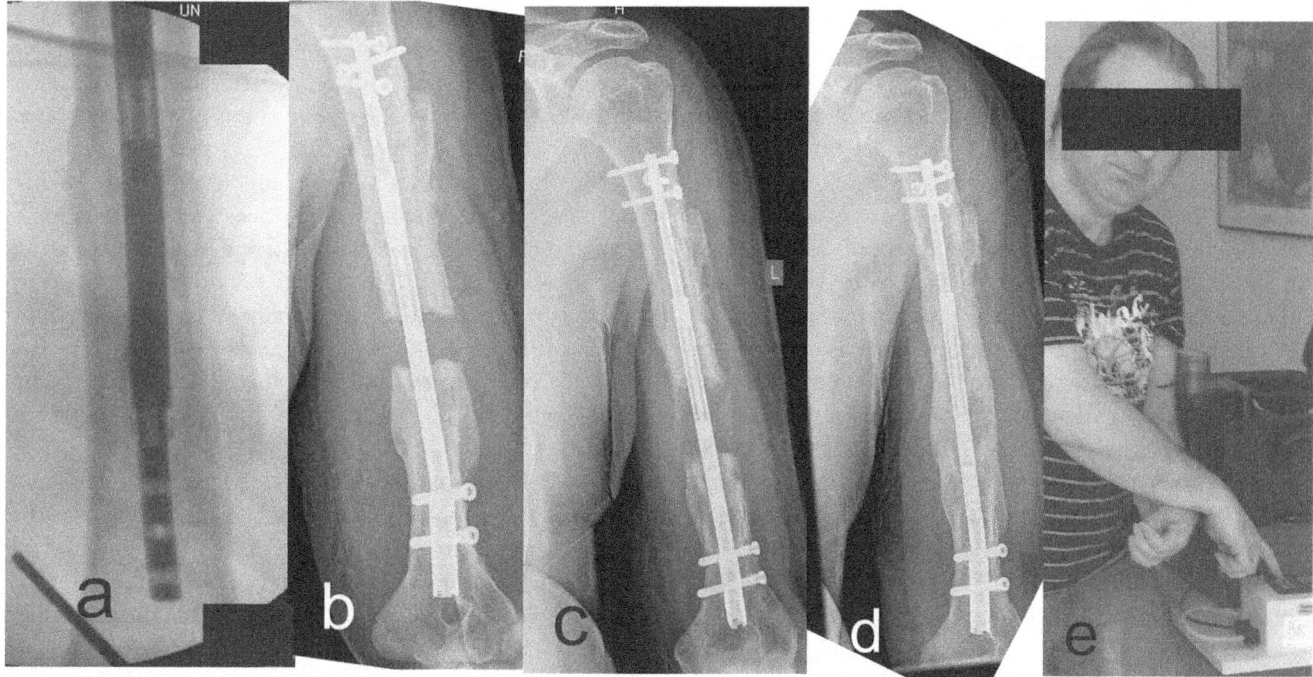

Fig. 3 a Intraoperative radiograph of crown breakage of patient G.K.; **b–d** radiographs during the lengthening progress with the new PRECICE P2.1; **e** positioning of the external remote controller for lengthening

Patient M.J. showed no change in elbow motion. Shoulder abduction decreased 20° and flexion decreased 10°.

Patient T.K. improved elbow extension 10° after Z-plastic of the biceps tendon and botox injections two times. Shoulder motion did not change. There was an intended acute external rotation at the osteotomy of 10°.

Patient G.K. showed 5° decreased elbow extension, but shoulder abduction and flexion increased 10°.

Complications

Irritation and pain caused by the cord, penetrating the rotator cuff, led to its removal in patient Y.G.

Lengthening in patient M.J. had to be stopped due to proximal migration of the humeral head and reduced shoulder function.

Reduction in elbow extension led to botox injections and a Z-plastic of the biceps tendon in patient T.K.

The first lengthening approach in patient G.K. failed after 10 mm of lengthening due to breakage of the crown (PRECICE P2) (see Fig. 2). After consolidation the implant was removed and a new osteotomy was performed 10 mm proximal to the regenerate. The nail was replaced by a 10 mm predistracted nail of the technically improved PRECICE P2.1 nail using the same locking options. At the beginning a transient radial nerve paralysis occurred, which recovered to the preoperative status. During the second lengthening approach, distraction progress declined in the radiographic controls compared to the controller. This can be related either to lack of transmission or to increase in resistance (early consolidation). We increased the distraction rate to 1.5 mm/day for 1 week. Finally, full lengthening was achieved, without facing other complications.

Further outcome parameters

All patients achieved full consolidation. In the frontal and sagittal plane, no axis deviation was introduced by lengthening. We achieved one intended, but no unintended change in humeral torsion. Although no scoring system was used to precisely quantify the effect of treatment, all patients reported they were satisfied with the outcome. Patients reported about reduced neck pain and improved function in performing daily activities such as clothing and personal hygiene; resting arms at the table; improved function in type writing on the computer and improved function in steering the bicycle. The implant removal of two FITBONE nails (patients M.J. and T.K.) and of the first used PRECICE nail (patient G.K.) was carried out without any problems. Implant removal of one FITBONE nail (patient Y.G.) and the second PRECICE nail (patient G.K.) is planned for the near future.

Discussion

Until now distraction osteogenesis for the humerus was only done by external fixation. Our report shows that lengthening of the humerus through intramedullary lengthening nails is possible. Evaluating the results we must consider the small sample size and our learning curve. Comparing with results of external lengthening, patients

age must also be taken into account as most of the existing data are on lengthening the humerus in children or adolescents [4–6, 9].

Due to an implant failure of the PRECICE nail, one patient sustained early consolidation. Crown breakage of the PRECICE nail second generation P2 was reported in several oral presentations and once in literature [10]. The overall incidence of such crown breakage is not reported. The manufacturer solved this problem in a timely manner with a new design of the nail P2.1 which was released in December 2014.

The FITBONE nail showed one minor implant-related complication with following removal of the cable that connected the nail and subcutaneous receiver. Further possible risks of the FITBONE nail are breakage and running back of the telescopic part [16, 19]. The risk is higher in the lower limb due to weight bearing, but we recommend a close radiographic follow-up during lengthening and consolidation [16]. Close aftercare for adjusting the lengthening due to reduced distraction rate was important in the second lengthening approach (PRECICE P2.1) of patient G.K. As this problem was solved by increasing the daily distraction rate for 1 week, it seemed to be related to higher resistance likely caused by early consolidation. Not only early consolidation like in this case is a possible risk during lengthening, we also must be aware of regenerate insufficiency. Here the PRECICE nail brings one main advantage. The callus can be compressed easily by changing the lengthening direction without further operation and can then be lengthened again. This so-called accordion maneuver improves callus formation in distraction osteogenesis with external fixation and in the animal model [20]. We successfully applied it several times using the PRECICE in intramedullary lengthening of the lower limb.

Reduced range of motion in the adjacent joints was a major problem in our patients during the lengthening phase.

Two patients lost shoulder function. This may be due to the antegrade approach and a violation of the rotator cuff as it is described in fracture treatment [21, 22]. In fracture treatment loss of range of motion is described in antegrade nails for the shoulder and in retrograde nails for the elbow joint [23]. Both patients with a loss of shoulder abduction had change in shoulder anatomy due to Erb–Duchenne palsy. The preexisting shoulder instability might have allowed for the proximal migration of the humeral head resulting in loss of shoulder motion. By using a retrograde approach in lengthening, the violation of the rotator cuff can be prevented and the osteotomy can be performed distally to the insertion of the M. deltoideus, so that its function can be possibly maintained. It might be that the technical more challenging retrograde approach would have prevented loss of shoulder function. But if retrograde nailing is chosen great care must be taken to prevent secondary fractures, which is a frequently mentioned complication (2–10%) in retrograde fracture nailing [23].

Elbow motion can also be reduced by the entry point in retrograde nailing and due to increased biceps tension and less motion in the joint during the lengthening process. Additional procedures like botox injections or Z-plastic of the biceps tendon can help to restore or improve the elbow motion. Reduced range of motion in the adjacent joints can compromise the final lengthening result and points out the importance of intensive physiotherapy during the lengthening process.

Compared to reports regarding external lengthening of the humerus, we had a similar consolidation index (33 vs. 27–32 days/cm) [4–6, 8]. Reports with external Ilizarov ring fixation report about reduced shoulder or elbow motion in up to 7% of the cases [4]. Lengthening with monolateral fixation improved the function of the upper limb [8]. Fixation time varied between 7 and 9 months in case series with external fixation. Refracture rate after removal of the fixation was between 10 and 16% [4–6, 8]. Superficial pin track infections are common in external fixation with a risk up to 100%, but the risk of deep infection is low [24]. By using internal lengthening we need no external apparatus and avoid pin track infections, but the risk of deep infections in internal lengthening is not yet quantified. Additionally, the urge for removal of the internal implants is less than for external fixation which might lower the risk of refracture. However, the reduction in function in the adjacent joints was more pronounced with internal lengthening, and we had two implant-related interventions.

For both nails, breakage or malfunction has been reported [10, 19]. The FITBONE has a longer clinical history of more than 20 years. It is reported to unintentional backtrack and has the disadvantage of an additional cable [16, 19]. The PRECICE nail has thinner options (min. 8.5 mm) and the additional option for shortening (accordion-manoeuver) without further surgery [10, 25]. But no information exists about failure rates of the actual available PRECICE P2.1.

Conclusions

Both implants (FITBONE and PRECICE) are possible options for intramedullary humerus lengthening and have different advantages and disadvantages. Reduced range of motion in the adjacent joints can be a problem during the lengthening. Both the entry point for the nail and the lengthening procedure can lead to reduced motion. As there are only few reports on humeral lengthening, we need more

data for further evaluation. In the hands of an experienced surgeon, familiar with intramedullary lengthening devices the described techniques might be valuable treatment options in deformity correction of the upper limb.

Funding No financial support or grants were received for this study.

Informed consent Informed consent was obtained from all individual participants included in the study.

References

1. Ilizarov GA (1990) Clinical application of the tension–stress effect for limb lengthening. Clin Orthop Relat Res 250:8–26
2. Tetsworth K, Krome J, Paley D (1991) Lengthening and deformity correction of the upper extremity by the Ilizarov technique. Orthop Clin North Am 22:689–713
3. Dick HM, Tietjen R (1978) Humeral lengthening for septic neonatal growth arrest. Case report. J Bone Jt Surg Am 60:1138–1139
4. Cattaneo R, Villa A, Catagni MA, Bell D (1990) Lengthening of the humerus using the Ilizarov technique. Description of the method and report of 43 cases. Clin Orthop Relat Res 250:117–124
5. Hosny GA (2005) Unilateral humeral lengthening in children and adolescents. J Pediatr Orthop Part B 14:439–443
6. Kashiwagi N, Suzuki S, Seto Y, Futami T (2001) Bilateral humeral lengthening in achondroplasia. Clin Orthop Relat Res 391:251–257
7. McCarthy JJ, Ranade A, Davidson RS (2008) Pediatric deformity correction using a multiaxial correction fixator. Clin Orthop Relat Res 466:3011–3017
8. Pawar AY, McCoy TH, Fragomen AT, Rozbruch SR (2013) Does humeral lengthening with a monolateral frame improve function? Clin Orthop Relat Res 471:277–283
9. Balci HI, Kocaoglu M, Sen C, Eralp L, Batibay SG, Bilsel K (2015) Bilateral humeral lengthening in achondroplasia with unilateral external fixators: is it safe and does it improve daily life? Bone Jt J 97-B:1577–1581
10. Paley D (2015) PRECICE intramedullary limb lengthening system. Expert Rev Med Devices 12:231–249
11. Betz A, Baumgart R, Schweiberer L (1990) First fully implantable intramedullary system for callus distraction–intramedullary nail with programmable drive for leg lengthening and segment displacement. Principles and initial clinical results. Chir Z Für Alle Geb Oper Med 61:605–609
12. Cole JD, Justin D, Kasparis T, DeVlught D, Knobloch C (2001) The intramedullary skeletal kinetic distractor (ISKD): first clinical results of a new intramedullary nail for lengthening of the femur and tibia. Injury 32(Suppl 4):SD129–SD139
13. Hankemeier S, Pape H-C, Gosling T, Hufner T, Richter M, Krettek C (2004) Improved comfort in lower limb lengthening with the intramedullary skeletal kinetic distractor. Principles and preliminary clinical experiences. Arch Orthop Trauma Surg 124:129–133
14. Guichet J-M, Deromedis B, Donnan LT, Peretti G, Lascombes P, Bado F (2003) Gradual femoral lengthening with the Albizzia intramedullary nail. J Bone Jt Surg Am 85-A:838–848
15. Kenawey M, Krettek C, Liodakis E, Wiebking U, Hankemeier S (2011) Leg lengthening using intramedullary skeletal kinetic distractor: results of 57 consecutive applications. Injury 42:150–155
16. Thaller PH, Zoffl F, Delhey P (2010) Comparison between fully implantable monitorized and mechanical distraction nails—a

matched-pairs analysis. In 3rd world congress on external fixation and 6th congress of the ASAMI international presented at: podium session 37: bone reconstruction 6, Barcelona

17. Thaller PH, Fürmetz J, Wolf F, Eilers T, Mutschler W (2014) Limb lengthening with fully implantable magnetically actuated mechanical nails (PHENIX(®))-preliminary results. Injury 45(Suppl 1):S60–S65

18. Rozbruch S, Hamdy R. Limb lengthening and reconstruction surgery case Atlas [internet]. http://www.springer.com/cn/book/9783319036380

19. Krieg AH, Lenze U, Speth BM, Hasler CC (2011) Intramedullary leg lengthening with a motorized nail. Acta Orthop 82:344–350

20. Makhdom AM, Cartaleanu AS, Rendon JS, Villemure I, Hamdy RC (2015) The accordion maneuver: a noninvasive strategy for absent or delayed callus formation in cases of limb lengthening. Adv Orthop 2015:912790

21. Euler SA, Hengg C, Kolp D, Wambacher M, Kralinger F (2014) Lack of fifth anchoring point and violation of the insertion of the rotator cuff during antegrade humeral nailing pitfalls in straight antegrade humeral nailing. Bone Jt J 96-B:249–253

22. Scheerlinck T, Handelberg F (2002) Functional outcome after intramedullary nailing of humeral shaft fractures: comparison between retrograde Marchetti-Vicenzi and unreamed AO antegrade nailing. J Trauma 52:60–71

23. Rommens PM, Kuechle R, Bord T, Lewens T, Engelmann R, Blum J (2008) Humeral nailing revisited. Injury 39:1319–1328. doi:10.1016/j.injury.2008.01.014

24. Jauregui JJ, Bor N, Thakral R, Standard SC, Paley D, Herzenberg JE (2015) Life- and limb-threatening infections following the use of an external fixator. Bone Jt J 97-B:1296–1300

25. Kirane YM, Fragomen AT, Rozbruch SR (2014) Precision of the PRECICE internal bone lengthening nail. Clin Orthop Relat Res 472:3869–3878

13

Shaped graft for aneurysmal bone cyst of upper limb bones

Mohamed F. Mostafa[1] · Yasser Y. Abed[1] · Sallam I. Fawzy[1]

Abstract The optimal treatment of aneurysmal bone cyst remains challenging. The aim of this prospective study was to evaluate the results of using bone grafts shaped to the defects caused by aneurysmal bone cysts of upper limb bones. Fifteen patients (12 males and 3 females) with an average age of 12 years (range 6–16 years) were treated for aneurysmal bone cysts of upper limb bones by intralesional resection, argon beam coagulation and shaped bone graft. The grafts were harvested from 14 patients (11 fibulas and 3 iliac bones) and from the mother of one patient (proximal fibula). Osteosynthesis was required to stabilize the graft in four cases. The modified Enneking's scoring system was used for functional evaluation. One patient developed partial recurrence at 6 months and required reoperation. Superficial wound infection was encountered in one patient. Shortening of the humeral segment was seen in two patients (1 and 1.5 cm) but without angular deformity. After a mean follow-up of 45 months (range 24–68 months), the mean functional score was 97.3%. This technique proved to be reliable in obtaining a well reconstructed and growing bone with no or minimal deformity and good function.

Keywords Aneurysmal · Bone cyst · Shaped graft

✉ Mohamed F. Mostafa
thabetortho20032003@yahoo.com

[1] Orthopedic Oncology Unit, Department of Orthopedic Surgery, Mansoura University Hospital, 36 Al-Gomhoria Street, P.O. Box 35516, Mansoura, Egypt

Introduction

Aneurysmal bone cyst (ABC) is an uncommon benign tumor-like lesion of unknown origin that may present a diagnostic and therapeutic dilemma [1]. There is controversy as to whether it is a distinct radiological and pathological entity or a pathophysiological change superimposed on a pre-existing lesion [2]. The original suggestion by Lichtenstein [3] favoring a local circulatory disturbance leading to the blow-out expansion of the bone is still popular. This suggestion is further emphasized by Mirra [4] who noted that the lesion is probably a periosteal to intraosseous arteriovenous malformation. The identification of a consistent t (16; 17) chromosomal translocation in primary cases suggests a de novo tumor [5].

Lack of understanding about its origin and growth makes treatment empirical. The most common treatment has been intralesional excision and bone grafting with a substantial rate of recurrence ranging from 10 to 44% [6–8]. Abrasions of all surfaces using a high-speed burr and local adjuvant such as phenol, liquid nitrogen or polymethylmethacrylate (PMMA) have been tried to lower the rate of recurrence. However, the use of these adjuvants is much controversial because firm evidence that they are effective is lacking and their use entails considerable risk. Argon beam coagulation has been used as an adjuvant avoiding complications of other adjuvants [9–11].

The commonly used filling materials such as autogenous cancellous or corticocancellous bone graft, allogenic freeze-dried cancellous and cortical bone graft, PMMA and bone substitutes usually take the shape of the lesion resulting in a deformed bone with the possible limitation of function especially in the upper limb [12–14]. The current prospective study was conducted to evaluate the results of using bone grafts shaped to the original bone after extended curettage and argon beam coagulation of ABC in upper limb bones.

Materials and methods

Between May 2005 and September 2011, 15 patients with ABCs of the upper limb bones were selected and treated at Orthopaedic Oncology Unit, Mansoura University Hospital, Egypt. For inclusion in the study which was approved by the institutional ethical research committee, all patients were briefed about the planned procedure and its possible complications and had to declare an informed consent to participate. Patients with acute pathological fracture through the cyst or secondary aneurysmal bone cyst were excluded from the study. Only patients with primary ABC of upper limb bones were included. There were 12 males and three females with an average age of 12 years (range

6–16 years) at time of surgery (Table 1). The diagnosis had been made on radiological and histological examination. Plain radiographs were performed for all cases to reveal the expanded multilocular lytic lesions. Computed tomography (CT) scan was done in 10 cases to evaluate the lesion for subtle cortical destruction or fracture. Additionally, magnetic resonance imaging (MRI) was performed in eight cases to identify the characteristic double density fluid levels and septations as well as the extension to the epiphysis. Tissue for histological examination was obtained by trephine biopsy. Two patients with recurrent lesions were biopsied preoperatively to confirm diagnosis. The presence of blood-filled cystic spaces separated by fibrous septa (membranes) of mononuclear stromal cells containing scattered multinucleated giant cells and less commonly reactive bone was suggestive of diagnosis.

The lesion was located in proximal humerus in eight patients, distal humerus in three, shaft humerus in two and

Table 1 Details and results in 15 patients with aneurysmal bone cysts of upper limb bones

Case no.	Age	Gender	Location	Stage	Size (cm^3)	Follow-up (month)	Time to consolidation (week)	Score[a]	Complications
1	6	Female	distal Radius	Stage 3	48	68	16	97	No complication
2	12	Male	Distal humerus	Stage 3	60	60	20	100	No complication
3	15	Male	Distal humerus	Stage 2	30	55	16	100	No complication
4	16	Female	Distal humerus	Stage 3	60	52	18	100	No complication
5	8	Male	Proximal humerus	Stage 3	66	50	18	97	Partial recurrence
6	10	Male	Proximal humerus	Stage 2	60	54	12	97	Superficial infection
7	11	Male	Proximal humerus	Stage 2	40	45	16	100	No complication
8	16	Male	Proximal humerus	Stage 3	150	50	22	90	Shortening of humerus
9	14	Male	Shaft humerus	Stage 2	72	41	20	100	No complication
10	7	Male	Distal radius	Stage 2	30	40	12	97	No complication
11	11	Male	Shaft humerus	Stage 2	99	39	14	100	No complication
12	13	Male	Proximal humerus	Stage 3	105	35	20	97	No complication
13	14	Male	Proximal humerus	Stage 2	60	29	16	97	No complication
14	15	Female	Proximal humerus	Stage 3	240	25	22	87	Shortening of humerus
15	10	Male	Proximal humerus	Stage 2	52	24	14	100	No complication

[a] Enneking scoring system (rating percentage of normal) [16]

distal radius in two. The approximate volume of the cyst was calculated using plain radiograph and more accurately CT scan by multiplying the maximum length and breadth in anteroposterior projection and the depth in lateral projection. Staging was accomplished using the criteria defined by Enneking [15]. Operative treatment consisted of a wide window, extended curettage, argon beam coagulation and graft insertion. Curved small curettes were helpful to reach small pockets and slits especially near the diaphyseal side. Care was taken while curetting the lesion close to the physis. A power burr was used to extend the margin of excision and to open the medulla in some cases but was avoided at the broached areas of physis. Argon beam coagulator (Birtcher 6000 Electrosurgical Generator + Argon Beam Coagulator, Irvine California, USA) was used like a paint brush throughout the entire inner wall and at a minimum near the physis. This produced a thin layer of eschar due to deposition of black carbonized debris (Fig. 1). Simultaneous irrigation and suction was helpful to clear debris and eschar, prevents contamination and allows for improved visualization. The sequence of curettage,

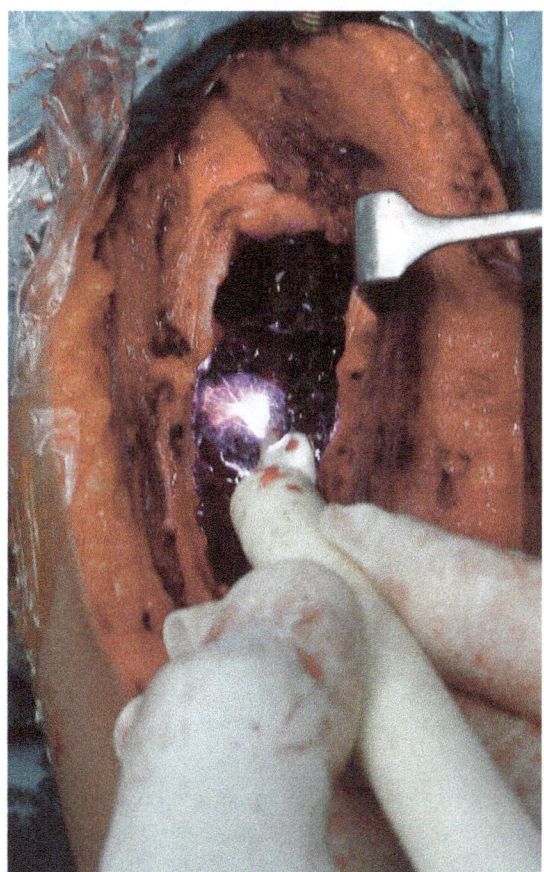

Fig. 1 An intraoperative photograph showing the argon beam coagulator wand used as a paint brush with eschar formation throughout the entire inner wall

argon beam coagulation and lavage was repeated three to four times before application of the graft.

After careful measuring the defect preoperatively and intra-operatively, the graft was harvested from the patient (proximal fibula = 9, shaft fibula = 2, iliac bone = 3) and from the patient's mother (proximal fibula = 1). Proximal fibular grafts taken from the patients provided a smooth cancellous surface for the exposed areas of proximal humeral physis (Fig. 2). The proximal fibular graft harvested from the mother of a 6-year-old girl (case 1) was cleaned from soft tissue, washed thoroughly with saline and reshaped before placement in the defect caused by ABC of the distal third radius. In this case, the proximal smooth cancellous surface was applied against the growth plate and the distal cortical part was internally fixed to the radius with plate and screws (Fig. 3). The fibular shaft graft was inserted retrograde into the proximal humerus then impacted back into the distal part in cases with diaphyseal lesion (Fig. 4). One of the two patients with diaphyseal ABCs developed intraoperative humeral shaft fracture during graft insertion and required internal fixation with plate and screws. A composite of synthetic bone substitute (ceraform; calcium phosphate hydroxyapatite 65% and tricalcium phosphate 35%, Teknimed S.A. France) and bone marrow aspirate was used to fill the remaining gaps around the graft. The distal humeral lesions were eccentric involving medial condyle in two patients and lateral condyle in one patient. These patients were older enough to obtain autogenous bone graft from their iliac bone. The graft was shaped and placed with the thick portion of the iliac crest at the periphery representing the medial or lateral column and the thin portion centrally toward the thin area of distal humerus where olecranon and coronoid fossae meet (Fig. 5). Smooth Kirschner wires were used to stabilize the graft in two patients. The expanded outer shell was collapsed manually and gently over the graft.

Patients with humeral lesions were instructed to keep the limb in arm sling till suture removal then started early passive range of motion (ROM) of shoulder, elbow and wrist. Isometric strengthening exercises and active ROM were postponed till complete healing of the lesion. For cases with distal radial lesions, a below elbow plaster cast was applied for 5–6 weeks. All patients were allowed to start finger movement early after surgery guided by pain. The mean duration of follow-up was 45 months (range 24–68 months). Patients were evaluated radiologically by plain radiographs every 4–6 weeks for progression of healing, local recurrence and deformity resulting from partial fusion of the epiphysis. After radiographic healing, patients were assessed clinically every 3 months for the first year and every 6 months during the 2nd year then yearly thereafter. Clinical assessment was done for pain, deformity, limitation of joint movement and complications

Fig. 2 a–c Diagrams showing
the selected part of the proximal
fibula placed after extended
curettage of a proximal humeral
lesion, the expanded outer
cortex was gently collapsed and
composite bone substitute was
used to fill the gaps. **d** The
proximal fibular graft provides a
smooth cancellous surface.
e After placement of the graft
with the cancellous surface
opposite the broached area of
the physis

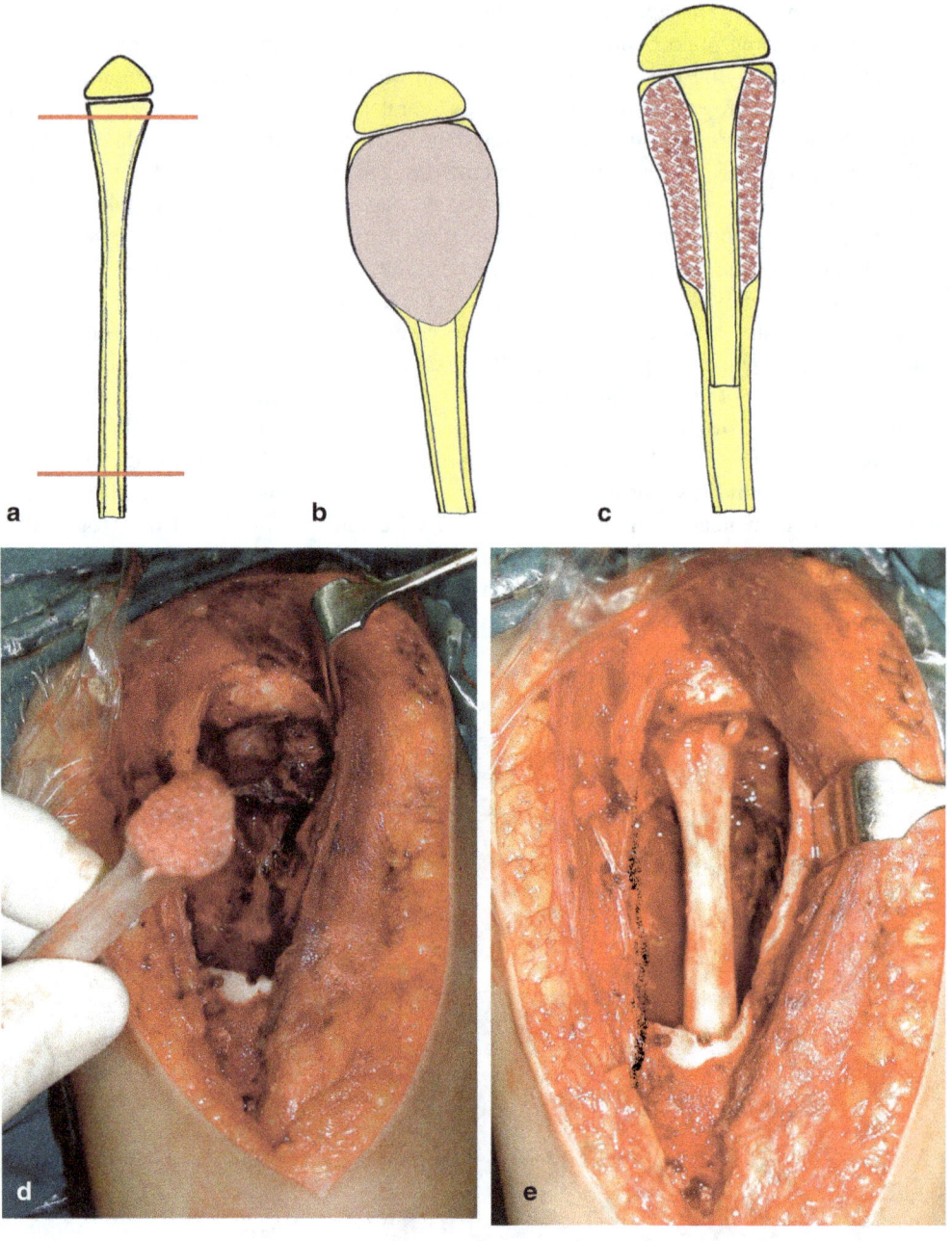

at the donor site. The modified Enneking scoring system [16] was used for functional evaluation at the time of final follow-up.

Results

The main presenting symptoms were pain and discomfort associated with swelling in 11 patients. The remaining four patients had repeated pathological fractures of a stage 3 proximal humeral lesions. One of them had significant varus deformity with limitation of abduction and was corrected at the time of surgery. There were eight lesions stage 2 and seven stage 3 with a mean size of 78 cm^3 (range 30–240 cm^3).

All lesions healed uneventfully after a mean time of 17 weeks (range 12–22 weeks). Only one patient (case 5) developed partial recurrence at 6 months that required reoperation. The collapsed outer shell disappeared with the progress of healing. The rapid healing of the lesion was closely related to the young age of patients, the small size and the less aggressive (stage 2) lesions. Most of patients (83.3%) with open physis and juxta-physeal lesions had continued growth in length and width as evidenced by absence of deformity or shortening and maintained open physis. The patient who received fibular graft from her

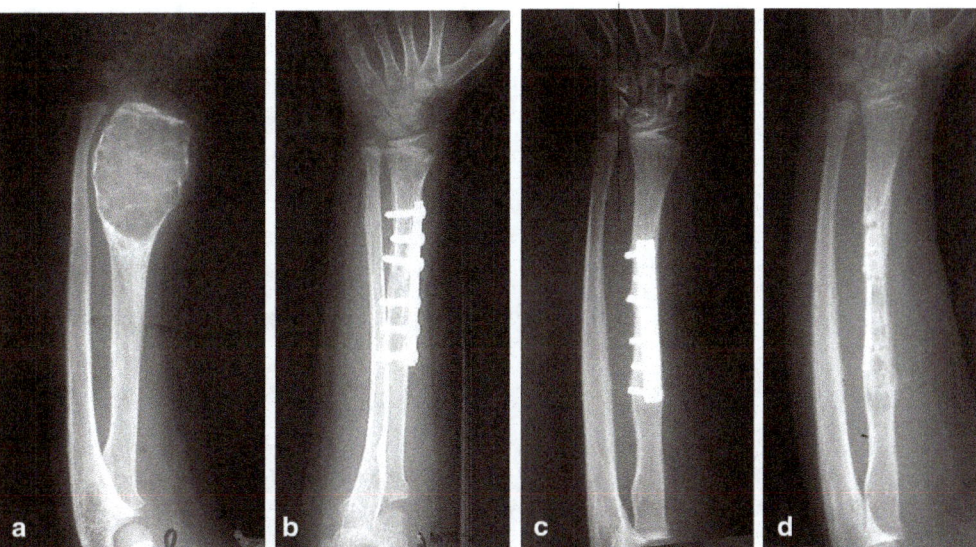

Fig. 3 a Anteroposterior radiograph of a 6-year-old girl with ABC destructing the distal one-third of left radius (Case 1). **b** Proximal fibular graft was harvested from her mother, shaped and stabilized with plate and screws. **c** Follow-up radiograph showing continued growth of the graft and maintained open physis. **d** 5 years after surgery with continuing growth and no deformity

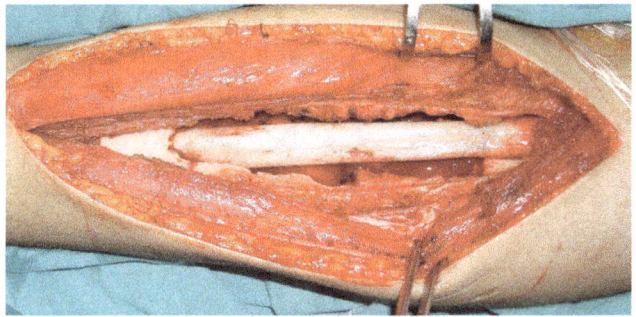

Fig. 4 Photograph showing fibular shaft graft placed intramedullary in humeral diaphyseal lesion

mother showed complete incorporation and remodeling of the graft with continued growth of the radius and no deformity. Only two patients (16.7%) developed shortening of the humeral segment (1 and 1.5 cm) due to premature fusion of the proximal humeral epiphysis but without angular deformity. These two patients had large size lesions (mean 195 cm^3) of the proximal humerus with marked broaching of the physis.

There were no cases of deep infection, nerve deficit or pathological fracture. Superficial infection of the operative wound was seen in one patient and was controlled with repeated dressing and systemic antibiotics. The mean functional score (rating percentage of normal) at treatment completion was 97.3% (range 87–100%). There were no complications related to the donor site. Subperiosteal harvesting of the fibular graft allowed regeneration of a new fibula. Postoperative pain, abductor dysfunction and limping after harvesting iliac bone graft could be avoided by proper soft tissue repair.

Discussion

ABC is one of the aggressive benign bone tumors. Despite being described for more than 60 years back, still there is controversy about its nature, pathophysiology and optimal treatment. Appropriate treatment can be made only after the exclusion of an underlying lesion particularly giant cell tumor [17]. The use of physical adjuvants such as phenol, liquid nitrogen and polymethylmethacrylate (PMMA) has been advocated to extend the surgical margin. These adjuvants produce chemical or thermal necrosis and microvascular damage to the walls of the physically excised cyst aiming to decrease the chance of recurrence. However, phenol and liquid nitrogen could penetrate tissues making the neurovascular structures at high risk. Also, liquid nitrogen can make the bone more brittle and increase the risk of fracture [6].

Lower recurrence rates can also be achieved by marginal or wide resection, but this entails loss of the supporting function of bone and the need for reconstructive surgery [18, 19]. Furthermore, others do not believe it is necessary to perform wide excision to eradicate the disease [20, 21]. In the current study, the cyst walls were not excised, instead allowed to collapse over the implanted graft to provide the new periosteum for growth in width. Local recurrence was seen only in one patient (7%) and was partial at the periphery of a large stage 3 proximal humeral lesion. In agreement with Gitelis and McDonald [22], local recurrence depends mainly on the adequacy of the tumor removal rather than the type of adjuvant used. This is achieved by making a large window to expose the whole cavity, using different sizes curettes, good visualization of

Fig. 5 a–c Diagrams of an
eccentric distal humeral ABC,
the planned area of iliac bone
graft and placement of the graft
with the thick portion (*x–*
y) laterally and the thin apex
(*z*) centrally toward the area
where coronoid and olecranon
fossae met. **d** An intraoperative
photograph showing the iliac
bone graft shaped to the defect
in the medial humeral condyle
(Case 4). **e** The graft in place

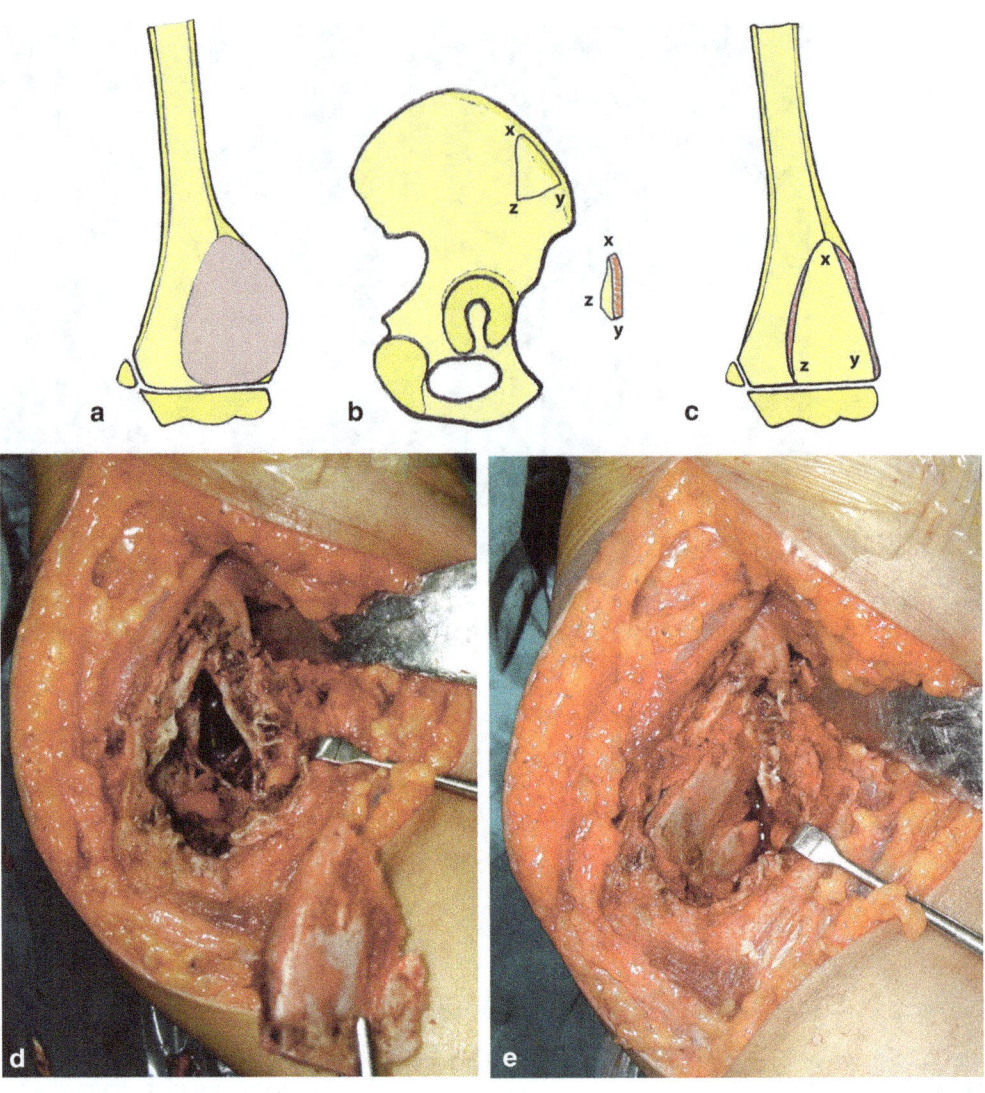

the inner walls with the help of a small light source fixed to
the suction nozzle and the use of power burr. The use of a
high-speed burr has been suggested to reduce the rate of
recurrence [23]. However, Lin et al. [21] detected no difference in recurrence rate with or without the use of high-
speed burr. On the other hand, high-speed burr could not be
used at the open physis, as this could destroy the growing
cells and cause cessation of growth. It is believed that
meticulous curettage with small curettes is preferred for the
physeal borders.

Argon beam coagulator is a monopolar coagulator
which utilizes a beam of argon gas to deliver a radiofre-
quency electric current to the tissues. The jet of gas blows
blood and debris away and allows the inner surface of the
cavity to be covered with a thin layer of eschar causing
coagulation of blood in the lumen of small vessels and
capillaries. The electrical current flows through the gas in
arcs that are distributed uniformly across the tissue in depth
and area, with tissue effects depending on the power setting

and duration of application. The temperature of the tissue
reaches a maximum of 205 °C when the spray passes over
the tissues. The residual tumor cells in the cavity are
destroyed by this thermal effect. Compared with other
adjuvant treatments, the limited beam length and area and
the directional nature of the beam make this technique
simple to use, precise and safe if the nearby neurovascular
bundles are protected [10]. Cummings et al. [9] in a preliminary study found that argon beam coagulation after
curettage provided improved local control of ABCs compared with curettage without adjuvant or with phenol and
not associated with an increase in the operative complications. In the current study, argon beam coagulation was
used as an adjuvant in all cases and there were no difficulties with its use or postoperative complications related
to it.

It is noted that the final shape of the new bone will
correspond to the one developed by the cyst at the time of
surgery. Stuffing the expanded lesion with the commonly

Table 2 Reported studies using different adjuvant agents compared with the current study

Study	Number of patients	Treatment	Adjuvant	Number of recurrence (%)	Mean functional score[a]	Complications
Ozaki et al. [12]	14	Curettage	PMMA in 5	2 (14%)	NS[b]	1 fracture 3 joint stiffness
Dormans et al. [27]	45	Curettage	Cauterization Phenol Hydrogen peroxide	8 (18%)	NS	–
Basarir et al. [28]	56	Curettage Resection	Cauterization Embolization	9 (16%)	NS	4 deformities 2 limb inequalities 1 infection
Peeters et al. [29]	80	Curettage Bone graft in 73	Liquid nitrogen	4 (5%)	97.3%	1 postoperative fracture 1 wound infection 3 transient nerve palsy
Cumming et al. [9]	29	Curettage Resection	Argon beam coagulation in 17	4 (14%)	NS	1 physeal arrest
Current study	15	Curettage Bone graft	Argon beam coagulation	1 (7%)	97%	1 superficial wound infection 2 shortening of humeral segment

[a] Modified Enneking scoring system [16]

[b] NS not stated

used filling materials such as autogenous cancellous or corticocancellous bone grafts, allogenic cancellous or cortical bone graft or bone substitutes including PMMA usually result in a bulky and deformed bone with possible premature fusion of the nearby epiphysis and shortening [24]. In the present cases, bone graft was intra-operatively shaped with the smooth cancellous surface placed opposite the exposed area of the physis allowing a regular enchondral ossification. This was evidenced by the maintained open physis, continued growth in length and absence of deformity. Furthermore, the expanded outer cortex was collapsed gently providing the graft its new periosteum for increase in width.

Autogenous bone graft remains the gold standard as a filler for cavity defects. It demonstrates a high degree of osteoinduction from surface osteoblasts in the host bone, circulating osteoprogenitor cells and donor cells that survive transplantation. In addition fresh transplanted autogenous bone exhibits no immune response and undergoes rapid revascularization. However, autogenous bone graft is sometimes not available in sufficient quantity and its harvest has the potential complications of pain, blood loss, increased operative time, infection and donor site instability [25]. No perioperative or postoperative complications were encountered with harvesting bone graft in the current study. The morbidity could be avoided or minimized if the graft harvesting technique is properly planned and performed. In our study, one young girl received fibular strut

graft from her mother and showed complete healing without any evidence of immunological reaction or rejection. The graft was transplanted fresh without processing other than removal of soft tissues and washing with saline. In agreement with Weber et al. [26], syngenesioplastic graft obtained from immediate relatives of the patient could be a reasonable alternative to autogenous bone graft for small children. The main weakness of this study was the limited sample size. Despite this recurrence rate, complications and functional results at the final follow-up were comparable to that of other studies using different methods of treatment and adjuvants (Table 2).

ABC remains an enigma not only regarding origin but also diagnosis and optimal treatment. The use of a shaped strut bone graft after meticulous curettage and argon beam coagulation is a reliable technique to obtain a well reconstructed and growing bone with minimal or no deformity and good function for ABCs of the upper limb bones. It is not necessary to perform wide excision to eradicate the disease. Great care should be exercised while removing the tumor near the physeal cartilage to avoid injury to the growing cells and premature epiphyseal fusion. Considering the limited quantity and the morbidities of harvesting autogenous bone graft, the author is looking forward for a shaped bone substitute that can be mixed with bone marrow as a source of osteogenic cells to aid in healing of such lesions.

Informed consent Informed consent was obtained from individual participants included in the study.

References

1. Schreuder HW, Veth RP, Pruszczynski M, Lemmens JA, Koops H, Molenaor WM (1997) Aneurysmal bone cysts treated by curettage, cryotherapy and bone grafting. J Bone Joint Surg Br 79:20–25
2. Kransdorf MJ, Sweet DE (1995) Aneurysmal bone cyst: concept, controversy, clinical presentation and imaging. AJR Am J Roentgenol 164:573–580
3. Lichtenstein L (1957) Aneurysmal bone cyst: observation on fifty cases. J Bone Joint Surg Am 39:873–882
4. Mirra JM (1989) Aneurysmal bone cyst. In: Mirra JM, Picci P, Gold RH (eds) Bone tumors: clinical, radiologic and pathologic correlations, 2nd edn. Lea and Febiger, Philadelphia, pp 1267–1311
5. Oliveira AM, Perez-Atayde AR, Inwards CY, Medeiros F, Derr V, His BL, Gebhardt MC, Rosenberg AE, Fletcher JA (2004) USP6 and CDH11 oncogenes identify the neoplastic cell in primary aneurysmal bone cysts. Am J Pathol 165:1773–1780
6. Marcove RC, Sheth DS, Takemoto S, Healey JH (1995) The treatment of aneurysmal bone cyst. Clin Orthop Relat Res 311:157–163
7. Mankin HJ, Hornicek FJ, Ortiz-Cruz E, Villafuerte J, Gebhardt MC (2005) Aneurysmal bone cyst: a review of 150 patients. J Clin Oncol 23:6756–6762
8. Cottolorda J, Bourelle S (2007) Modern concepts of primary aneurysmal bone cyst. Arch Orthop Trauma Surg 127:105–114
9. Cummings JE, Smith RA, Heck RK Jr (2010) Argon beam coagulation as adjuvant treatment after curettage of aneurysmal bone cysts. Clin Orthop Relat Res 468:231–237
10. Lewis VO, Wei A, Mendoza T, Primus F, Peabody T, Simon MA (2007) Argon beam coagulation as an adjuvant for local control of giant cell tumor. Clin Orthop Relat Res 454:192–197
11. Takeda N, Kobayashi T, Tandai S, Matsuno T, Shirado O, Watanabe T, Minami A (2009) Treatment of giant cell tumors in the sacrum and spine with curettage and argon beam coagulator. J Orthop Sci 14:210–214
12. Ozaki T, Hillmann A, Lindner N, Winkelmann W (1996) Aneurysmal bone cysts in children. J Cancer Res Clin Oncol 122:767–769
13. Malawer MM, Dunham W (1991) Cryosurgery and acrylic cementation as surgical adjuvants in the treatment of aggressive (benign) bone tumors: analysis of 25 patients below the age of 21. Clin Orthop 262:42–57
14. Schindler OS, Cannon SR, Briggs TWR, Blunn GW (2008) Composite ceramic bone graft substitute in the treatment of locally aggressive benign bone tumors. J Orthop Surg 16(1):66–74
15. Enneking WF (1986) A system of staging musculoskeletal neoplasms. Clin Orthop Relat Res 204:9–24
16. Enneking WF, Dunham W, Gebhardt MC, Malawer M, Pritchard DJ (1993) A system for the functional evaluation of reconstructive procedures after surgical treatment of tumors of the musculoskeletal system. Clin Orthop Relat Res 286:241–246
17. Martinez V, Sissons HA (1988) Aneurysmal bone cyst: a review of 123 cases including primary lesions and those secondary to other bone pathology. Cancer 61:2229–2304
18. Campanacci M, Capanna R, Picci P (1986) Unicameral and aneurysmal bone cysts. Clin Orthop 204:25–36
19. Cole WG (1986) Treatment of aneurysmal bone cysts in childhood. J Pediatr Orthop 6:326–329
20. Cottalorda J, Kohler R, Chotel F, de Gauzy JS, Lefort G, Louahera D, Bourelle S, Dimeglio A (2005) Recurrence of aneurysmal bone cysts in young children: a multicenter study. J Pediatr Orthop B 14:212–218
21. Lin PP, BrownC Raymond AK, Deavers MT, Yasko AW (2008) Aneurysmal bone cysts recur at juxtaphyseal locations in skeletally immature patients. Clin Orthop Relat Res 466:722–728
22. Gitelis S, Mc Donald DJ (1998) Curettage. In: Simon MA, Springfield D (eds) Surgery for bone and soft tissue tumors. Lippincott-raven, East Washington Square, pp 133–157
23. Gibbs CP Jr, Hefele MC, Peabody TD, Montag AG, Aithal V, Simon MA (1999) Aneurysmal bone cyst of the extremities: factors related to local recurrence after curettage with a high-speed burr. J Bone Joint Surg Am 81:1671–1678
24. Delloye C, De Nayer P, Molghem J, Noel H (1996) Induced healing of aneurysmal bone cysts by demineralized bone particles. A report of two cases. Arch Orthop Trauma Surg 116:141–145
25. Perry CR (1999) Bone repair techniques, bone graft and bone graft substitutes. Clin Orthop 360:71–86
26. Weber U, Pteifer G, Mahn I, Schulz G (1977) Immunological aspects of syngenesioplastic bone transplantation in treatment of infantile bone tumors. Arch Orthop Unfallchir 90(2):213–231
27. Dormans JP, Hanna BG, Johnston DR, Khurana JS (1986) Surgical treatment and recurrence rate of aneurysmal bone cysts in children. Clin Orthop Relat Res 204:9–24
28. Basarir K, Piskin A, Guclu B, Yildiz Y, Saglik Y (2007) Aneurysmal bone cyst recurrence in children: a review of 56 patients. J Pediatr Orthop 27:938–943
29. Peeters SP, Van der Geest IC, de Rooy JW, Veth RP, Schreuder HW (2009) Aneurysmal bone cyst: the role of cryosurgery as local adjuvant treatment. J Surg Oncol 100(8):719–724

14

Midshaft clavicle fractures treatment: threaded Kirschner wire versus conservative approach

Valentino Coppa[1] · Luca Dei Giudici[1] · Stefano Cecconi[2] · Mario Marinelli[2] ·
Antonio Gigante[1]

Abstract Clavicle fractures are common, accounting for 2.6 to 10% of all fractures. Treatment of these fractures is usually non-surgical. Recent evidence, however, reveals that the final result of non-surgically midshaft clavicular fractures, particularly those with quite large displacements or shortening, is not like that which was previously thought. This study evaluated retrospectively all patients presented with a clavicle fracture at Emergency Department of our Institution, between January 2006 and December 2011. Fractures were classified according to Allman's radiographic classification system, modified by Nordqvist and Petersson. Patients were distinguished into two groups: one that underwent conservative treatment with a "figure-of-8" orthosis and one that underwent surgery with reduction in fracture and fixation with intramedullary threaded Kirschner wire. Pin removal was performed after 4 weeks of rest in Gilchrist bandage, after clinical and radiographic evaluation demonstrating the bone healing. The QuickDASH score and the Constant Murley Shoulder Score were used to evaluate the clinical outcomes. The radiographic outcome was evaluated at 1 and 6 months of follow-up. Database review provided a final cohort of 58 patients, with similar demographic features. There was no significant difference in qDASH and CS between the two groups. The results of qDASH and CS evaluated in function of the radiographic outcome show a statistically significant correlation between the worst qDASH and CS results and the grade of malunion in both groups. In particular, we have found unsatisfactory results when final shortening of the clavicle was 20 mm or more. On radiographic evaluation, surgical treatment demonstrated a greater efficacy in reducing initial shortening of the fractured bone; this is in opposition to conservative treatment that results very often in malunion, shortening, anatomic alterations and loss of functionality. The use of intramedullary threaded Kirschner wire for fixation of midshaft clavicle fractures is a safe procedure and is recommended in case of shortening greater than 2 cm in high-function-demand patients.

Keywords Clavicle fracture · Midshaft · Conservative treatment · Clavicle pinning · Mini invasive

Introduction

Clavicle fractures are common lesions, ranging from 2.6 to 10% of all fractures and up to 44.1% of the fractures involving the upper girdle [1]. Males are generally more affected, with sport injuries representing the most described traumatic pattern in young patients, while falling on the ground is the most common in adults. A direct hit on the shoulder is the most common cause of midshaft clavicle fractures [2].

Traditionally, midshaft clavicular fractures have been managed non-operatively, even when substantially displaced [3, 4], with good to excellent results [5, 6]. Recent evidence, however, reveals that the final result of non-surgically midshaft clavicular fractures, particularly those with quite large displacements or shortening, is not like

✉ Valentino Coppa
  coppa.valentino@gmail.com

[1] Clinical Orthopaedics, Department of Clinical and Molecular Science, School of Medicine, Università Politecnica delle Marche, Via Tronto, 10/A, 60126 Ancona, Italy

[2] Clinic of Adult and Paediatric Orthopaedic, Azienda Ospedaliero-Universitaria, Ospedali Riuniti di Ancona, Ancona, Italy

that which was previously thought, demonstrating higher rates of delayed union, non-union, shoulder weakness and residual pain [7, 8]. Several recent articles have characterized the symptoms reported with clavicular malunion, which is associated with substantial degrees of skeletal deformity, especially shortening of ≥ 2 cm [9].

Although many methods have been described for closed reduction in displaced clavicular shaft fractures, none has been consistently reliable in achieving and maintaining reduction. Thus, displaced midshaft fractures of the clavicle typically heal in approximately the same position as that seen on initial radiographs [9]. The limits associated with non-operative treatment are, in fact the risk of non-union, malunion, altered biomechanics of the upper girdle, deformity with unsatisfactory cosmetic results, and upper extremity weakness [7, 10–12]. These factors have caused an increase in the indications for surgical treatment [11, 13, 14].

Surgery finds absolute indication in the presence of open fractures, high comminution and dislocation of the fragments, high risk for in–out skin wounds, a shortening superior to 20 mm, floating shoulder and neurovascular lesions. Relative indications are polytraumas, painful malunions or non-unions [15, 16].

Operative treatment of displaced MSCFs can be achieved successfully using plates or intramedullary (IM) implants like Rush pins, Kirschner wires, or nails, but an optimal surgical technique is still not identified [4].

Aim of the present paper is to clinically evaluate the outcomes of two groups of patients suffering from displaced midshaft clavicle fracture, treated by conservative and by surgical treatment, depicting every possible association.

Materials and methods

This study evaluated all patients presented at our Emergency Department with a clavicle fracture in a time frame ranging from 1 January 2006 to 31 December 2011.

Data about patients were gathered by retrospectively reviewing hospital records. Triage Informatic Records were reviewed first, filtering records for clavicle fracture only. The results of patients were evaluated according to the inclusion and exclusion criteria (shown below) to include those in the study. The enrolled patients were then reviewed on the Surgical Procedures Registry to divide surgical patients from non-surgical ones. Lastly, a double check was performed through the analysis of Radiological Imaging Database for a specific patient, from the time of admittance at the emergency department onward, to confirm surgical and non-surgical patients.

In regards to Institute's Privacy Policy, it must be noted that every reported system and records provided were sorted by an anonymous identification number assigned at the admittance to the hospital.

Clavicle fractures were defined as displaced according to Postacchini et al. [17], therefore considering the distance between the inferior border of one bone fragment and that of the corresponding border of the other fragment at the fracture site if exceeding 3 mm on radiographs with a 1:1 magnification. Identified fracture was then classified according to Allman's radiographic classification system [18], modified by Nordqvist and Petersson [1, 10, 19]. This system was chosen for its simplicity compared to other classification systems and for the proper prognostic predictively.

This classification sets 3 groups and 3 subgroups of fractures. Group I fractures include fractures of middle third. Group II and group III include fracture of lateral and medial third, respectively. Subgroups a, b, and c include undisplaced, displaced, and multifragmentary fracture, respectively [1].

We also divided the patients on the amount of the shortening evaluated at XR before and after treatment (group A: shortening less than 1 cm; group B: shortening more than 1 cm but less than 2 cm; and group C with shortening greater than 2 cm).

For every patient, a clinical assessment was performed, along with a standard biprojective XR of the affected shoulder girdle.

Patient's inclusion criteria were fracture's types IB and IC according to Nordqvist and Petersson, age ranging from 14 years old to 65 years old, a complete file record, the completion of the rehabilitation programme and the voluntary positively response to the last follow-up.

Exclusion criteria were fractures types II and III and IC with high comminution (more than four fragments), polytrauma, open or pathological fractures, infective or systemic disease, previous surgeries on the affected shoulder, floating shoulder, anatomical variations in respect of normal anatomy, previous traumas and previous rehabilitation treatments on the affected joint.

Study cohort was determined according to the diagram provided in Fig. 1.

Concordance between observers, in regard of the treatment performed, was re-evaluated at the end of the study, obtaining a K coefficient >0.85.

Non-operative treatment

Patients treated conservatively were managed with a "figure-of-8" orthosis. After its application, the patient underwent a plain radiograph to check the alignment of the fragments; patients were also instructed on its use, on how

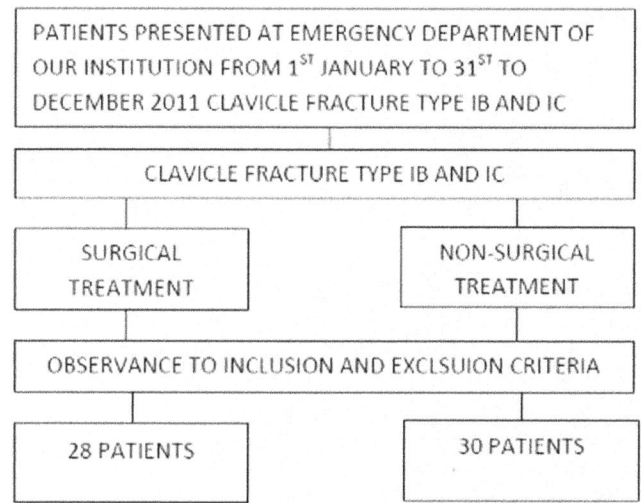

Fig. 1 Algorithm used to determine the study cohort

to maintain its correct position, how to re-tension and avoid axillary decubitus ulcers and compression of the neurovascular bundle.

All patients treated non-operatively have been invited, in the first phase, to avoid all active movements of shoulder and to perform slight mobilization movements of the hand and the elbow without load to prevent joint contractures and oedema.

After 4 weeks of treatment, patients were asked to remove the bandage and start to perform rehabilitation programme.

Surgical technique

The patient candidates for surgical treatment were subjected to the reduction in fracture and fixation with intramedullary threaded Kirschner wire (K-wire) with a procedure similar to the Murray method [20].

The patients underwent general anaesthesia. The technique (Fig. 2) provides the patient in the supine position on a radiolucent surgical table with a slight overflow of the arm out from the edge of the bed and with a slight inclination of the trunk to ensure freedom of movement of the arm.

A small incision (3–4 cm) (Fig. 2 b, c) was made at the level of the fracture in line with its major axis of the clavicle. After a blunt dissection of the soft tissue, the fracture site is reached. A 2.5-mm drilling bit is used to open the intramedullary canal (Fig. 2d, e). The threaded Kirschner wire (from 2 to 3 mm diameter according to the size of the intramedullary canal) was advanced in the lateral bone fragment intramedullary canal till the K-wire exits throughout the postero-lateral skin (Fig. 2f) and then (Fig. 2g) it is advanced in the medial bone fragment

intramedullary canal (in–out technique). The advancement of the K-wire was controlled with an image intensifier.

To provide the best reduction, the bone nearby the fracture site was gently deperiosted, facilitating the alignment of the bone ends. A cerclage with a high strength non-absorbable suture #2 (FiberWire®, Arthrex, Naples U.S.) was performed in the presence of a third fragment, or multifragmentary fracture.

At the end of the procedure, the K-wire folded and cut close to the exit point in order to minimize irritation of the soft tissues, but leaving a sufficient part for an easier removal afterwards (Fig. 2h). A control radiography was performed at the end of the procedure (Fig. 3). A Gilchrist bandage was applied for 4 weeks postoperatively. Acetaminophen use was suggested in case of persistent pain, usually in the first postoperative days. Pin removal was allowed after 4 weeks of rest in an outpatient setting without any anaesthesia.

Outcome measure

The Quick Disabilities of the Arm, Shoulder and Hand (qDASH) score [21, 22] score and the Constant Murley Shoulder (CS) score [23] were used to evaluate the clinical outcomes. The minimal detectable change at the 95% confidence level (MDC95%) ranged from 16 to 20 QuickDASH points (with a mean of 18) [22]. The MIC 95% limit of CS was found at a mean change of 24 points [24].

The radiographic outcome was determined by a pre-treatment, post-treatment and at 1 and 6 months of follow-up standard posteroanterior thorax radiograph according to Smekal et al. [25]. Post-treatment radiographs were firstly evaluated for the presence of delayed union, non-union and malunion. Union was defined as bony bridging over the fracture gap [26]. The malunion is evaluated by calculating the results in shortening in centimetres compared to the contralateral side. The images were all analysed using an open-source software (OsiriX, v5.0.2) in terms of mean displacement and shortening.

Statistical analysis

The two groups have been compared with the Fisher's exact test to confirm the homogeneity about age, gender, side affected, fracture type according to Allman's Classification modified by Nordqvist and Petersson [18, 19] and displacement grade of the fracture before treatment.

The results of the qDASH and CS were analysed in function of the treatment performed (surgical or non-surgical) by the Wilcoxon test.

In patients who have undergone surgery, the results of qDASH and CS were analysed in function of radiographic

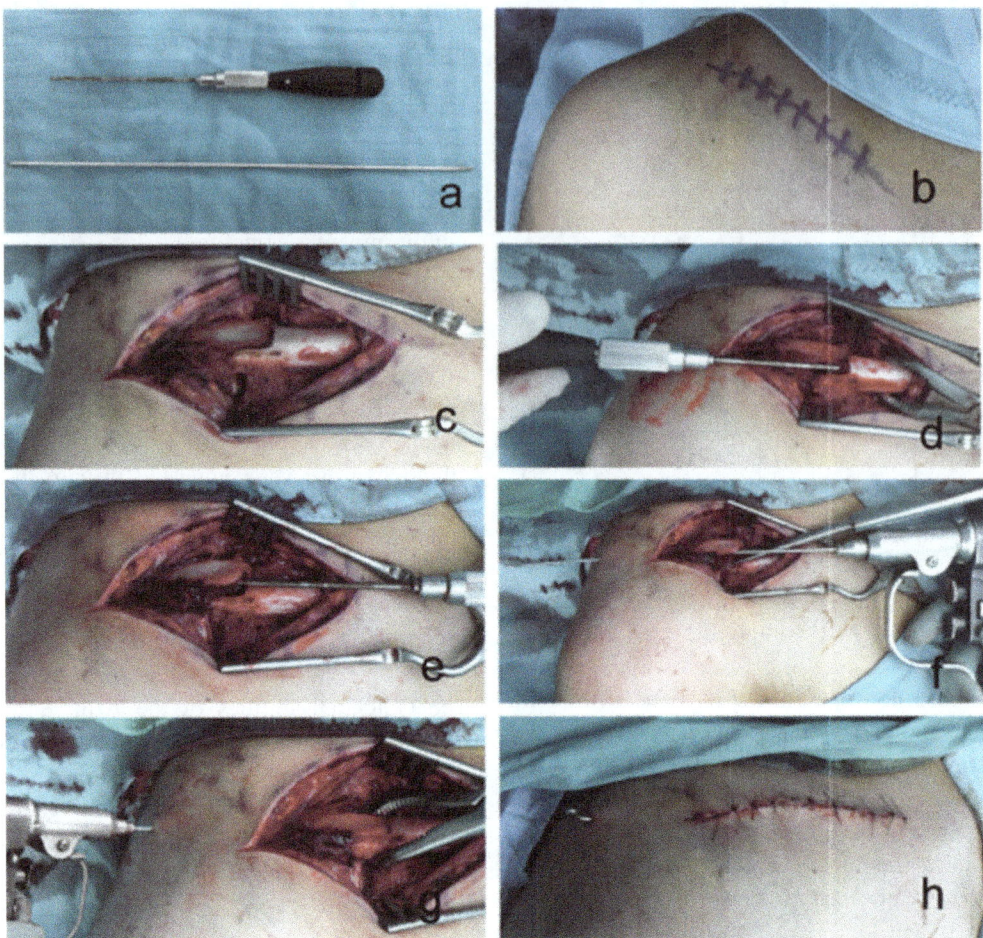

Fig. 2 Figure shows the essential surgical instruments and the main steps of our technique

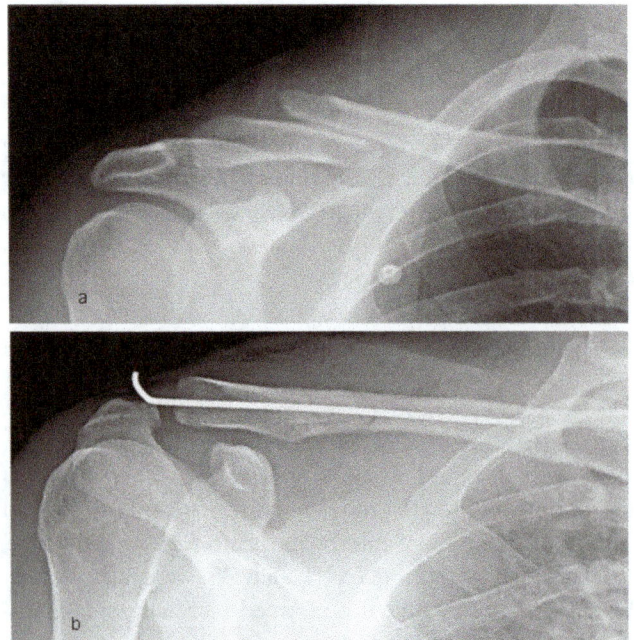

Fig. 3 Figure shows the radiography of midshaft clavicle fracture **a** before and **b** after the surgical treatment

outcome by Wilcoxon test. In patients treated non-operatively, the same evaluation has been performed by Kruskall–Wallis test. Post-hoc power analysis on the two groups constituting the cohort has been performed.

The radiographic outcomes were evaluated in function of the treatment by the Student's t test.

Results

Database review provided a total of 243 patients with clavicular fractures of which 174 were excluded because they matched one of the exclusion criteria and 11 were eligible to be included in the study but lost to follow-up (dropouts). Of these, 4 were unreachable, 3 were off site and 4 have refused to be included in the study for personal reasons.

A final cohort of 58 patients (51 males, 7 females; man age 38.35 years old; median 35.64 years old) who met the inclusion and exclusion criteria was enrolled to constitute two groups: one of 30 patients that underwent conservative treatment and one of 28 patients that underwent surgical treatment. Out of these, we found a total of 25 fractures on the right side and 33 on the left side. The two groups were significantly homogeneous concerning age, gender, side, fracture subtype, and displacement extent before treatment (analysed by Fisher's exact test, respectively, with $p = 1$, $p = 0.595$, $p = 0.706$, $p = 0.802$, Table 1).

According to Nordqvist and Petersson classification, a total of 19 fractures were classified as type IB and 39 as type IC [1, 10, 18, 19].

Functional outcomes were analysed at a mean follow-up of 48 months (range 28.32–74.52 months) for the surgical-treated group and 45 months (range 22.68–73.92 months) for the non-surgical-treated group.

Operative versus non-operative group

The results of qDASH and CS obtained after treatment have showed no statistically significant difference between the two groups (Fig. 4a, b).

Clinical outcome in function of radiographic outcome

The results of qDASH evaluated in function of the radiographic outcome (Fig. 5I, II) showed a statistically significant correlation between the worst (lower) qDASH results and the grade of radiograph shortening in both groups (respectively, Wilcoxon test $p = 0.002$ in surgically treated group and Kruskall–Wallis test $p = 0.018$ in non-operative treated group).

Table 1 Demographic data, fracture classification and initial clavicle shortening

	Surgical group	Non-surgical group
Total	28	30
Age (years)	39.5 ± 15.7	37.4 ± 15.5
Sex		
Male	26 (92.9%)	25 (83.3%)
Female	2 (7.1%)	5 (16.7%)
Affected side		
Right	12 (42.9%)	13 (43.3%)
Left	16 (57.1%)	17 (56.7%)
Fracture classification		
1b	9 (32.1%)	10 (33.3%)
1c	19 (67.9%)	20 (66.7%)
Initial shortening		
a (<1 cm)	9 (32.1%)	10 (33.33%)
b (1/2 cm)	10 (35.7%)	10 (33.33%)
c (>2 cm)	9 (32.1%)	10 (33.33%)
Follow-up (years)	4 ± 1.9	3.8 ± 1.5

In particular, in the group non-operatively treated the difference between the medians of the results of the qDASH of patients with shortening <2 cm and those with shortening greater than 2 cm was approximately 25 points.

In the group surgically treated, instead, there is a difference of about 20 points in the median of the results of the qDASH of patients without shortening and those with shortening <2 cm.

The results of CS evaluated in function of the radiographic outcome (Fig. 5III, IV) have shown a statistically significant correlation between the worst CS results and the grade of shortening in both groups (respectively, Wilcoxon test $p < 0.001$ in surgically treated group and test Kruskall–Wallis $p = 0.005$ in non-operatively treated group).

In the group surgically treated, there is a difference of about 20 points between the medians of the CS results of patients without shortening (median of 100 points) and those with shortening of less than 2 cm (median of 80 points). In the group treated non-operatively, the difference between the medians of the CS results of patients with shortening of less than 2 cm and those with shortening greater than 2 cm is about 30 points (in patients without shortening the median is 100 points, in those with shortening of less than 2 cm the median is 90 points in the patients with shortening greater than 2 cm the median is 60 points).

Radiographic outcome

In the group of patients surgically treated, a reduction in displacement was observed in 25 (89.29%) cases and not in 3 (10.71%) cases. The improvement was statistically significant ($p = 0.032$). In particular, there were no patients with a shortening greater than 2 cm at the end of treatment.

In non-operatively treated group, the improvement in radiographic outcome was not statistically significant ($p = 0.464$) with 23 cases (76.67%) in which there was no improvement of the shortening and only 6 cases (20.69%) in which was obtained an improvement of the fracture displacement by the figure-of-8 orthosis application. One case (3.33%) showed a worse radiographic outcome than pre-treatment.

Complications

No iatrogenic lesions have been reported after both treatment options. No implant failure occurred. Superficial infection at the site of the surgical approach for the fracture reduction was seen in 1 patient (3.57%) with hypertrophic scar formation. Three patients (10.71%) of the surgical groups have complained to feel pain in case of touch at the level of the previous fracture zone.

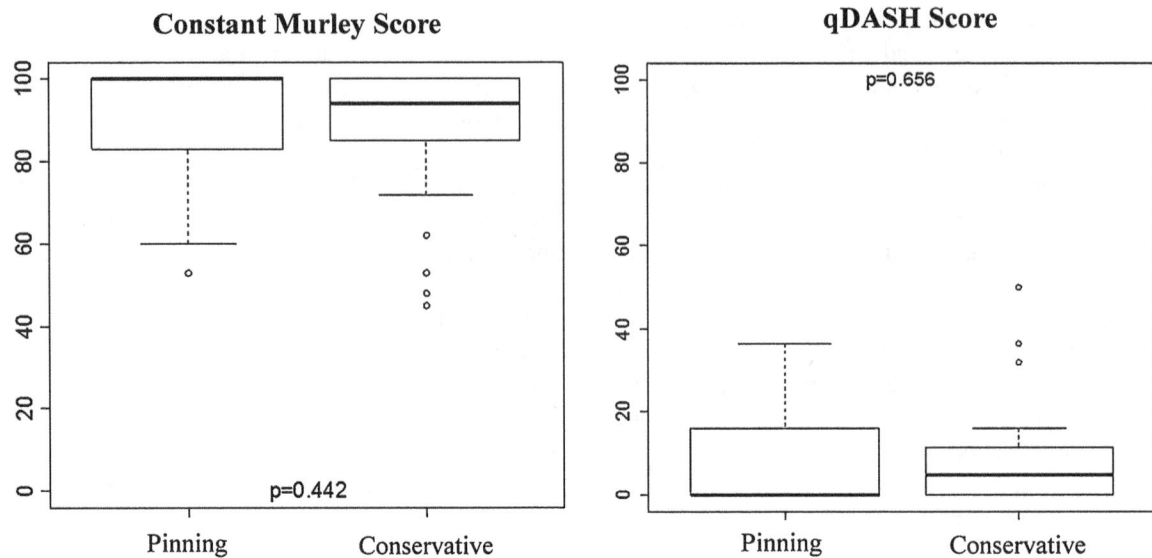

Fig. 4 *Box plot* with outcomes of **a** constant score (best score = 0), **b** qDASH score (best score = 0) compared by the type of treatment

We found one (3.33%) non-union in the non-operative-treated group and none in the surgical-treated group.

Discussion

Aim of our study was to evaluate, on a mid- to long-term follow-up, two different treatments for midshaft clavicular fractures, underlining any possible difference in terms of functional and radiographic outcomes, and non-union rates.

Our results showed that there are no significant differences between qDASH and CS in the two groups at the latest follow-up. We hypothesize this is due to the fact that not all types of clavicle fractures require surgical treatment and have a good outcome both with a surgical treatment and a conservative one. This is confirmed by the study of Nordqvist and Petersson [10].

In this study, of 225 patients with midshaft clavicle fracture treated conservatively, 185 were asymptomatic. Canadian Orthopaedic Trauma Society (COTS) (2007) [27] reported better results, evaluated by DASH score, in favour of the surgical group at all-time points. The magnitude of the difference, however, was less than 10 points, which is not considered a clinically relevant difference [21, 28].

A particular correlation was found statistically and clinically significant between the functional outcomes and the entity of displacement observed at follow-up, with worst and lower scores associated to a greater shortening. In those patients, surgical treatment with elastic stable intramedullary nailing (ESIN) performed significantly better compared to conservative treatment [29]. This is supported by the results of Ledger et al. [12] and Ristevski et al. [30].

They have shown in their patients that an average shortening, respectively, of 21.4 mm and 21.1 mm, is associated with an alteration of the normal anatomy of the scapular girdle with a worsening of shoulder function. Our results are in line with those of Hill et al. [7] who reported unsatisfactory results in 31% of patients when the final shortening of the clavicle was 20 mm or more. Lazarides et al. [31] showed similar results: out of all evaluated patients in their study (132), 34 (25.8%) were dissatisfied. They found that the increase in the shortening associated with accumulation and final clavicular shortening of more than 18 mm in male patients, and of more than 14 mm in female patients, was significantly associated with an unsatisfactory result.

Oroko et al. [32] found 3 of 41 patients with shortening of 15 mm or more who had low Constant disability scores, but this could be attributed to other factors. Smekal et al. [26] evaluated ESIN versus non-operative with randomized, controlled, clinical trial. These Authors showed a significant positive correlation between DASH score at endpoint and definite shortening, and between patient satisfaction and definite shortening. Furthermore, patients suffering from sequelae after 2 years had an average shortening of 6.1% (65.2%).

Rasmussen et al. [33], however, advocate conservative treatment of midshaft clavicle fractures with a shortening of 20 mm or more. They have clinically evaluated 130 patients treated conservatively. They have found patients with a shortening less than 20 mm had a mean difference in the Constant–Murley Score of 7.2. Mean difference between the two groups was 0.7 with no correlation between shortening of the clavicle and the clinical

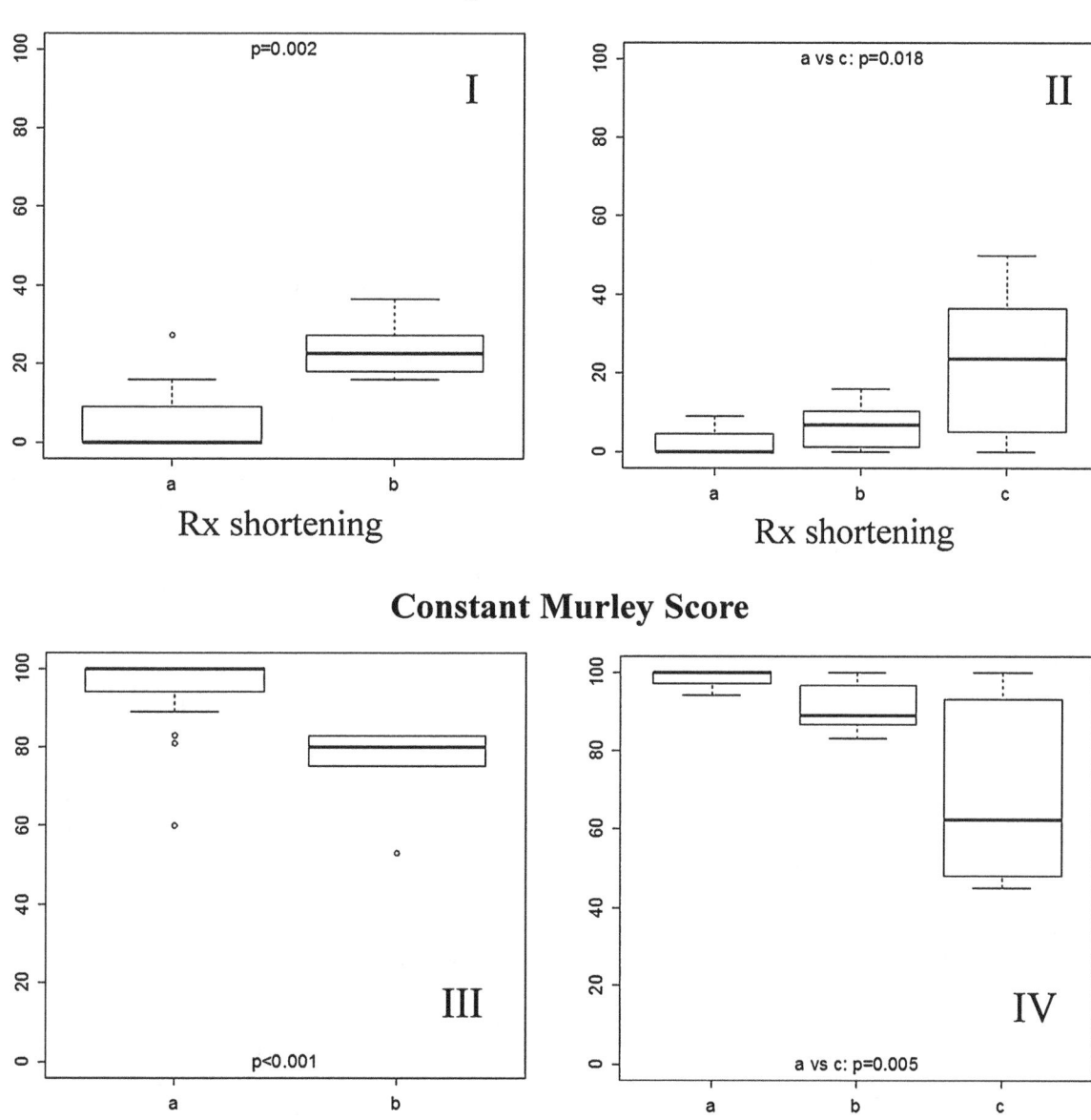

Fig. 5 *Box plot* of DASH (*I, II*) score and constant score divided (*III, IV*) by treatment (*I, III* surgical treatment; *II, IV* conservative treatment and radiograph shortening

outcome. They have concluded a shortening of more than 20 mm was not associated with a poorer clinical outcome.

Nordqvist et al. [10] have found that comminuted fractures (1C) do not behave significantly worse than do non-comminuted fractures (1B) and they have suggested that selection for surgical treatment cannot be based on the appearance of the fracture. However, Nowak et al. have shown that comminution in clavicle fractures is a negative prognostic indicator [14]. O'Neill et al. [1] in their series have found 6.2% of displaced simple fractures (1B) and 11.2% of comminuted fractures reach out to non-union.

On radiographic evaluation, surgical treatment demonstrated a great efficacy in reducing initial shortening of the fractured bone; this is in opposition to conservative treatment that, according also to other results showed in the literature, results very often in malunion, shortening, anatomic alterations and loss of functionality [7, 12, 31, 34].

Moreover, the vast majority of our surgically treated patients has reported a faster recovery, with a mean time of 3 months to return to full activities, while the non-surgical patients needed a mean time of 6 months; this results is in accordance with the data shown by Naveen et al. [35].

Non-union incidence in our study was 3.33% in the non-surgical-threaded group and is lower than was stated in the literature for the type of fractures studied that is usually over 10% [7, 26–28]. Our opinion about it is that in our study are excluded patients with high fracture comminution and other factors which are associated with clavicular non-union. In literature, indeed, it is reported that factors which predisposed to non-union include open fractures, refractures, associated multiple injuries, significant displacement, high comminution and inadequate immobilization [13] and it is suggested by several Authors [14, 15, 35] that patients with non-union risk factors aforementioned, in particular high comminution, should be surgically treated by open reduction and internal fixation (ORIF) by plating.

Among complications of surgical treatment, the most common one associated with nailing is the medial migration with skin irritation [36–38]. None of our patients reported such complication. This could be explained by the usage of a threaded Kirschner wire that has its medial extremity threaded that can provide higher stability of the construct, especially to telescopic forces. This finding is supported by results provided by Frigg et al. [39] that showed a reduction in medial migration when using an end cap for titanium elastic nail (TEN).

Biomechanically, plate fixation is superior to intramedullary fixation because it better resists the bending and torsional forces that occur during elevation of the upper extremity above shoulder level [40]. Patients treated with plate fixation can be allowed full range of motion once their soft tissues have healed. Disadvantages of plate fixation include the slightly higher infection rates, soft tissue irritation due to plate decubitus, and the risk of refracture after plate removal [8, 27].

The patients undergoing plating the implant removal need another surgery done under general anaesthesia, with a large-sized incision, while the intramedullary devices can be removed as outpatients with or without local anaesthesia [8]. In our experience, to obtain an anatomic reduction of clavicular fracture and application of treated k-wire, in particular in case of severe displacement of the fragments, is required an exposure similar to ORIF by plating (Fig. 2c–g) but the removal of threaded k-wire is easier than plate and it was performed in outpatient setting without any anaesthesia in all cases.

This paper presents some limitations. In first place, it is a retrospective analysis, without treatment randomization, limiting its power; this study design also presents only one follow-up at 46 months. This could obviously lead to a loss of information about trends and minor details that could have arose during the interval between treatment and follow-up, but one of the strongest points of the study groups is the completeness of the records that therefore limits the bias due to the design to a minimum, giving a precise picture of the outcome of the patient. A minor limitation could be the number of patients analysed, but even if other papers evaluated bigger groups, the statistical analysis performed allowed to state that the 58 patients included represent an adequate cohort in order to obtain statistical significance. Another bias could be the radiographic methods to evaluate the clavicle shortening. In fact, some recent studies have shown that plain radiograph-based measurements of midshaft clavicle shortening are precise, but inaccurate [41] and there is only a low correlation between X-ray and CT measurement [42]. However, Smekal et al. [25] have demonstrated that it is possible to obtain a result comparable to CT images with a posteroanterior thorax radiograph. Furthermore, it is our opinion, always in agreement with the same Authors, that the CT should not be used to evaluate an acute fracture since the supine position may change the fracture displacement and shortening.

In conclusion, with this study, we can assert that patients who would benefit more from an intramedullary synthesis in case of midshaft fracture of the clavicle are patients with a high degree of initial displacement, particularly if shortening greater than 2 cm.

We also noticed that when surgical treatment is performed, to achieve the best clinical results, it is necessary to obtain an anatomic reduction, in particular in relation to the length.

Surgeon should also investigate the real patient's needs, in particular in workers and sportsman, as the surgical treatment is able to ensure a return to complete activity of the upper limb more quickly.

The patient's profile related to fracture is, in our opinion, a new way to look after the surgical indications: the fracture characteristic in itself should not be the only landmark, but understanding the patient's abilities and demands should rule the surgeon decision-making.

Informed consent Informed consent was obtained from all individual participants included in the study.

References

1. O'Neill BJ, Hirpara KM, O'Briain D, McGarr C, Kaar TK (2011) Clavicle fractures: a comparison of five classification systems and their relationship to treatment outcomes. Int Orthop 35:909–914. doi:10.1007/s00264-010-1151-0
2. Stanley D, Trowbridge EA, Norris SH (1988) The mechanism of clavicular fracture. A clinical and biomechanical analysis. J Bone Joint Surg Br 70:461–464
3. Xu JJ, Xu L, Xu W, Gu Y, Xu JJ (2014) Operative versus non-operative treatment in the management of midshaft clavicular fractures: ameta-analysis of randomized controlled trials. J Shoulder Elb Surg 23:173–181. doi:10.1016/j.jse.2013.06.025

4. Hübner EJ, Hausschild O, Südkamp NP, Strohm PC (2011) Clavicle fractures—is there a standard treatment? Acta Chir Orthop Traumatol Cech 78:288–296

5. Neer CS (1960) Nonunion of the clavicle. J Am Med Assoc 172:1006–1011

6. Rowe CR (1968) An atlas of anatomy and treatment of mid-clavicular fractures. Clin Orthop Relat Res 58:29–42

7. Hill JM, McGuire MH, Crosby LA (1997) Closed treatment of displaced middle-third fractures of the clavicle gives poor results. J Bone Jt Surg 79:537–539. doi:10.1302/0301-620X.79B4.7529

8. Narsaria N, Singh AK, Arun GR, Seth RRS (2014) Surgical fixation of displaced midshaft clavicle fractures: elastic intra-medullary nailing versus precontoured plating. J Orthop Traumatol 15:165–171. doi:10.1007/s10195-014-0298-7

9. McKee MD, Pedersen EM, Jones C, Stephen DJG, Kreder HJ, Schemitsch EH, Wild LM, Potter J (2006) Deficits following nonoperative treatment of displaced midshaft clavicular fractures. J Bone Joint Surg Am 88:35–40. doi:10.2106/JBJS.D.02795

10. Nordqvist A, Petersson CJ, Redlund-Johnell I (1998) Mid-clavicle fractures in adults: end result study after conservative treatment. J Orthop Trauma 12:572–576

11. Nowak J, Holgersson M, Larsson S (2005) Sequelae from clavicular fractures are common A prospective study of 222 patients. Acta Orthop 76:496–502. doi:10.1080/17453670510041475

12. Ledger M, Leeks N, Ackland T, Wang A (2005) Short malunions of the clavicle: an anatomic and functional study. J Shoulder Elb Surg 14:349–354. doi:10.1016/j.jse.2004.09.011

13. Wick M, Müller EJ, Kollig E, Muhr G (2001) Midshaft fractures of the clavicle with a shortening of more than 2 cm predispose to nonunion. Arch Orthop Trauma Surg 121:207–211. doi:10.1007/s004020000202

14. Nowak J, Holgersson M, Larsson S (2004) Can we predict long-term sequelae after fractures of the clavicle based on initial findings? A prospective study with nine to ten years of follow-up. J Shoulder Elb Surg 13:479–486. doi:10.1016/j.jse.2004.01.026

15. van der Meijden OA, Gaskill TR, Millett PJ (2012) Treatment of clavicle fractures: current concepts review. J Shoulder Elb Surg 21:423–429. doi:10.1016/j.jse.2011.08.053

16. Lenza M, Belloti JC, Gomes Dos Santos JB, Matsumoto MH, Faloppa F (2009) Surgical interventions for treating acute fractures or non-union of the middle third of the clavicle. Cochrane Database Syst Rev. doi:10.1002/14651858.CD007428.pub2

17. Postacchini F, Gumina S, De Santis P, Albo F (2002) Epidemiology of clavicle fractures. J Shoulder Elbow Surg 11:452–456

18. Allman FL (1967) Fractures and ligamentous injuries of the clavicle and its articulation. J Bone Joint Surg Am 49:774–784

19. Nordqvist A, Petersson C (1994) The incidence of fractures of the clavicle. Clin Orthop Relat Res 300:127–132

20. Geckeler EO (1951) Fractures of the clavicle in adults. Am J Surg 81:333–335. doi:10.1016/0002-9610(51)90237-1

21. Gummesson C, Ward MM, Atroshi I (2006) The shortened disabilities of the arm, shoulder and hand questionnaire (Quick-DASH): validity and reliability based on responses within the full-length DASH. BMC Musculoskelet Disord 7:44. doi:10.1186/1471-2474-7-44

22. Mintken PE, Glynn P, Cleland JA, Mintken PE, Glynn P, Cleland JA (2009) Psychometric properties of the shortened disabilities of the Arm, Shoulder, and Hand Questionnaire (QuickDASH) and Numeric Pain Rating Scale in patients with shoulder pain. J Shoulder Elbow Surg 18:920–926. doi:10.1016/j.jse.2008.12.015

23. Constant CR, Murley AH (1987) A clinical method of functional assessment of the shoulder. Clin Orthop Relat Res 160–4

24. Holmgren T, Oberg B, Adolfsson L, Björnsson Hallgren H, Johansson K (2014) Minimal important changes in the Constant–Murley score in patients with subacromial pain. J Shoulder Elb Surg. doi:10.1016/j.jse.2014.01.014

25. Smekal V, Deml C, Irenberger A, Niederwanger C, Lutz M, Blauth M, Krappinger D (2008) Length determination in midshaft clavicle fractures: validation of measurement. J Orthop Trauma 22:458–462. doi:10.1097/BOT.0b013e318178d97d

26. Smekal V, Irenberger A, Struve P, Wambacher M, Krappinger D, Kralinger FS (2009) Elastic stable intramedullary nailing versus nonoperative treatment of displaced midshaft clavicular fractures-a randomized, controlled, clinical trial. J Orthop Trauma 23:106–112. doi:10.1097/BOT.0b013e318190cf88

27. Society COT (2007) Nonoperative treatment compared with plate fixation of displaced midshaft clavicular fractures. A multicenter, randomized clinical trial. J bone Jt Surg Am 89:1–10. doi:10.2106/JBJS.F.00020

28. Lenza M, Buchbinder R, Johnston R, Belloti J, Faloppa F (2013) Surgical versus conservative interventions for treating fractures of the middle third of the clavicle (Review). Cochrane database Syst Rev Online. doi:10.1002/14651858.CD009363.pub2. Copyright

29. Smekal V, Irenberger A, El Attal R, Oberladstaetter J, Krappinger D, Kralinger F (2011) Elastic stable intramedullary nailing is best for mid-shaft clavicular fractures without comminution: results in 60 patients. Injury 42:324–329. doi:10.1016/j.injury.2010.02.033

30. Ristevski B, Hall JA, Pearce D, Potter J, Farrugia M, McKee MD (2013) The radiographic quantification of scapular malalignment after malunion of displaced clavicular shaft fractures. J Shoulder Elb Surg 22:240–246. doi:10.1016/j.jse.2012.04.011

31. Lazarides S, Zafiropoulos G (2006) Conservative treatment of fractures at the middle third of the clavicle: the relevance of shortening and clinical outcome. J Shoulder Elb Surg 15:191–194. doi:10.1016/j.jse.2005.08.007

32. Oroko PK, Buchan M, Winkler A, Kelly IG (1999) Does shortening matter after clavicular fractures? Bull Hosp Jt Dis 58:6–8

33. Rasmussen JV, Jensen SL, Petersen JB, Falstie-Jensen T, Lausten G, Olsen BS (2011) A retrospective study of the association between shortening of the clavicle after fracture and the clinical outcome in 136 patients. Injury 42:414–417. doi:10.1016/j.injury.2010.11.061

34. McKee MD, Wild LM, Schemitsch EH (2003) Midshaft malunions of the clavicle. J Bone Joint Surg Am 85–A:790–797

35. Naveen BM, Joshi GR, Harikrishnan B (2017) Management of mid-shaft clavicular fractures: comparison between non-operative treatment and plate fixation in 60 patients. Strateg Trauma Limb Reconstr 12:11–18. doi:10.1007/s11751-016-0272-4

36. Andermahr J, Jubel A, Elsner A, Johann J, Prokop A, Rehm KE, Koebke J (2007) Anatomy of the clavicle and the intramedullary nailing of midclavicular fractures. Clin Anat 20:48–56. doi:10.1002/ca.20269

37. Kettler M, Schieker M, Braunstein V, König M, Mutschler W (2007) Flexible intramedullary nailing for stabilization of displaced midshaft clavicle fractures: technique and results in 87 patients. Acta Orthop 78:424–429. doi:10.1080/17453670710014022

38. Wijdicks FJG, Houwert RM, Millett PJ, Verleisdonk EJJM, Van Der Meijden OAJ (2013) Systematic review of complications after intramedullary fixation for displaced midshaft clavicle fractures. Can J Surg 56:58–64. doi:10.1503/cjs.029511

39. Frigg A, Rillmann P, Perren T, Gerber M, Ryf C (2009) Intramedullary nailing of clavicular midshaft fractures with the titanium elastic nail: problems and complications. Am J Sports Med 37:352–359. doi:10.1177/0363546508328103

40. Golish SR, Oliviero JA, Francke EI, Miller MD (2008) A biomechanical study of plate versus intramedullary devices for midshaft clavicle fixation. J Orthop Surg Res 3:28. doi:10.1186/1749-799X-3-28

15

Distal femoral flexion deformity from growth disturbance treated with a two-level osteotomy and internal lengthening nail

Austin T. Fragomen[1,2] · Fiona R. Fragomen[2]

Abstract Salter Harris fractures of the distal femur can lead to growth disturbance with resulting leg length inequality and knee deformity. We have looked at a case series (3) of patients who presented with a distal femur flexion malunion and shortening treated with a distal femoral osteotomy and plating and a proximal femoral osteotomy with a magnetic internal lengthening nail. Does a two-level osteotomy and internal fixation approach provide a reliable result both radiographically and functionally? The average knee extension loss was 12°, LLD 47 mm, PDFA 65°, MAD 2 mm. The patients were treated with an acute, posterior, opening wedge osteotomy of the distal femur stabilized with a lateral plate and screws and grafted with cancellous chips and putty. A second osteotomy was made proximally in the femur percutaneously, and the internal lengthening nail was inserted. Lengthening was done at approximately 1 mm/day. The average extension gain was 12°; amount of lengthening at the proximal site was 40 mm, LLD was 3 mm. The average PDFA was 81°, and MAD 3 mm. There were no complications. Functional results were excellent. Bone healing index was 24 days/cm. The average distance from the distal osteotomy to the joint line was 57 mm. The technique of two-level femur osteotomy stabilized with a plate and lengthening nail yielded excellent results with acceptable correction of deformity, full knee extension, and improved function. There were no complications including implant failure, infection, need for blood transfusion, knee stiffness, nonunion, compartment syndrome, or malunion.

Keywords Magnetic internal lengthening nail · Precice · TomoFix · Osteotomy · Deformity · Limb lengthening

Introduction

Salter Harris fractures of the distal femur can lead to a high rate of growth disturbance [1]. The combination of the fracture and the physeal injury can result in leg length inequality and distal femoral deformity. Most deformity that is noticeable lies in the coronal plane with sagittal (flexion) deformity going underappreciated [1]. If diagnosed early, anterior physeal stapling can reduce the degree of flexion deformity [2, 3] but cannot correct the limb shortening. The apex of the flexion deformity, typically very close to the knee joint, influences treatment options. Anterior closing wedge distal femoral osteotomy with plate fixation has been used for treatment of knee flexion deformities in cerebral palsy [4] and polio [5] with success but at the expense of limb length [6]. Treatment by distal femoral osteotomy and a hexapod external fixator (or monolateral frame) can correct both deformity and length [7–10], but associated problems include knee stiffness [9, 11–14], pin infections [7–9], pain, difficulty sitting and sleeping, and difficulty controlling the sagittal plane with residual flexion deformity [8, 10, 15, 16]. External fixation has been shown to have a higher complication rate when compared with the internal lengthening nail (ILN) techniques [17]. Improved patient satisfaction with internal fixation has also pushed surgeons to seek surgical solutions without the use of external fixation [18]. The lengthening and then plating technique reduces time in the frame but is

✉ Austin T. Fragomen
FragomenA@hss.edu

[1] Weill Medical College, Cornell University, 535 East 70th Street, New York, NY 10021, USA

[2] Hospital for Special Surgery, 535 East 70th Street, New York, NY 10021, USA

associated with plate failure, malunion, need for further surgery, and a risk of deep infection [19].

The ILN has solved many problems that were associated previously with external fixation. The problem with using the ILN and a single osteotomy approach to correct this distal femoral flexion deformity is that a very distal osteotomy (less than 7 cm from the joint line) is needed at apex of the deformity, making intramedullary (IM) nail fixation, lengthening over nail (LON), and ILN corrections less reliable. Furthermore, retrograde ILN is associated with risk of increased flexion deformity at the osteotomy site which would threaten to undo any correction initially obtained [20, 21]. Performing the osteotomy more proximally to allow for proper IM nail fixation would require excessive posterior translation of the distal fragment precluding IM nailing or, without the translation, result in under-correction of the flexion deformity.

We reviewed a case series of skeletally mature patients who presented with a distal femur flexion malunion and shortening. All patients were treated with a two-level osteotomy technique including a distal femoral osteotomy (DFO) using acute correction and plating and a proximal femoral osteotomy used for lengthening with a magnetic ILN. The question asked was: does a two-level osteotomy and all-internal fixation approach provide a reliable result both radiographically and functionally?

Materials and methods

Three patients presented between 2014 and 2016 with complaints of a knee flexion deformity, shortening of the femur, with hip, knee, and low back pain. All patients had sustained an injury to the right femur during adolescence that involved damage to the distal femoral physis (Table 1). The resultant growth disturbance created the identical deformity pattern of distal femoral procurvatum and shortening (Fig. 1a, b). Patients underwent physical examination, including prone rotational profile and radiographic evaluation. The average knee extension loss was

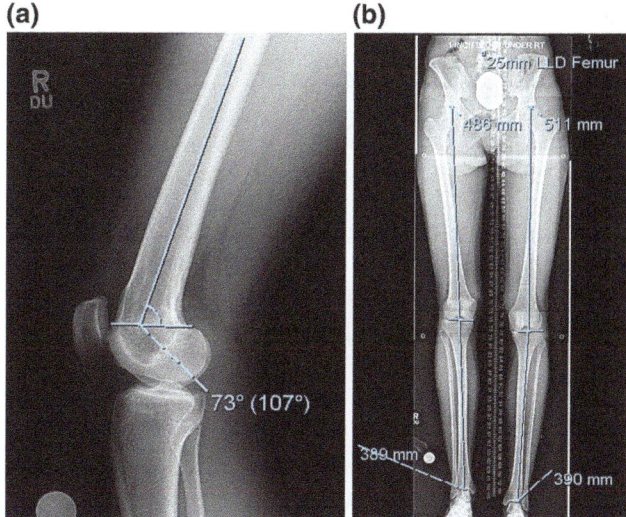

Fig. 1 a This lateral radiograph of the knee shows a distal femoral flexion deformity of 10°. The posterior distal femoral angle (PDFA) measures 73° with the normal averaging 83°, **b** a 51 in., standing, bipedal radiograph with a 25-mm block under the right foot demonstrates a 25 mm leg length discrepancy originating from the right femur

12°, leg length discrepancy (LLD) was 47 mm, posterior distal femoral angle (PDFA) was 65°, and mechanical axis deviation (MAD) was 2 mm lateral (Table 2). Deformity planning indicated that the apex of the deformity was at the level of the distal epiphyseal scar in all cases (Fig. 2a–c). The magnitude of bony deformity was considered in the context of the physical exam. In case 3, for example, the patient lacked 15° of knee extension but had a bony deformity of 30°. The bone was corrected by 15° to achieve full knee extension without hyperextension.

One gramme of Tranexamic acid was administered intravenously at the time of the incision and 3 h later to prevent blood loss and haematoma. The deformities were corrected with an acute, posterior opening wedge osteotomy of the distal femur at the level of the trochlea and posterior condyles (a more distal osteotomy was not possible without cutting into the trochlea or condyles). The anterior cortex was maintained intact to increase the

Table 1 Patient injury details

Patient	Age at the time of injury (years)	Mechanism of injury	Nature of fracture	Initial treatment
1	13	Soccer	Distal femur growth plate closed SH	Closed reduction and casting
2	11	Motor vehicle accident	Distal femur growth plate closed SH	Closed reduction and casting
3	9	Motor vehicle accident	Distal femur growth plate closed SH	Closed reduction, percutaneous pinning, and casting. Later, osteotomy and plating for deformity correction

SH Salter Harris (SH grade is unknown by patient history)

Table 2 Patient demographics

Patient	Age at surgery	Laterality	Sex	Max knee ext (deg)	LLD (mm)	PDFA (deg)	MAD (mm)	LDFA (deg)
1	25	R	Female	− 10	25	73	0	84
2	16	R	Female	− 12	40	70	3 lateral	94
3	35	R	Male	− 15	75	52	3 lateral	93
Average	25	R		− 12	47	65	2 lateral	90

Knee extension measurements were obtained through physical exam

R right, *Ext* extension (a "−" sign indicated a lack of knee extension = flexion deformity), *LLD* leg length discrepancy, *PDFA* posterior distal femoral angle, *MAD* mechanical axis deviation, *LDFA* lateral distal femoral angle (ref-Paley)

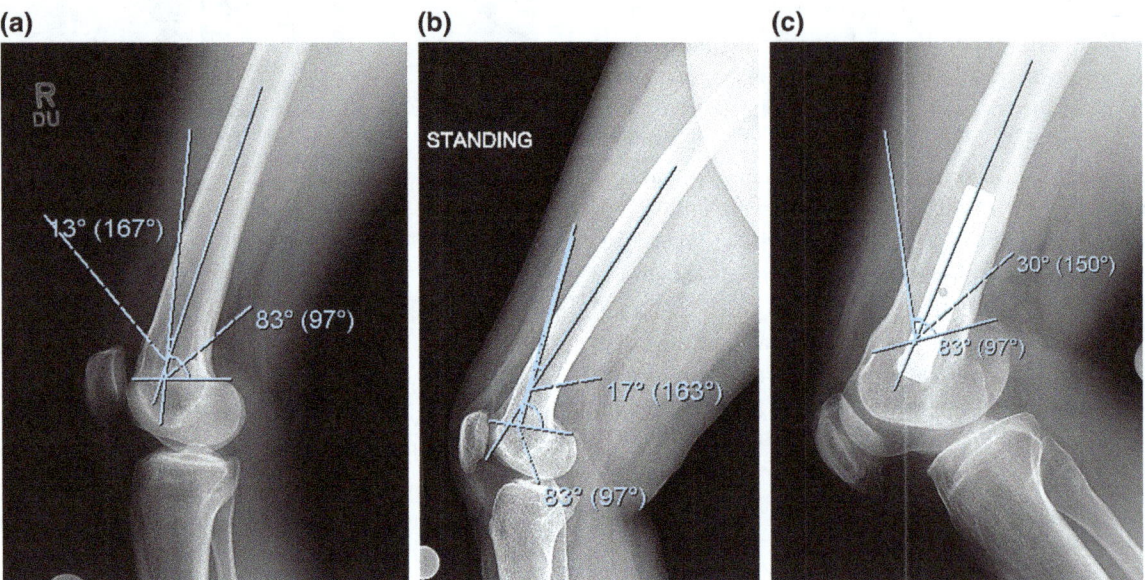

Fig. 2 a The lateral radiograph of patient 1 shows the apex of deformity lies just proximal to the posterior condyles and has a magnitude of 13°, **b** the lateral radiograph of patient 2 shows the apex of deformity lies slightly more proximal than patient 1 and has a magnitude of 17°, **c** the lateral radiograph of patient 3 shows the apex of deformity lies at the level of the posterior condyles and has a magnitude of 30°

stability of the osteotomy site. Maintaining an intact anterior cortex was thought to prevent the introduction of coronal plane deformity and improve healing of the osteotomy. The posterior soft tissue was carefully dissected with the knee flexed. The osteotomy was performed with a micro-saw and osteotomes, ensuring division of the medial cortex. A laminar spreader was used to open the posterior cortex and correct the deformity (Fig. 3a–c). An anteriorly based closing wedge osteotomy could have been used as well but we were more comfortable with the opening wedge method. The osteotomy was then stabilized with a TomoFix (Synthes, West Chester, PA) titanium lateral plate and screws and grafted with allograft cancellous freeze-dried chips and demineralized bone matrix putty (Fig. 4). The femoral rotation was then marked with half pins. Two 6-mm pins were placed separately in the lesser trochanter and into the distal femur, posterior to the plate. These pins were used to control the fragments after

osteotomy and set the rotational alignment. A second osteotomy was made proximally in the femur using a percutaneous technique employing multiple drill holes followed by a corticotomy. The Precice (NuVasive, San Diego, CA) internal lengthening nail was inserted using a piriformis fossa entry portal (Fig. 5). The ILN was 10.7 or 12.5 mm diameter and 245–275 mm in length. The length of the nail was selected pre-operatively and based on the position of the plate. The longest nail that would not touch the screws within the plate was utilized. The site of the osteotomy needed to be 8 cm+ the proposed lengthening (in centimetres) proximal to the distal tip of the nail. This would ensure that enough of the thick portion of the nail remained in the distal femur at completion of lengthening. In Case 2, an acute rotational correction of 15° was performed, correcting a retroversion malunion (Fig. 6). This was assisted with the posterior half pins inserted previously.

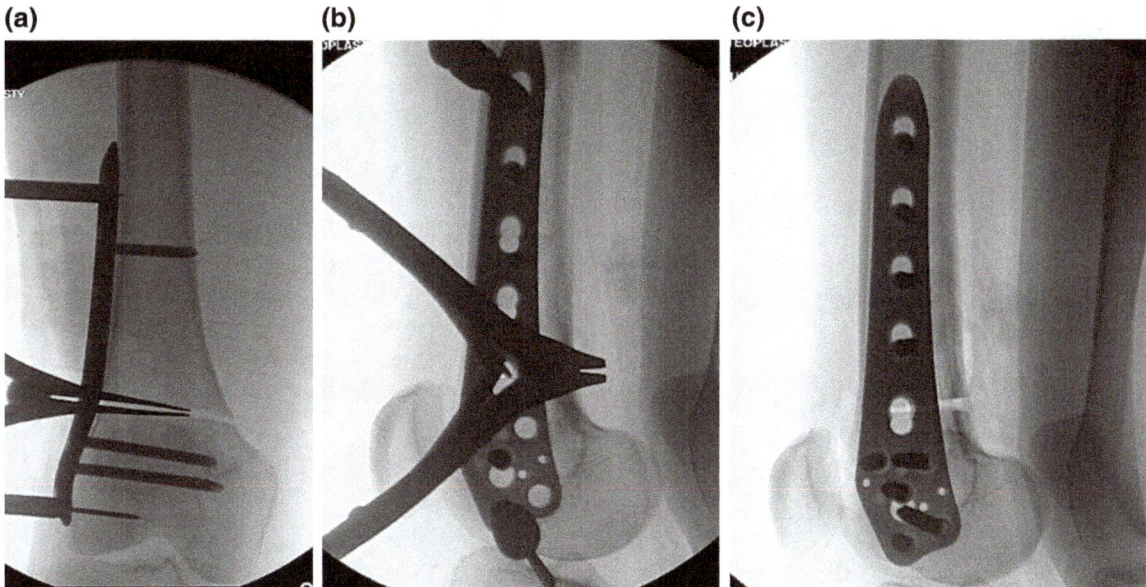

Fig. 3 **a** An AP view of the posterior opening wedge osteotomy in patient 1 with the laminar spreader inserted centrally in the posterior cortex. Care is taken to avoid eccentric placement of the laminar spreader which could lead to unwanted varus–valgus deformity, **b** a lateral intraoperative view of the laminar spreader is seen holding the bony correction during plating, and **c** the final result of the posterior opening wedge correction after plating is seen on this lateral radiograph

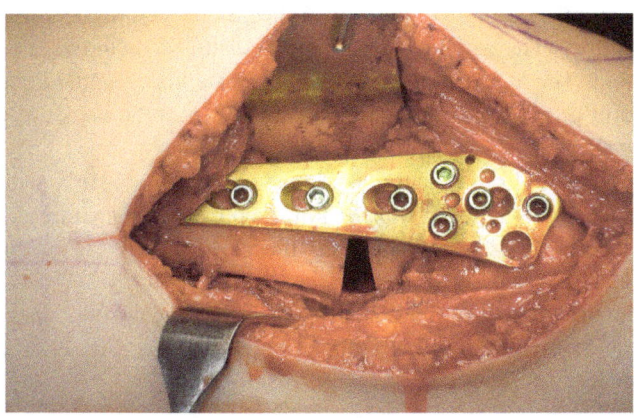

Fig. 4 This intra-op radiograph from patient 2 shows the open posterior cortex prior to grafting with the plate secured

Post-operatively Rivaroxaban was started on day 2 and continued for 2 weeks to prevent VTE as per our post-limb deformity surgery protocol. Instructions for magnet use were taught to the patients during the admission. Lengthening began on post-operative day 4. It was done at 0.33 mm four times per day for 4 days and then three times per day until the desired length was obtained.

Patients were allowed 30 lbs. weight bearing immediately after surgery as determined by the plate rather than the ILN which allows 50–70 lbs. Weight-bearing restrictions were maintained for 3 months at which point the distal femoral osteotomy was healed; thereafter, the quality of proximal regenerate became the determining factor. Once two cortices of bone were seen on orthogonal X-rays, then weight bearing as tolerated was allowed.

Follow-up visits were conducted every 2 weeks with radiographs and the quality of the regenerate assessed (Fig. 7a, b). In Case 3, it was noted that the amount of bone lengthening was less than expected on post-op day 30 and the patient at risk for premature consolidation. The patient admitted to missing several adjustments and to smoking marijuana daily. He then proceeded with 0.99 mm per day lengthening with normal regenerate formation.

The primary outcome measures were: (a) an ability to achieve full knee extension; (b) the PDFA, MAD and the LLD measurements and; (c) the BHI (bone healing index). The MAD and PDFA measurements were made on 51 in., standing, bipedal radiographs taken 10 feet away from the patient and using a calibration ball. Outcome scores used the Knee Injury and Osteoarthritis Outcome Score (KOOS) [22]. Although the KOOS score is used primarily for knee osteoarthritis, it was selected in this study since it measures knee disability from acute injury as well. For a patient without arthritis, it is possible to score 100% once the acute injury has resolved. Complications including infection, a need for blood transfusion, knee stiffness, nonunion, compartment syndrome, and malunion were recorded.

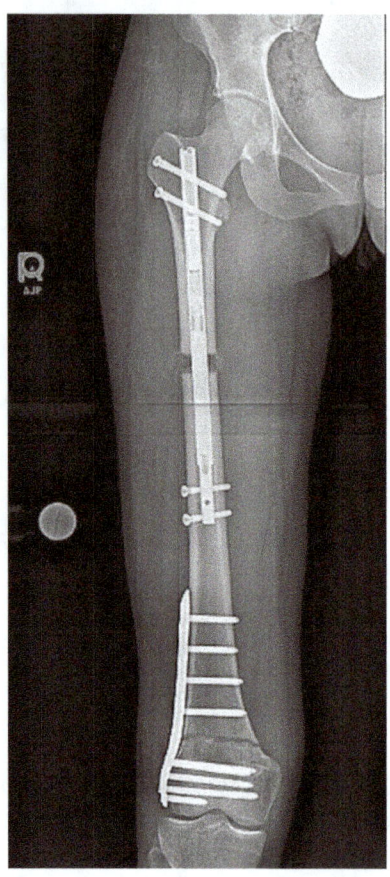

Fig. 5 This post-operative radiograph demonstrates the entire construct including the piriformis entry ILN and the distal plate. This needs to be planned well to ensure the proper nail length and osteotomy location are selected so that the nail is long enough to control the lengthening bone but short enough to not interfere with the plate. The concern about a stress riser between the nail and the plate has not been an issue in this young adult population

Results

Outcomes were divided into functional, implant-related, and bone (radiographic) results. Follow-up was 19 months (range 12–33). The average knee extension gain was 12° with all patients achieving full extension and none losing flexion (Table 3). Functional results, as measured by the KOOS, were excellent with average improvement in knee symptoms of 41%, knee pain of 29%, sports function of 32%, and quality of life 67% (Table 4). There were no implant-related failures.

Radiographic assessment showed the average amount of lengthening at the proximal osteotomy site was 40 mm (there was additional lengthening that occurred at the distal osteotomy site), and the residual LLD was 3 mm with the right leg shorter. The average post-op PDFA was 81° and MAD was 3 mm medial (Fig. 8a, b; Table 5). Bone healing index (days to consolidation from osteotomy date/cm lengthening) average was 24 days/cm (Table 5). All distal

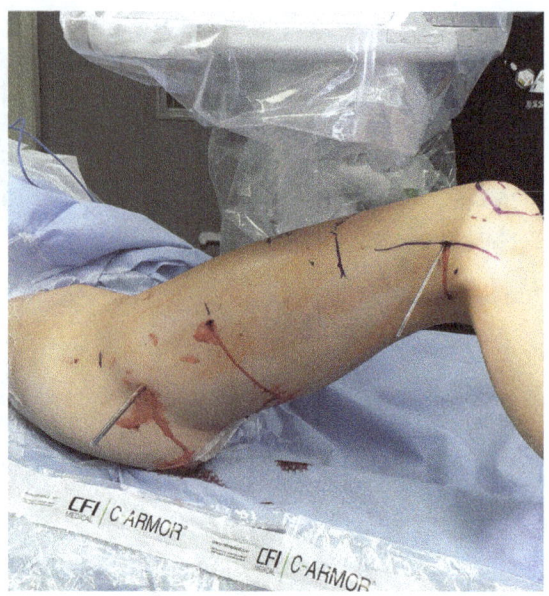

Fig. 6 This intraoperative photograph shows the concept of using pins to mark the femoral rotation and, specifically, using a 6 mm half pin in the lesser trochanter to control the proximal fragment during nail preparation and insertion

femoral osteotomy sites were healed at 3 months post-surgery. The distal osteotomy was located close to the knee joint. The average distance from the osteotomy to the knee joint line was 57 mm, and the distance from the osteotomy to the notch was 47 mm (Table 6).

Potential complications of post-operative anaemia with a need for blood transfusion, compartment syndrome, fracture of the femur between the plate and the tip of the IM nail, excessive stress on the distal osteotomy site from the proximal lengthening causing displacement of the distal osteotomy, venous thromboembolism (VTE), and knee stiffness were not seen.

Discussion

The technique of two-level femur osteotomy stabilized with a DFO plate and ILN yielded a full range of knee motion which helped to provide improved outcome scores. Patients had excellent outcomes on the KOOS which improved an average of 8–66% depending on the subscale item (Table 4) All patients had knee pain and a lack of full extension pre-operatively which the KOOS was able to capture. They also complained of pre-surgery low back and hip pain during activities, presumably from the limb length inequality, which resolved completely after treatment.

On radiographs the PDFA improved to the normal range and the average amount of clinical correction of knee flexion deformity was 12° with a maximum of 15° in patient 3. In that case the final lateral radiograph showed

(a) **(b)**

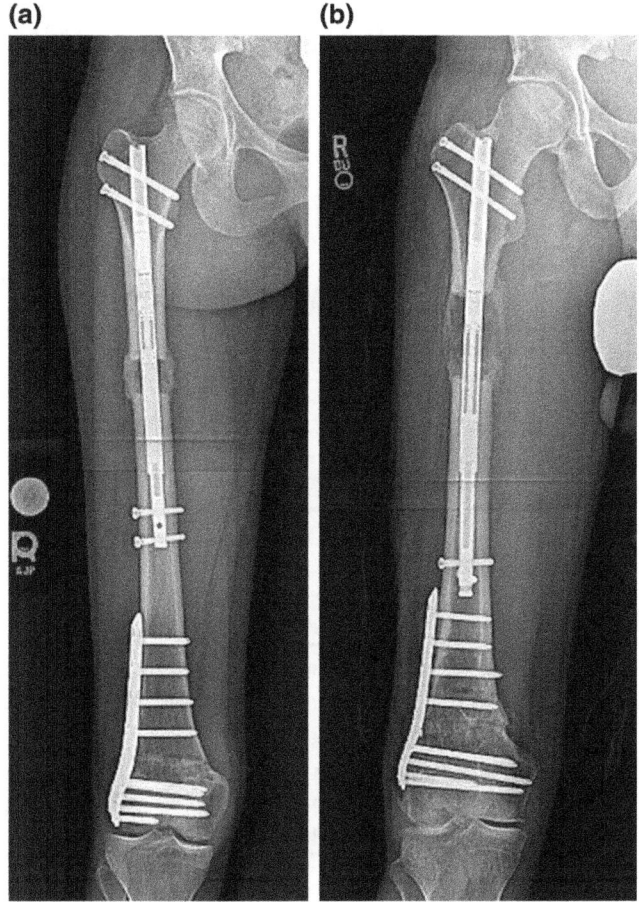

Fig. 7 a This post-operative radiograph of patient 1 shows a consolidating proximal regenerate with bicortical bridging callus during the consolidation phase of lengthening, **b** this post-operative X ray of patient 3 shows a healthy regenerate during the distraction phase of lengthening. The rate of distraction was not altered after this appointment

some anterior translational deformity of the distal fragment relative to the proximal fragment, which was without any negative functional impact, but suggests that a correction of a flexion deformity larger than 15° may be best accomplished by completion of the osteotomy through the anterior cortex, allowing for posterior translation of the distal fragment. A closing wedge technique may provide a better strategy as well (Fig. 9). The LLD decreased from 47 mm pre-op to 3 mm post-op as measured on standing radiographs. The patient with the largest residual LLD (5 mm, patient 3) was secondary to the patient feeling his limb was too long and refusing to do more lengthening. In all cases, the ILN was capable of more length and it was with the surgeon's agreement to stop lengthening slightly short of the actual LLD to avoid the patient's sense of over-lengthening. There was a minimal change in the MAD for patients 1 and 2. Patient 3 had a larger change in the MAD. This may have been due to an inability to accurately measure the actual distal femoral deformity (LDFA) pre-operatively secondary to the large flexion deformity and dysplastic distal femur. Alternatively, the large correction of flexion may have introduced varus into the distal osteotomy. The anterior cortex may have been too compromised (after 15° of opening) to maintain coronal plane alignment. The danger of a using a lateral approach, with lateral soft tissue stripping and insertion of instrumentation from the lateral side, was introducing an unintentional varus deformity.

The effect of lengthening the femur along the anatomic axis is to lateralize the mechanical axis [23], but this seemed to have no radiographic or clinical impact on outcome due to the modest amount of lengthening done in these cases. The BHI was low (24 days/cm), which was in keeping with observations from multiple studies on the ILN in femur reconstruction [21, 24, 25].

The average distance from the intercondylar notch to the distal osteotomy site was 47 mm. This is less than is considered the minimum acceptable distance for the ILN to succeed. Few studies on retrograde ILN have documented the distance of the distal femoral osteotomy to the intercondylar notch. One study reported an average distance of 81 mm [24]. Krieg et al. [25] explain that a limitation of retrograde ILN surgery is the need for a distance of 70–110 mm from the joint line to the osteotomy site, the variation being due to differences in femur length between patients. The authors add that an apex of deformity far distal from this osteotomy site may require excessive translation precluding use of the nail [25]. A review of our surgeries utilizing a single osteotomy with a retrograde ILN to correct distal femoral deformity yielded an average distance of 85 mm (with a minimum distance of 77 mm) from the osteotomy to the intercondylar notch. For the Precice ILN, the

Table 3 Knee ROM

Patient	Pre-knee ext (deg)	Post-knee ext (deg)	Pre-knee flex (deg)	Post-knee flex (deg)
1	− 10	0	140	140
2	− 12	0	130	130
3	− 15	0	120	130
Average	− 12	0	130	133

ROM range of motion, *Pre* pre-operative, *Post* post-operative, *ext* extension, *flex* flexion, *deg* degrees

Table 4 KOOS scores

Patient	Subscale items	Pre (%)	Post (%)
1	KOOS symptoms/stiffness	71.43	100
	KOOS pain	83.33	100
	KOOS function (daily living)	91.18	100
	KOOS function (sports and recreational actives)	55.00	100
	KOOS quality of life	37.50	100
2	KOOS symptoms/stiffness	85.71	100
	KOOS pain	80.56	100
	KOOS function (daily living)	82.35	100
	KOOS function (sports and recreational actives)	50	100
	KOOS quality of life	25	100
3	KOOS symptoms/stiffness	67.86	100
	KOOS pain	50	100
	KOOS function (daily living)	100	100
	KOOS function (sports and recreational actives)	100	100
	KOOS quality of life	37.5	100

Average	Subscale items	Pre (%)	Post (%)	Average improvement (%)
	KOOS symptoms/stiffness	58.92	100	41.08
	KOOS pain	71.29	100	28.71
	KOOS function (daily living)	91.18	100	8.82
	KOOS function (sports and recreational actives)	68.33	100	31.67
	KOOS quality of life	33.33	100	66.67

KOOS Knee Injury & Osteoarthritis Outcome Score

(a)   **(b)**

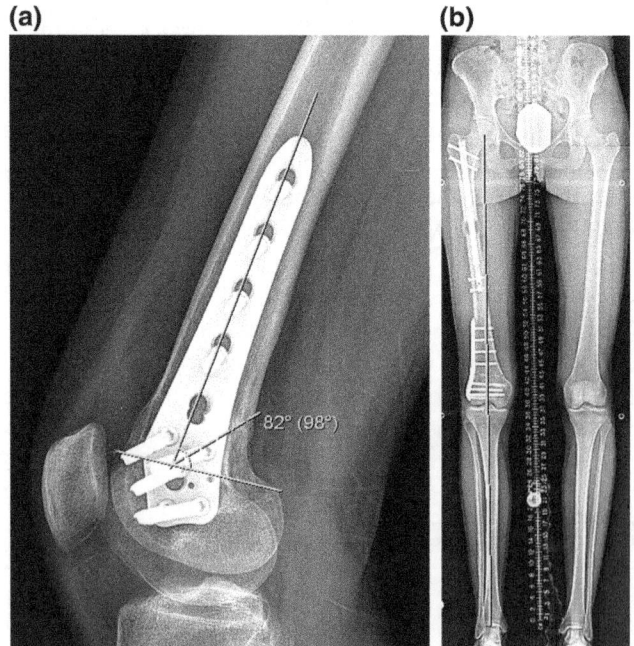

Fig. 8 a This lateral femoral radiograph of patient 1 shows a PDFA of 82°, **b** this 51 in. standing film of patient 1 shows a MAD of 0 mm

distance from the tip of the IM nail to the top of the most proximal distal locking hole is 48 mm. This would indicate that a minimum of at least 60 mm from the notch should be used to have both locking screws in bone with a margin of bone between the screw and the osteotomy to offer minimum control. It would be useful to define a zone of deformity in the distal femur ("a far-distal femoral deformity") that lies between the joint line and, approximately, 70 mm proximally where an ILN will not have sufficient control of the distal fragment. This threshold needs to be further studied.

There were no true complications including need for additional surgery for knee contracture (a common problem after LON). The implant company guidelines require removal of the ILN which was done concomitantly with the plate removal. Patients did have pain over the lateral knee which was relieved by plate removal. The need to remove the plate due to pain could be considered a complication, but this was a possibility the patient was informed of prior to surgery.

Table 5 Radiographic results

Patient	Pre-LLD (mm)	Post-LLD (mm)	Proximal osteotomy length achieved (mm)	Distal osteotomy length achieved (mm) (calculated)	Pre-MAD (mm)	Post-MAD (mm)	BHI (days/cm)
1	25	2	21	2	0	0	26
2	40	3	34	3	3 lateral	0	28
3	75	5	65	5	3 lateral	9 medial	19
Average	47	3	40	4	2 lateral	3 medial	24

Pre pre-operative, *Post* post-operative, *LLD* limb length discrepancy, *MAD* mechanical axis deviation, *BHI* bone healing index

Table 6 Distance to distal femoral osteotomy from the knee joint line and from the supracondylar notch

	Dist (mm) to osteotomy from joint	Dist (mm) to osteotomy from notch
1	50	43
2	56	44
3	66	56
Average	57	47

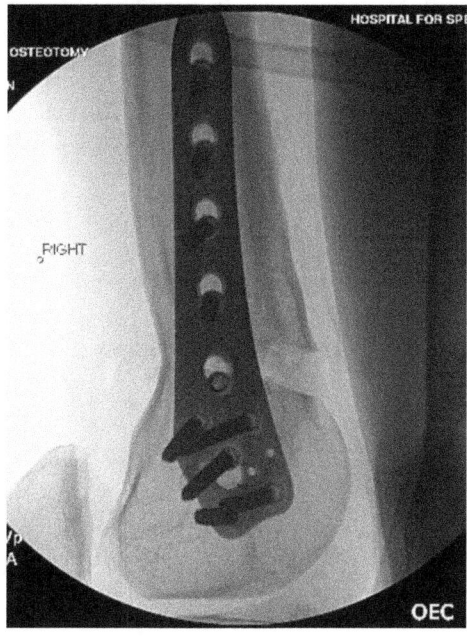

Fig. 9 This intraoperative fluoroscopy film shows the obligate anterior translational deformity of the distal femoral fragment created by leaving the anterior cortex intact. This was felt to be clinically insignificant but was recognized

Conclusion

We recommend a two-level osteotomy for distal femoral deformities where the apex of deformity is very distal and is associated with shortening. An acute distal femoral osteotomy with plating will correct the sagittal plane deformity as was shown in this case series. A correction of over 12° may affect the coronal plane alignment and will cause some anterior translation of the distal fragment in the sagittal plane. Rotational correction can be performed acutely through the proximal osteotomy. It is unlikely the patient will need a blood transfusion if tranexamic acid is used intraoperatively and we no longer recommend cross-matched blood to be available. Knee range of motion will improve in extension and remain unchanged in flexion if the amount of lengthening is modest.

Informed consent Informed consent was obtained from all individual participants included in the study.

References

1. Basener CJ, Mehlman CT, DiPasquale TG (2009) Growth disturbance after distal femoral growth plate fractures in children: a meta-analysis. J Orthop Trauma 23(9):663–667
2. Spiro AS, Stenger P, Hoffmann M, Vettorazzi E, Babin K, Lipovac S, Kolb JP, Novo de Oliveira A, Rueger JM, Stuecker R (2012) Treatment of fixed knee flexion deformity by anterior distal femoral stapling. Knee Surg Sports Traumatol Arthrosc 20(12):2413–2418. doi:10.1007/s00167-012-1915-8
3. Klatt J, Stevens PM (2008) Guided growth for fixed knee flexion deformity. J Pediatr Orthop 28(6):626–631
4. de Morais Filho MC, Neves DL, Abreu FP, Juliano Y, Guimarães L (2008) Treatment of fixed knee flexion deformity and crouch gait using distal femur extension osteotomy in cerebral palsy. J Child Orthop 2(1):37–43
5. de Moraes BarrosFucs PM, Svartman C, de Assumpção RM (2005) Knee flexion deformity from poliomyelitis treated by supracondylar femoral extension osteotomy. Int Orthop 29(6):380–384
6. Grant AD, Small RD, Lehman WB (1982) Correction of flexion deformity of the knee by supracondylar osteotomy. Bull Hosp Joint Dis Orthop Inst 42(1):28–38
7. Kocaoglu M, Eralp L, Bilen FE, Balci HI (2009) Fixator-assisted acute femoral deformity correction and consecutive lengthening over an intramedullary nail. J Bone Joint Surg Am 91(1):152–159

8. McCarthy JJ, Ranade A, Davidson RS (2008) Pediatric deformity correction using a multiaxial correction fixator. Clin Orthop Relat Res 466(12):3011–3017

9. Zarek S, Macias J (2002) The Ilizarov method in the treatment of postinflammatory deformites of the distal epiphysis of the femur. Ortop Traumatol Rehabil 4(3):341–347

10. Kawoosa AA, Wani IH, Dar FA, Sultan A, Qazi M, Halwai MA (2015) Deformity correction about knee with Ilizarov technique: accuracy of correction and effectiveness of gradual distraction after conventional straight cut osteotomy. Ortop Traumatol Rehabil 17(6):587–592

11. Pallaro J, Angelliaume A, Dunet B, Lavoinne N, Tournier C, Fabre T (2015) Reconstruction of femoral bone loss with a monoplane external fixator and bone transport. Orthop Traumatol Surg Res 101(5):583–587. doi:10.1016/j.otsr.2015.04.001

12. Khakharia S, Fragomen AT, Rozbruch SR (2009) Limited quadricepsplasty for contracture during femoral lengthening. Clin Orthop Rel Res 467(11):2911–2917

13. Hosalkar HS, Jones S, Chowdhury M, Hartley J, Hill RA (2003) Quadricepsplasty for knee stiffness after femoral lengthening in congenital short femur. J Bone Joint Surg Br 85(2):261–264

14. Koczewski P, Shadi M (2005) Repair of the knee extension apparatus in the treatment of knee extension contracture after femoral lengthening. Chir Narz Ruchu Ortop Pol 70(2):91–96

15. Georgiadis AG, Rossow JK, Laine JC, Iobst CA, Dahl MT (2017) Plate-assisted lengthening of the femur and tibia in pediatric patients. J Pediatr Orthop 37(7):473–478

16. Iobst CA, Dahl MT (2007) Limb lengthening with submuscular plate stabilization: a case series and description of the technique. Pediatr Orthop 27(5):504–509

17. Black SR, Kwon MS, Cherkashin AM, Samchukov ML, Birch JG, Jo CH (2015) Lengthening in congenital femoral deficiency: a comparison of circular external fixation and a motorized intramedullary nail. J Bone Joint Surg Am 97(17):1432–1440

18. Landge V, Shabtai L, Gesheff M, Specht SC, Herzenberg JE (2015) Patient satisfaction after limb lengthening with internal and external devices. J Surg Orthop Adv 24(3):174–179

19. Harbacheuski R, Fragomen AT, Rozbruch SR (2012) Does lengthening and plating shorten duration of external fixation? Clin Orthop Relat Res 470(6):1771–1781

20. Baumgart R, Betz A, Schweiberer L (1997) A fully implantable motorized intramedullary nail for limb lengthening and bone transport. Clin Orthop 343:135–143

21. Kirane Y, Fragomen A, Rozbruch SR (2014) Precision of the PRECICE internal bone lengthening nail. Clin Orthop Rel Res 472(12):3869–3878

22. Roos EM, Roos HP, Lohmander LS, Ekdahl C, Beynnon BD (1998) Knee Injury and Osteoarthritis Outcome Score (KOOS)—development of a self-administered outcome measure. J Orthop Sports Phys Ther 28(2):88–96

23. Burghardt RD, Paley D, Specht SC, Herzenberg JE (2012) The effect on mechanical axis deviation of femoral lengthening with an intramedullary telescopic nail. J Bone Joint Surg Br 94(9):1241–1245

24. Kucukkaya M, Karakoyun O, Erol MF (2016) The importance of reaming the posterior femoral cortex before inserting lengthening nails calculation of the amount of reaming. J Orthop Surg Res 11:11

25. Krieg AH, Lenze U, Speth BM, Hasler CC (2011) Intramedullary leg lengthening with a motorized nail. Acta Orthop 82(3):344–350

16

Multiple osteochondromas (MO) in the forearm: a 12-year single-centre experience

John Ham[1] · Mark Flipsen[1] · Marianne Koolen[1] · Arnard van der Zwan[1] ·
Konrad Mader[2,3]

Abstract Multiple osteochondromas (MO) are a rare autosomal dominant disorder characterized by the presence of osteochondromas located on the long bones and axial skeleton. Patients present with growth disturbances and angular deformities of the long bones as well as limited motion of affected joints. Forearm involvement is found in a considerable number of patients and may vary from the presence of a simple osteochondroma to severe forearm deformities and radial head dislocation. Patients encounter a variety of problems and symptoms e.g., pain, functional impairment, loss of strength and cosmetic concerns. Several surgical procedures are offered from excision of symptomatic osteochondromas to challenging reconstructions of forearm deformities. We describe visualizing, planning and treating these forearm deformities in MO and, in particular, a detailed account of the surgical correction of Masada type I and Masada type II MO forearm deformities.

Keywords Multiple hereditary exostoses (MHE) ·
Multiple osteochondromas (MO) · Masada classification ·
Forearm reconstruction · Corrective osteotomy · External
fixation · Review

✉ Konrad Mader
    konrad.mader@outlook.com

[1] Orthopædic Department, Expertise Center MO, OLVG,
    Amsterdam, The Netherlands

[2] Section Upper Extremity, Department of Orthopaedic,
    Trauma and Spine Surgery, Asklepios Klinik Altona,
    22763 Hamburg, Germany

[3] Berliner Freiheit 9, Aalto- Hochhaus 14/9, 28327 Bremen,
    Germany

Introduction

Multiple osteochondromas (MO), also known as multiple hereditary exostoses (MHE), are disorder of endochondral bone growth producing abnormal metaphyseal bony prominences capped with cartilage. It is accompanied by defective metaphyseal remodelling and asymmetrical retardation of longitudinal bone growth [1]. MO is a rare, monogenetic, autosomal dominant disorder with an estimated prevalence of 1: 50,000 according to the older literature and 1:20,000–30,000 in more recent publications for the Dutch population [2, 3]. It is caused by loss of function mutations in either the exostosin-1 (EXT1 on chromosome 8) or exostosin-2 (EXT2 on chromosome 11) gene [4]. EXT1 and EXT2 mutations are found in over 90 % of all MO cases [5]. Whilst in 10 % of cases no EXT1 or EXT2 gene mutation is found, a third EXT loci has not been identified. A family history of MO exists in approximately 70–80 % of affected individuals, whereas 20–30 % of the cases are spontaneous mutations [3].

The forearm is involved in MO often, and osteochondromas are found most notably in the distal radius and ulna. Deformities of the forearm are reported in approximately 40–80 % of the patients and can be unilateral or bilateral, whereas one forearm is usually more severely affected than the other [1, 6–9]. Wrist osteochondromas and the developmental deformity give rise to complaints of pain and or progressive limitation of forearm rotation during growth. It has been suggested that the severity of forearm deformity correlates with overall disease severity and the risk of malignant degeneration [8].

The most common forearm deformities are:

1. a combination of relative shortening of either (usually the ulna) or both forearms

2. bowing of either one or both forearm bones
3. increased ulnar tilt of the distal radial epiphysis
4. ulnar deviation of the hand
5. progressive ulnar translocation of the carpus and
6. dislocation of the radial head [1, 6, 10–13].

The different deformities of the forearm are often classified according to the Masada deformity scale [11]; (Fig. 1). The treatment of these forearm deformities is difficult, and there is no consensus to overall management.

This report describes the strategies evolved by a MO-study group treating a large population of children with this disease in the Netherlands over the last 12 years.

The Amsterdam MO database

In the Netherlands, the OLVG (Amsterdam) is regarded an expert centre for MO. Almost 600 patients with MO have been entered into a prospective database for various studies including a large series of 120 patients with forearm osteochondromas and deformities (140 forearms, surgically treated since 2002 by three surgeons AvdZ, JH and KM). Surgical procedures performed included excision of osteochondromas, ulnar lengthening, radial corrective

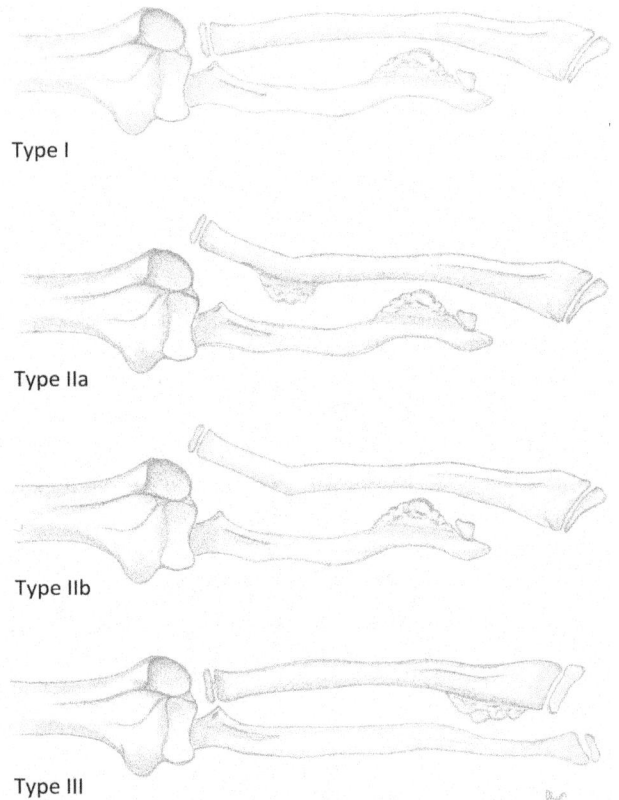

Type I

Type IIa

Type IIb

Type III

Fig. 1 Schematic drawing of the Masada classification for forearm deformity in patients with MO [drawing by M.F., modified after 8]

osteotomy (proximal and distal), and excision of the radial head and neck (as a salvage procedure). A combination of procedures has been performed, e.g., corrective osteotomies of the radius (with plates) and lengthening of the ulna using hydroxyapatite-coated pins in a monolateral external fixator. All patients were counselled and provided informed consent to a structured treatment plan (Fig. 4). This is the strategy for treatment of forearm involvement in MO, and we describe the surgical technique for the extensive combined procedures performed in patients with severe forearm deformities and impaired function.

Fundamentals of MO in the forearm

The Masada classification for forearm deformity from MO has been used since 1989 [11]. The classification is based on the morphological characteristics of the deformity on plain radiographs (Fig. 1). Three types are identified:

Type I The main osteochondroma formation is located in the distal portion of the ulna. The ulna is shortened, and there is bowing of the radius. However, the radial head is not dislocated (this is the most common type in 55–61 % of cases).

Type II In addition to ulnar shortening, the radial head is dislocated (22–33 % of patients). Bowing of the radius is less pronounced than in type I, and this could be an effect of the dislocation. In *subtype IIA*, the radial head is dislocated because of an additional osteochondroma at the proximal metaphysis of the radius. In *subtype IIB*, whilst there are osteochondromas at the distal ulna, there are none detectable in this region. Dislocation of the radial head leads to rotational impairment of pronation in general.

Type III The main osteochondroma formation is in the metaphysis of the distal radius, and there is relative shortening of the radius.

According to Masada et al. [11], this classification indicates both the severity of the forearm deformity and the functional disabilities. Forearm rotation is most severely impaired in type I, whereas elbow motion is normal. Type II shows restriction of both elbow movement and forearm rotation. Radial deviation of the wrist is severely restricted in both subtypes. Type III retains most forearm and elbow movement, but ulnar deviation of the wrist is restricted and painful often.

Diagnosis and imaging

Anteroposterior radiographs of the entire forearm in full supination and pronation, completed with a lateral view are necessary to:

- visualize the presence of symptomatic and function-limiting osteochondromas
- to define the deformities in both forearm bones
- image all four joints (elbow, wrist, distal- and proximal radioulnar joints)
- to determine the centre of rotation and angulation (CORA) in case osteotomies have to be planned
- to locate the most appropriate site for ulnar lengthening (Fig. 2).

PA or AP radiographs can be obtained with the arm placed on the imaging plate with the shoulder at 90° of abduction and the elbow at 90° of flexion and for as far as is tolerable within patients' range of motion. The beam is orthogonally directed towards the forearm in neutral position in the PA direction. Several angles and other variables can be measured on the radiographs and form the basis for follow-up during growth or outcome after forearm reconstruction. The two most important radiographic measurements are the radial articular angle (RAA) and the carpal slip (CS). These measurements are used frequently in the assessment, classification and follow-up of forearm deformities and were first described by Fogel et al. [14]. The RAA is the angle between two lines: one along the articular surface of the radius and the other perpendicular to a line from the centre of the radial head to the radial edge of the radial epiphysis. The normal value of the RAA is between 15 and 30° (Fig. 2) [14, 15]. The CS is measured as the percentage of the lunate in contact with the joint surface of the distal radius, using a line drawn from the centre of the olecranon through the ulnar edge of the radial epiphysis. This line bisects the lunate normally which makes the CS abnormal if ulnar displacement of the lunate is more than 50 % [11, 16]. These measurements are of interest since both have implications for loads across the lunate. An increase of CS or a decrease of RAA will intensify the radio-carpal force, with potential links to arthritic changes, pain and loss of range of motion. MRI can provide additional information on the extent of osteochondromas, the width of the cartilage cap, and the relation to or involvement of neurovascular structures. It can show changes in the ligamentous structures in both the joints and the intraosseous membrane, visualize the pathoanatomy of the soft tissues in chronic radial head dislocations and display the organization of the distal radioulnar joint (DRUJ) in complex ulnar-minus variants.

CT scans display the distorted anatomy at different angles as well in 3D and are useful in surgical planning. These images are very informative and helpful during the counselling of the patient and their relatives. CT images give more insight into joint anatomy and may visualize (early) degenerative changes. Special scanning protocols

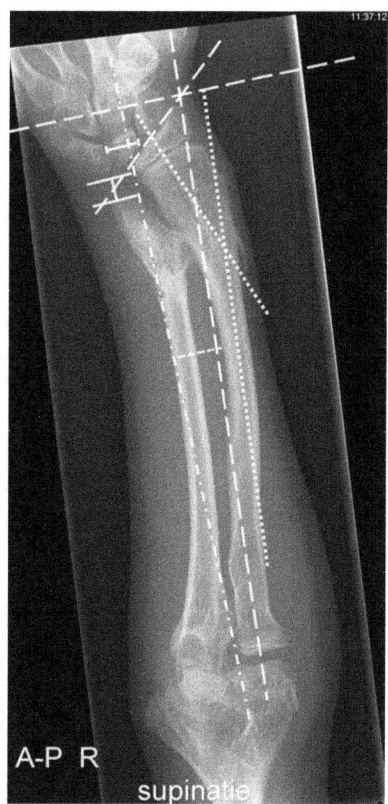

Fig. 2 AP X-ray of the right forearm in a 14-year-old patient from the OLVG MO forearm database with Masada type I deformity: measurement of the RAA, CS, UV, RB and CORA [13]. *Dashed dotted lines* radial articular angle (RAA) between (1) a line perpendicular to a line that bisects the head of the radius and passes through the radial edge of the distal radial epiphysis and (2) a line along the articular surface of the distal radius. Normal values are defined between 15° and 30° by Fogel et al. [1]. Value measured: 43.1°. ⊢—⊣ Carpal slip (CS) percentage of the lunate surface in contact with the radius, as limited by the axial line drawn from the ulnar edge of the radial head through the ulnar edge of the radial epiphysis. This line normally bisects the lunate. Normal values for CS are >50 %. Value measured: 38 %. ⊤ Ulnar variance (UV) distance between the distal end of the ulna to the ulnar border of the distal radial epiphysis measured along the axial line. Normal values <15 mm. Value measured: 8.8 mm. *Dashed lines* radial bowing (RB) greatest distance between the radial diaphysis and the axial line. Normal values are defined as <12 mm. Value measured: 17.2 mm. *Dotted lines* centre of rotation of angulation (CORA) the intersection of the proximal axis and distal axis of a deformed bone

with the neighbouring joints can be used for computerized planning templates.

Should MO forearm deformities be operated on and, if so, when?

Despite the 25 years following the original paper by Masada, the optimal treatment for an individual patient with MO of the forearm is unresolved. Published studies in the past are critiqued for being poorly designed, being retrospective case series with short follow-up, lacking detailed descriptions of the types of deformations (Masada-types) treated, using different indications for surgery (if mentioned at all), using different surgical procedures, and lacking outcome measurements. A lack of information on external validity items and well-defined outcomes can lead to difficulties in extrapolating the results of a study to other MO-patients with forearm deformities. Although the review performed on the outcome of surgical treatment by this study group showed an overall benefit from surgery, there was no control group for a comparison to the natural history of the condition [17]. Data on this are lacking and as such a comparison to those treated difficult [18].

The age reconstructive surgery should be performed in children is debatable. There are two opposing opinions in the literature. Several authors recommend early surgical intervention, but in their report the mean follow-up is short and appears insufficient to assess for recurrence [10]. The second view, represented by Akita et al., proposes a less aggressive approach involving surgical interventions towards the end of the growth spurt. The longer-term follow-up (13 years) of their study revealed recurrence in children who underwent surgery too early [1]. We share the same experience; we counsel and follow the patients, if possible, until the age of 13–15 years and recommend intervention then and as one correction.

As with Litzelmann et al., we see radial head instability to be a major prognostic factor as this is associated with symptoms frequently. If progressive radial head dislocations are detected, ulnar lengthening by callus distraction and corrective osteotomy of the radius should be considered early. This is done to avoid development of pain or restriction of pronation and supination at the elbow level [10, 19]. The maintenance of a reduced radial head following these "levelling or rebalancing procedures" is, however, uncertain and a second (salvage) procedure necessary at a later stage.

MO-study group protocol

Specific indications for surgery are determined. Pain due to impingement of an osteochondroma, restriction of motion, functional deficits, loss of strength, severity of deformity and/or dislocation of the radial head are recorded. The Masada classification still forms the basis for surgery.

1. Patients with Masada type I deformity with mild radial bowing and mild symptoms will be counselled for conservative treatment and receive yearly follow-up. In patients with large osteochondromas which are painful despite minimal functional impairment,

elective removal of the symptomatic osteochondroma is recommended as are those which give rise to gradual erosion and deformity of the adjacent bone and limited rotation and pain.

2. Patients with advanced deformity and major functional impairment will be counselled to wait until the age of 13. Only if there is a large impact on daily living would a corrective osteotomy of the radius and lengthening with monolateral fixation, even at young age, be performed and with yearly follow-up. In patients with Masada type IIA deformity, removal of the proximal osteochondroma (as they are painful) and, in type IIB, removal of the ulnar osteochondroma is recommended. An expectant approach is carried out for Masada type II problems if symptoms are mild and the radial head is stable. If advanced functional impairment as well as instability and pain is present, we either plan a 2-stage procedure (first levelling of the forearm bones and, later, a radial head resection—rarely) or we advocate a complex correction with indirect reduction of the radial head using a ring fixator [20, 21].

3. In patients with type III deformity, we offer to remove the painful osteochondroma but counsel most patients to wait until growth is completed. Some patients in this group need treatment for their positive ulnar variance, usually by ulnar shortening osteotomy.

Correction in advanced MO Masada type I or levelling procedure in Masada IIB

Thorough counselling is recommended prior to a full treatment plan being advocated. These reconstructive procedures are elective, and a clinical benefit remains to be proven. In large deformities, we start with a corrective osteotomy of the radius (Fig. 3), but in those with a mild deformity of the radius, ulnar lengthening (often paired with slight translation of the distal ulnar segment to avoid impingement in the DRUJ) is possible. If using monolateral fixators, it is important to correct acutely the concomitant deformation of the ulna (bowing, rotation and adduction of the distal ulna due to tethering effect of the soft tissues and disorientation of the distal ulnar growth plate) through appropriate placement of the fixator pins (Fig. 3). The osteotomy is performed percutaneously using a sharp drill through a drill-guide with normal saline cooling and completion of the osteotomy with a sharp chisel. Care must be taken not to split the bone, especially in the area where an osteochondroma has been removed as the bone can be brittle. An intraoperative test for distraction is performed to ensure completion of the osteotomy. Distraction for

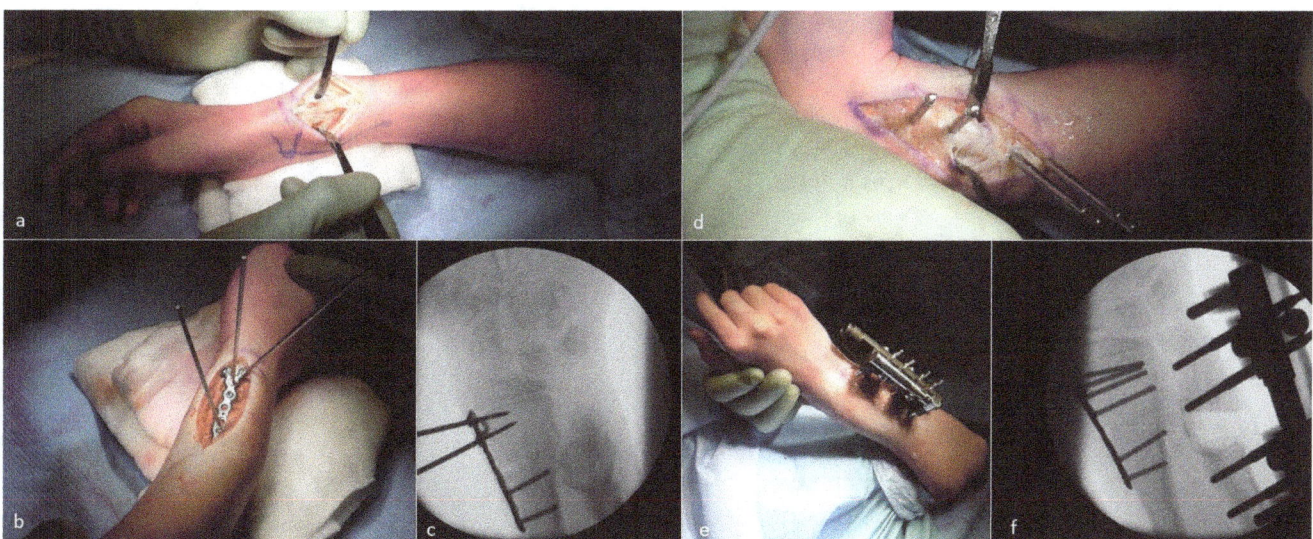

Fig. 3 Intraoperative images of a corrective osteotomy and ulnar lengthening fixator application at the right forearm with a Masada type I deformity (patient from Fig. 2). **a** clinical image of the right forearm, after marking of the CORA the osteotomy site at the radius is exposed; **b** a closing wedge osteotomy is performed (15°) using FFS (Orthofix®) for temporary fixation and a low profile plate (Medartis®); **c** fluoroscopic image showing correction of the radius and good positioning of the plate proximal to the growth plate; **d** via a direct ulnar approach 4 fixator pins are placed into the distal ulna, note the use of different angles both in rotation and abduction of the pins in order to correct the deformity of the ulna by pin placement; **e** the monolateral lengthening fixator is mounted, both radius and ulna are straightened; **f** fluoroscopy shows the radius osteotomy and a nice alignment of the ulna (under test distraction)

gradual lengthening starts after a latency period of a minimum of 5 days post-operatively with 3×0.25 mm lengthening per day until the target length (levelling) is reached.

Preoperative planning and the surgical technique

All surgeries for the past 14 years were performed with prior counselling of the patient and parent(s) and with full informed consent; special emphasis was made to consider the relative merits of operative and conservative treatment (Fig. 4). In all cases, the main indication for surgery was pain and/or functional impairment, documented as an active and passive motion of both the wrist and elbow using the neutral—0—method. Preoperative planning was an essential and integral part of deformity correction surgery. In all cases forearm radiographs, and later CT scan reconstruction images, were used for conceptual drawings of surgery and to formulate a structured treatment plan [21]; key information on the medical condition and treatment history, symptoms and functional impairment, the problems (deformity) to be addressed, the planning method used (conventional versus computerized), the surgical procedure (with the different operative steps), the equipment needed and potential obstacles during or after the surgery (Fig. 4). A basic stepwise approach was used for analysing the deformity. In cases of combined procedures (i.e., removal of one or more osteochondromas at the distal radius or ulna in conjunction with a corrective osteotomy

of the radius and monolateral lengthening of the ulna), the osteochondromas were removed first followed by an osteotomy of the radius at the CORA with the application of a monolateral lengthening fixator. In all cases, hydroxyapatite screws (Orthofix®) were used and the Pennig monolateral lengthener (Orthofix®).

All operations were performed by consultant orthopaedic surgeons, with a minimum of two surgeons assisting each other (JH, AvdZ, KM). Full general anaesthesia and a tourniquet (200 mmHg for a maximum of 90 min) and hand table were used. Fluoroscopy was used to mark the deformity, the CORA at the radius, the osteotomy level and pin insertion areas in the ulna.

A direct radial approach to the radius over the CORA was performed with the superficial branch of the radial nerve visualized and protected. In most cases, a closing wedge osteotomy was performed using the Fragment Fixation System (FFS; Orthofix®) for temporary fixation and a low profile plate (Depuy Synthes® or Medartis®) for definitive fixation. Great care was taken not to damage the distal growth plate of the radius (Fig. 3). From the preoperative planning, four fixator pins (typically 80 mm length with 20 mm thread length (conical blunt-tipped and hydroxyapatite coated, Orthofix®) were placed into the distal ulna through stab incisions. Using special screw and drill guides and with predrilling and cooling, different angles of pin placement with regard to rotation and abduction allowed for pre-emptive correction of the deformity of the ulna (Fig. 4). Meticulous care was taken

Fig. 4 Printout of a structured treatment plan for a 14-year-old patient with MO Masada I

Case 1. ♀ name of patient
(DOB) 14 years, R

Diagnosis: HME Masada I
Problems and complaints: Pain and forearm rotation impairment, elbow free, pain over osteochondroma
Carpal slip over 50%, RAA over 40°
Plan:
Excision osteochrondroma ulna
-    ulna lengthening
-    corrective osteotomy radius (closing wedge 15° at CORA)
Equipment: Mediartis plates, Pennig wrist monolateral lenghtening fixator, HA pins

Surgeon: John Ham
Assistant: Konrad Mader

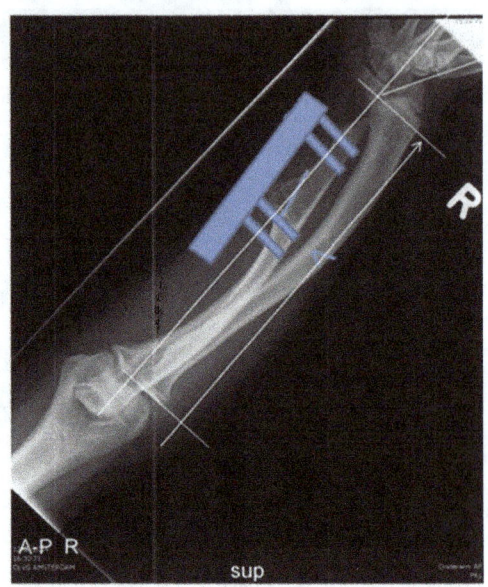

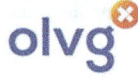

for good purchase and bicortical penetration of all pins, which was difficult due to previous or simultaneous resection of osteochondromas in the area. The osteotomy was performed using a sharp drill and a chisel whilst preserving the periosteum. The monolateral lengthening fixator was mounted, the acute re-alignment of the ulna was documented, and a test distraction performed (Fig. 3). Wounds were closed using resorbable subcutaneous and skin sutures. A posterior backslab cast with the wrist in neutral position was applied. After a waiting period of 5 days (usually), lengthening was performed following a written protocol (0.25 mm × 3 per day) until the required length was reached. The fixator was removed under light anaesthesia when callus maturation was documented by standard radiographs (three cortices visible).

Outcome

From a systematic review (unpublished) of 16 studies, both the ulnar lengthening procedure and a radial correction with ulnar lengthening improved clinical and radiographic parameters significantly [17]. All clinical and radiographic parameters of patients with MO of the forearm were worse than in healthy individuals before surgery; patients with worse baseline parameters benefited the most from surgery.

Ulnar lengthening with or without excision of osteochondroma(s) improved range of motion of the forearm and elbow, wrist radial deviation, the forearm bone length discrepancy (levelling), radial bowing, radial articular angle and carpal slip of the forearm. A radial osteotomy and or radial stapling with or without ulnar lengthening or excision of osteochondromas had the same improvement across the same parameters; there were fewer radial head dislocations after the procedure(s). Simple removal of osteochondromas seemed to improve the range of motion but without improvement of radiographic parameters (RAA, CS).

Post-surgical patient-reported outcomes were improved, but the complication rate of ulnar lengthening was high. Radial osteotomy and or radial stapling with or without excision of osteochondroma showed a lower complication rate but a higher risk of recurrence.

The internal and external validity of the included studies in the systematic review was low as important criteria were missing on different items. A lack of information on internal validity items, such as the representativeness of the study group, duration of follow-up, blind assessment of the outcome and adjustment for other factors could have led to invalid results. This demonstrated that the results of surgical management for forearm deformities in patients with multiple osteochondromas are, as yet, not yet clear.

A lack of evidence as to which procedure gives optimal results in forearm MO long-term prompted a review of our own data before starting a prospective trial. From retrospective studies in which the first 94 patients (125 forearms) operated on were included, we concluded that significant improvements were made in pain complaints and range of motion by excision of osteochondromas or corrective procedures in patients with forearm deformities in MO. Following the treatment protocol described, significant improvements were made for Masada type 0 (no deformities but only symptomatic osteochondroma(s) resulting in pain or functional loss) and type I patients in the parameters of pronation, supination, dorsal extension, and radial deviation after 2, 5 and 10 years. Additionally, for Masada type 0 and I patients pain improved significantly after excision of osteochondromas. Compared to Masada type 0 and I, Masada type II, patients tend to have lower preoperative DASH scores, more severe functional impairment and have from aesthetic concerns.

Conclusion

We present a summary of a treatment protocol and the basis for visualizing, planning and treating forearm deformities in MO. We have described our current method of surgical correction of Masada type I and the levelling procedure in Masada type II MO forearm deformities. Whilst initial results are encouraging, more research is needed for prognostic variables that might influence outcome and patient satisfaction in surgery for forearm abnormalities from multiple osteochondromas.

Informed consent Informed consent was obtained from all individual participants included in the study.

References

1. Akita S, Murase T, Yonenobu K, Shimada K, Masada K, Yoshikawa H (2007) Long-term results of surgery for forearm deformities in patients with multiple cartilagenous exostoses. JBJS AM 89:1993–1999
2. Schmale GA, Conrad EU III, Raskind WH (1994) The natural history of hereditary multiple exostoses. J Bone Joint Surg 76A:986–992
3. Goud AL, de Lange J, Scholtes VAB, Bulstra SW, Ham SJ (2012) Pain, physical and social functioning and quality of life in individuals with hereditary multiple exostoses in the Netherlands. A national cohort study. J Bone Joint Surg 94A:1013–1020
4. Wuyts W, van Hul W, Wauters J et al (1996) Positional cloning of a gene involved in hereditary multiple exostoses. Hum Mol Genet 5:1547–1557
5. Jennes I, Pedrini E, Zuntini M et al (2009) Multiple osteochondromas: mutation update and description of the multiple osteochondromas mutation database (MOdb). Hum Mutat 30:1620–1627
6. Westhoff B, Stefanovska K, Kraupse R (2014) Multiple kartilaginäre Exostosenkrankheit. Orthopäde 43:725–732
7. Shapiro F, Simon S, Glimcher MJ (1979) Hereditary multiple exostoses. Anthropometric, roentgenographic, and clinical aspects. J Bone Joint Surg Am 61(6A):815–824
8. Taniguchi K (1995) A practical classification system for multiple cartilaginous exostosis in children. J Pediatr Orthop 15(5):585–591
9. Ham SJ (2013) Multiple hereditary exostoses. Clinical problems and therapeutic solutions. Orthop Trauma 27:118–125
10. Litzelmann E, Mazda K, Jehanna P, Brasher C, Pennecot G-F, Ilarreborde B (2012) Forearm deformities in hereditary multiple exostosis: clinical and functional results at maturity. J Pediatr Orthop 32:1835–1841
11. Masada K, Tsuyuguchi Y, Kawai H, Kawabata H, Noguchi K, Ono K (1989) Operations for forearm caused by multiple osteochondromas. J Bone Joint Surg Br 71B:24–29
12. Shin EK, Jones NF, Lawrence JF (2006) Treatment of multiple hereditary osteochondromas of the forearm in children. J Bone Joint Br 88:255–260
13. Hill RA, Ibrahim T, Mann HA, Siapkara A (2011) Forearm lengthening by distraction osteogenesis in children: a report of 22 cases. J Bone Joint Surg Br 93:1550–1555
14. Fogel GR, McElfresh EC, Peterson HA, Wicklund PT (1984) Management of deformities of the forearm in multiple hereditary osteochondromas. J Bone Joint Surg Am 66-A:670–680
15. Burgess RC, Cates H (1993) Deformities of the forearm in patients who have multiple cartilaginous exostosis. J Bone Joint Surg Am 75-A:13–18
16. Mader K, Gausepohl T, Pennig D (2003) Shortening and deformity of radius and ulna in Children: correction of axis and length by callus distraction. J Pediatr Surg B 12:183–191
17. Koolen M, Flipsen M, Mader K, Ham J (2016) Evaluation of the surgical management of patients with multiple hereditary osteochondromata of the forearm: a systematic review. Bone Joint J
18. Noonan KJ, Levenda A, Snead J, Feinberg JR, Mih A (2002) Evaluation of the forearm in untreated adult subjects with multiple hereditary osteochondromatosis. J Bone Joint Surg Am 84-A(3):397–403
19. Beutel BG, Klifto CS, Chu A (2014) Timing of forearm deformity correction in a child with multiple hereditary exostosis. Am J Orthop 43:422–425
20. Song SH, Lee H, Youssef H, Oh SM, Park JH, Song HR (2013) Modified Ilizarov technique for the treatment of forearm deformities in multiple cartilaginous exostoses: case series and literature review. J Hand Surg Eur 38:288–296
21. Villa A, Paley D, Catagni MA, Cattaneo R (1990) Lengthening of the forearm by the Ilizarov technique. Clin Orthop Rel Res 250:125–137

17

Evaluation of the muscle morphology of the obturator externus and piriformis as the predictors of avascular necrosis of the femoral head in acetabular fractures

Lalit Maini[1] · Santosh Kumar[1] · Sahil Batra[1] · Rajat Gupta[1] · Sumit Arora[1,2]

Abstract Avascular necrosis (AVN) of femoral head is a recognised complication of fracture dislocation of the hip joint but is not studied frequently in relation to acetabulum fractures. The aim was to establish the relationship between obturator externus and piriformis muscle morphology in acetabulum fractures and potenital development of AVN of the femoral head. Twenty-five fractures were included in this prospective study and were subjected to radiological assessment and computed tomography of the pelvis. Magnetic resonance imaging (MRI) of the hip was performed to assess the morphology of obturator externus and piriformis, and findings were compared intraoperatively (in 15 cases). Serial radiographs were taken at monthly intervals to assess the development of avascular necrosis. The patients with no evidence of AVN on radiographs at 6 months had additional MRI scans to look for such changes. Three patients developed AVN of femoral head and two had complete tears of piriformis and/or obturator externus muscles on the pre-operative MRI with the findings confirmed intraoperatively ($p = 0.013$). None of the patients without changes of AVN at 6-month follow-up had complete tears of either or both muscles. Of these patients, there was one case each of T-type fracture, isolated posterior wall fracture with hip dislocation, and posterior wall with transverse fracture of the acetabulum. Complete tears of obturator externus and/or piriformis muscles are a strong predictor of future development of AVN of the femoral head.

Keywords Avascular necrosis · Femoral head · Acetabular fracture · Obturator externus · Piriformis

Introduction

Acetabular fractures result from high-energy trauma in which soft tissues around the involved hip are severely affected. These cases may, at times, be associated with dislocation of the hip joint and lead to avascular necrosis (AVN) of femoral head potentially. The incidence of AVN has been reported to be 0–11.8 % and attributed as a sequel of the initial dislocation or subsequent to surgery [1–10]. No study has been undertaken, to the authors' knowledge, to investigate femoral head AVN after acetabular fractures.

The relevant nutrient vessel to the femoral head in adults is the deep branch of the medial femoral circumflex artery (MFCA) [11]. It may be injured during the posterior approach to the hip and acetabulum. There are two central and five peripheral anastomoses of the MFCA [11]. All of the peripheral anastomoses have been observed to be extracapsular with the largest and the most consistent being a branch of the inferior gluteal artery which runs along the inferior border of piriformis. Gautier et al. [11] stated the piriformis branch might play a role in vascularisation of the femoral head after injury of the deep branch of the MFCA. They observed also the obturator externus muscle protects the MFCA when the hip is dislocated. Theoretically, an intact obturator externus tendon would imply a preserved blood supply to the femoral head if no additional intracapsular lesion of the MFCA is present.

✉ Sumit Arora
  mamc_309@yahoo.co.in

1 Department of Orthopaedic Surgery, Maulana Azad Medical College and Associated Lok Nayak Hospital, New Delhi 110002, India

2 C/o Mr. Sham Khanna, 2/2, Vijay Nagar, Delhi 110009, India

We sought to evaluate the possible association between the integrity of obturator externus and piriformis muscle and femoral head vascularity in acetabular fractures prospectively. We investigated the possible association of acetabular fracture pattern on development of AVN of the femoral head.

Patients and methods

The study was undertaken in a government-based tertiary care teaching hospital between July 2011 and April 2013. All consecutive patients presenting with acetabular fractures were evaluated by two authors (LM and SK) for possible inclusion in the study by the following criteria: (1) closed pelvic fractures; (2) age group 18–60 years; (3) injury less than 2 weeks old; (4) adequate pelvis radiographs and Judet views. All patients with pre-existing hip disease, ipsilateral fracture of the head and neck of the femur, inter-trochanteric fracture, or with any contraindication for an MRI examination were excluded. Those with fractures associated with life-threatening complications were excluded also. There were 25 patients who met the requirements. Written informed consent was obtained from each patient and approval from the Institutional Review Board granted.

These patients had non-contrast computed tomography (NCCT, with 3-dimensional reconstructions) and plain radiographs to evaluate the anatomy and type of fracture. Magnetic resonance imaging (MRI) of the pelvis and both hips were performed to assess the integrity of obturator externus and piriformis muscles. The scans were obtained with an advanced high-field 1.5-T scanner (Sonata Magnetom, Siemens) using the standard protocol. The muscle injury was graded as proposed by Rybak et al. [12]. The system included grade 1 (oedema only no discontinuity of fibres—contusion); grade 2 (partial tear); and grade 3 (complete tear) pattern of muscle injury.

The mode of treatment (non-operative or operative) was decided on an individual basis after evaluating the general condition, fracture displacement, hip joint stability, and congruity. All cases were operated by an experienced pelvi-acetabular trauma surgeon (LM). The appropriate surgical approaches were chosen based on the fracture pattern and surgeon's experience. The clinical morphology of obturator externus and piriformis could not be evaluated for the patients that were managed non-operatively or those operated with an anterior approach alone. Fracture fixation was done using a variety of 3.5-mm reconstruction plates, 6.5-mm cancellous lag screws, 4.0-mm cancellous lag screws, and 3.5-mm cortical screws (lengths up to 120 mm) and 6.5-mm fully threaded cancellous screws depending on fracture pattern. All the implants were made of titanium metal so that an MRI could be done 6 months post-operatively if required.

The reduction of the fracture fragments was evaluated post-operatively with similar antero-posterior and Judet view radiographs. The immediate post-operative reduction was evaluated and graded according to radiological grading as described by Matta and Merritt [13]. Patients were kept non-weight bearing for a period of 6–12 weeks depending on the stability of fixation. Full weight bearing was allowed after 12–20 weeks after surgery. Serial radiographs were taken at monthly interval to assess the fracture healing and detect the development of avascular necrosis of femoral head. All patients who had normal femoral head appearances on radiographs at the end of 6 months had further MRI evaluation for development of avascular necrosis of femoral head. The functional status was assessed at 6 months according to Merle d' Aubigne scoring system [14].

The analysis of data was performed using Statistical Package for Social Science (SPSS Inc. version 17.0 for windows) Chicago, Illinois. Fisher's exact test was used to examine the significance of association (contingency) between two groups. It was referenced for a two-tailed p value, and a 95 % confidence interval was constructed around sensitivity proportions using normal approximation method. A two-tailed p value of <0.05 was assumed to attain sufficient statistical significance.

Results

Twenty-five patients were evaluated in this present study and included 22 men and 3 women. The mean age of patients was 31.8 years (range 18–55 years). The most common fracture pattern was a T-type (eight patients, Table 1). Isolated posterior column and anterior wall fractures were not detected in any of the patients. Fifteen patients underwent surgery and 10 patients were treated non-operatively. The Kocher–Langenbeck approach was used in eight cases, the ilio-inguinal approach in five cases, and a combined approach for two cases. Intraoperatively, the morphology of piriformis and obturator externus was examined in 10 cases that were operated with Kocher–Langenbeck approach and the findings compared with the pre-operative MRI.

The MRI revealed complete tears of either or both piriformis and obturator externus in two patients, a partial tear of both muscles in nine patients, an isolated partial tear of obturator externus in two patients, and an isolated partial tear of piriformis in one patient. The remaining patients had intact or partially contused muscles (Table 1). Avascular necrosis was seen in both patients with complete tears of either or both piriformis and obturator externus.

Table 1 Detailed outline of all the 25 patients in our series

S no	# Type	Treatment	Delay in surgery (days)	Surgical approach	MRI findings	Intraoperative findings
1	Transverse	Operative	3	Posterior	Contusion/partial tear both muscles	Same
2	Transverse	Non-operative	–	–	Both intact	–
3	T-type	Operative	12	Ant + post	Complete tear either/both	Same
4	Ant + post hemi transverse	Operative	4	Anterior	Both intact	–
5	T-type	Operative	3	Anterior	Contusion/partial tear both muscles	–
6	Post wall	Operative	4	Posterior	Complete tear either/both	Same
7	Post wall	Non-operative	–	–	Both intact	–
8	Transverse	Operative	7	Anterior	Contusion/partial tear obturator externus	–
9	Posterior wall	Operative	5	Posterior	Both intact	Same
10	T-type	Operative	5	Posterior	Contusion/partial tear obturator externus	Same
11	Post wall + transverse	Operative	3	Posterior	Contusion/partial tear both muscles	Same
12	Bicolumnar	Operative	3	Posterior	Contusion/partial tear piriformis	Contusion/partial tear both muscles
13	Transverse	Operative	8	Posterior	Contusion/partial tear both muscles	Same
14	Transverse	Non-operative	–	–	Both intact	–
15	Ant column	Non-operative	–	–	Both intact	–
16	T-type	Operative	3	Posterior	Contusion/partial tear both muscles	Same
17	Ant column	Operative	8	Anterior	Contusion/partial tear both muscles	–
18	Bicolumnar	Operative	4	Anterior	Contusion/partial tear both muscles	–
19	T-type	Operative	7	Ant + post	Contusion/partial tear both muscles	Same
20	Ant column	Non-operative	–	–	Both intact	–
21	T-type	Non-operative	–	–	Both intact	–
22	Transverse	Non-operative	–	–	Both intact	–
23	T-type	Non-operative	–	–	Both intact	–
24	Post column + post wall	Non-operative	–	–	Both intact	–
25	T-type	Non-operative	–	–	Contusion/partial tear both muscles	–

Patient number 3, 6, and 11 developed AVN of the femoral head in follow-up

Table 2 Table showing detailed outlines of the patients that developed AVN of the femoral head in follow-up

No.	Age (Y)	Sex	Type of fracture	MRI status of obturator ext. and piriformis	Management	Time since injury to surgery (days)	Associated dislocation	Approach	Intraoperative muscle status
3	32	M	T-type (Fig. 1a–d)	Complete tear of obturator externus, partial tear of pyriformis	Operative	12	Posterior	Combined	Same as MRI findings
6	42	F	Post. Wall (Fig. 2a–d)	Complete tear of both the muscles	Operative	4	Nil	Posterior	Same as MRI findings
11	42	M	Post. wall + Transverse (Fig. 3a–d)	Partial tear of both the muscles	Operative	3	Central	Posterior	Same as MRI findings

However, only one patient developed avascular necrosis out of nine patients who had partial tear of both the muscles (Table 2). The remaining patients who had normal or partially contused muscles or partial tears of one of the muscles did not develop femoral head AVN. Of the remaining 22 patients who did not develop avascular necrosis of the femoral head, eight patients had contusion or partial tears of both piriformis and obturator externus

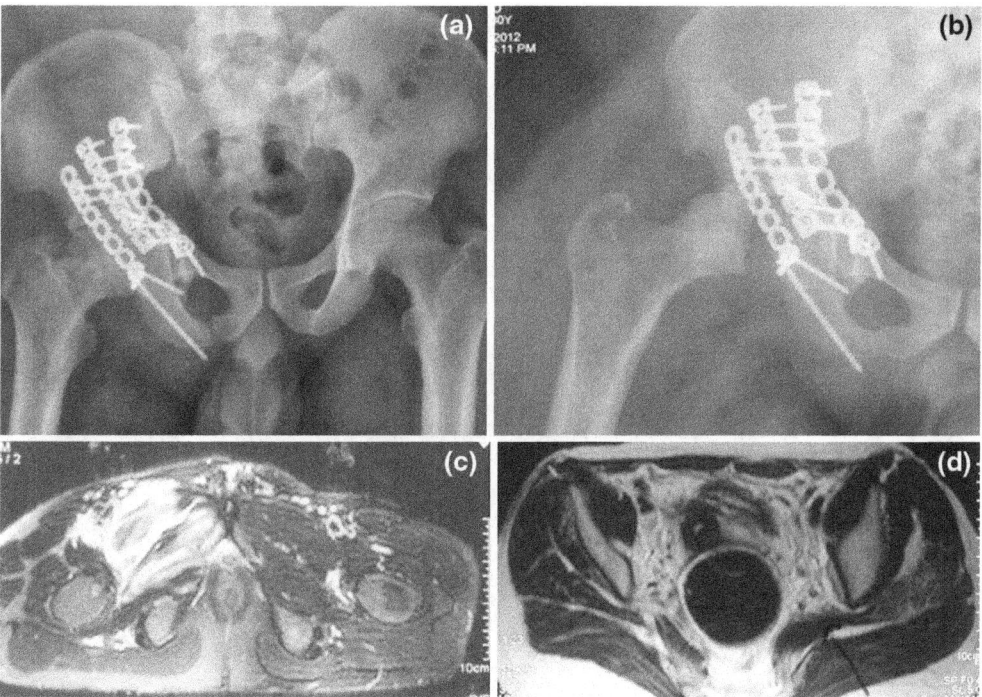

Fig. 1 Imaging of case 3 showing T-type acetabular fracture. **a** 2-month post-operative antero-posterior radiograph showing operative fixation of the fracture with reconstruction plates and normal femoral head; **b** 4-month post-operative radiograph showing features suggestive of avascular necrosis of femoral head with resorption; **c** pre-operative MRI of the patient had shown a complete tear of obturator externus; and **d** a partial tear of piriformis

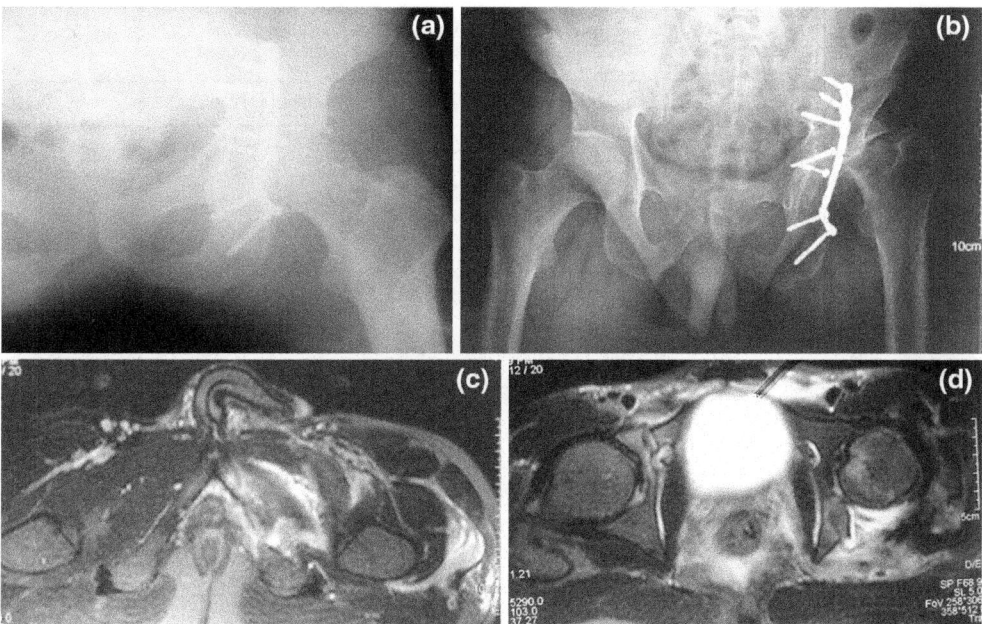

Fig. 2 Imaging of case 6 with posterior wall fracture. **a** 1-month post-operative antero-posterior radiograph showing operative fixation of the fracture with buttress reconstruction plate and normal femoral head; **b** 3-month post-operative radiograph showing avascular necrosis of femoral head with resorption; **c** pre-operative MRI of the patient had shown a complete tear of obturator externus; and **d** a complete tear of piriformis

muscles on MRI and half of these were confirmed intra-operatively. The other eight patients had both the muscles declared intact on MRI, but intraoperative confirmation of these findings was not possible as they were managed non-operatively. The pre-operative grading of obturator externus and piriformis tear as a predictor of future AVN of the

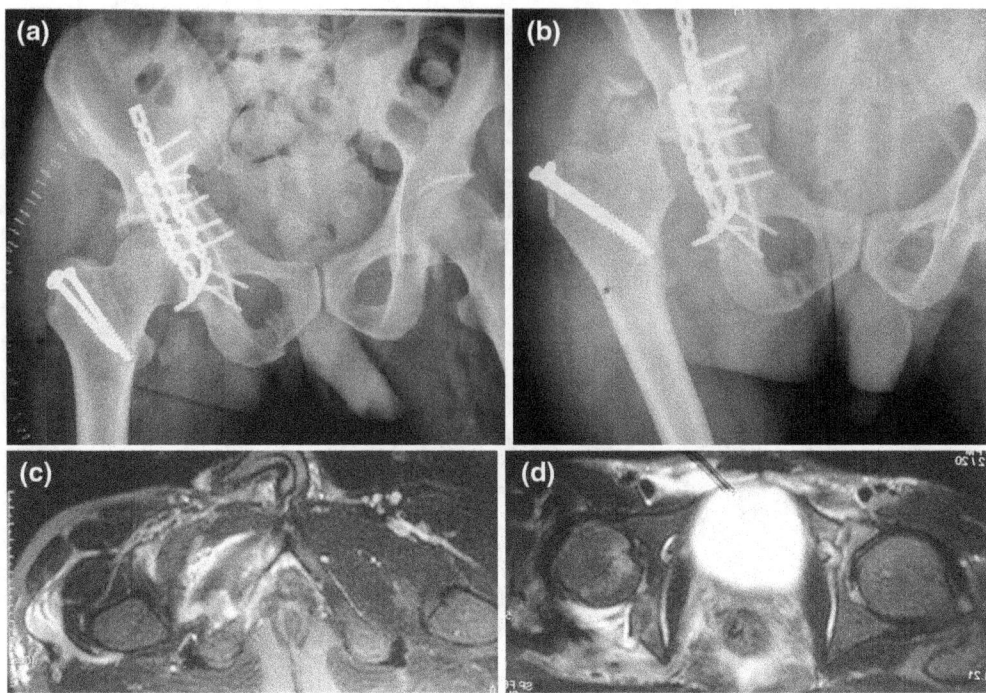

Fig. 3 Imaging of case 11 with transverse fracture with posterior wall fracture. **a** Immediate post-operative antero-posterior radiograph showing operative fixation of the fractures with reconstruction plates and normal femoral head; **b** 3-month post-operative radiograph showing evidence of avascular necrosis of femoral head with resorption; **c** pre-operative MRI of the patient had shown a partial tear of obturator externus; and **d** a partial tear of piriformis

Table 3 Various reported series on acetabular fractures with possible remarks on the development of AVN of the femoral head following this injury

S. no.	Author	Year	No. of cases	% with AVN	Hypothesis given	Remarks
1	Matta [18]	1988	121	0	No	–
2	Heeg [8]	1990	54	11.2	No	–
3	Mayo [3]	1994	163	0.6	No	–
4	Matta [2]	1996	259	3	No	–
5	Siebenrock [6]	2002	12	0	Yes	Obturator externus acts as a protector for deep branch of MCFA
6	Giannoudis [4]	2005	2010	5.6	No	–
7	Panagiotis [7]	2007	75	8	No	–
8	Hadjicostas [5]	2008	31	6.4	No	–
9	Tannast [1]	2010	60	0	Yes	Injury to MCFA
10	Naranje [9]	2010	18	5.5	No	–
11	Briffia [10]	2011	161	11.8	No	–
12	Uchida K [16]	2012	91	0.022	No	–
13	Mitsionis [17]	2012	19	0.053	Yes	Greater chance of AVN in isolated posterior dislocation of the hip than dislocation with fracture
						More chances of AVN if head is reduced late

femoral head was statistically significant ($p = 0.013$). Only one patient was found to have different muscle morphology intraoperatively in comparison with the pre-operative MRI.

An associated hip dislocation was found in seven patients of which two developed AVN of the femoral head. With the numbers available, hip dislocation as a predictor of future development of femoral head AVN was not statistically significant ($p = 0.18$). Of the three patients with posterior wall fractures, one developed AVN of the femoral head and one patient (out of eight) with T-type fractures developed this complication. The only patient in the study with a transverse with posterior wall fracture also developed AVN of the femoral head. Ten patients were managed non-operatively and none of them had evidence of AVN of the femoral head in follow-up. However, the mode of treatment as a predictor for future development of AVN was not statistically significant ($p = 0.25$).

Discussion

Avascular necrosis of the femoral head after acetabular fractures is a devastating outcome. There is little information on prognosis of this complication in this patient group. As was suggested from earlier studies [11], we agree that both piriformis and obturator externus muscles protect the MCFA which is the major blood supply to the head of the femur. In this study, both patients who had complete tears in either or both obturator externus and piriformis muscles developed AVN of the femoral head ($p = 0.013$). Thus, an injury to obturator externus and piriformis muscles may be indirect pointer for damage to the MCFA and, potentially, subsequent development of AVN of the femoral head.

Tannest et al. [15] performed MRI scans in the acute phase of posterior hip dislocation and suggested that an intact obturator externus tendon preserves the deep branch of MFCA to the femoral head. In accordance with this suggestion, we propose that early MRI evaluation may help detect injury to obturator externus or piriformis muscles and potential development of AVN of the femoral head at an early date and avoid the erroneous link to an iatrogenic complication of the surgical approach to the acetabulum [16]. Of the 10 patients treated conservatively, none developed avascular necrosis. This is in keeping with the earlier studies but, in this study, this mode of treatment as a predictor of avascular treatment was not statistically significant. In contrast, in the posterior approach to the hip and acetabulum where tenomyotomy of the external rotator muscles is done, this interrupts the anastomosis between the inferior gluteal artery and the deep branch of the MFCA and subjects the deep branch itself to risk.

The finding in all the cases that developed avascular necrosis of femoral head was of significant head resorption; this is not seen in a traumatic osteonecrosis of femoral head. Other causes which could lead to head resorption are occult fracture of femoral head or infection. However, in this study, an occult head fracture was ruled out in all cases since pre-operative CT and MRI evaluations were undertaken. Infection was ruled out by hip aspiration and culture

which was repeated when these patients had total hip replacements.

Previous studies [1–10, 17–19] on acetabular fractures reported the percentage of cases with avascular necrosis (Table 3). The majority did not comment as to what may have led to avascular necrosis and none noted the extensive head resorption. Further studies with larger sample sizes are needed to evaluate all possible predictors of AVN of the femoral head after acetabular fractures. We suggest pre-operative MRI scans of the pelvis may be considered for high-energy trauma cases that require operative stabilisation. Such an exercise may be helpful in pre-operative prognostication for the development of avascular necrosis of the femoral head.

Conclusion

We conclude that damage to obturator externus and piriformis is a possible predictor for consequent development of AVN of the femoral head which can be judged on pre-operative MRI scans. The type of acetabular fracture and associated dislocation of the hip, if present, may have a bearing on this complication but was not established in this sample studied.

Acknowledgments The authors did not receive grants from any commercial entity in support of this work.

Informed consent Informed consent was obtained from all individual participants included in the study.

References

1. Tannast M, Krüger A, Mack PW, Powell JN, Hosalkar HS, Siebenrock KA (2010) Surgical dislocation of the hip for the fixation of acetabular fractures. J Bone Joint Surg Br 92:842–852
2. Matta JM (1996) Fractures of the acetabulum: accuracy of reduction and clinical results in patients managed operatively within 3 weeks after the injury. J Bone Joint Surg Am 78:1632–1645
3. Mayo KA (1994) Open reduction and internal fixation of fractures of the acetabulum. Clin Orthop 305:31–37
4. Giannoudis PV, Grotz MRW, Papakostidis C (2005) Operative treatment of displaced fractures of the acetabulum: a meta-analysis. J Bone Joint Surg Br 87:2–9
5. Hadjicostas PT, Thielemann FW (2008) The use of trochanteric slide osteotomy in the treatment of displaced acetabular fractures. Injury 39:907–913
6. Siebenrock KA, Gautier E, Woo AKH, Ganz R (2002) Surgical dislocation of the femoral head for joint debridement and accurate reduction of fractures of the acetabulum. J Orthop Trauma 16:543–552
7. Panagiotis T, Elias P (2007) Long term results in surgically treated acetabular fractures through the posterior approaches. Trauma 62:378–382
8. Heeg M, Klasen HJ, Visser JD (1990) Operative treatment for acetabular fractures. J Bone Joint Surg Br 72:383–386

9. Naranje S, Shamshery P, Yadav CS (2010) Digastric trochanteric flip osteotomy and surgical dislocation of hip in the management of acetabular fractures. Arch Orthop Trauma Surg 130:93–101

10. Briffa N, Pearce R, Hill AM, Bircher M (2011) Outcomes of acetabular fracture fixation with 10 years follow-up. J Bone Joint Surg Br 93:229–236

11. Gautier E, Ganz K, Krugel N (2000) Anatomy of the medial femoral circumflex artery and its surgical implications. J Bone Joint Surg Br 82:679–683

12. Rybak LD (2003) Torriani M magnetic resonance imaging of sports related muscle injuries. Top Magn Reson Imaging 14:209–219

13. Griffin DB, Beaule PE, Matta JM (2005) Safety and efficacy of the extended ilio-femoral approach in the treatment of complex fractures of the acetabulum. J Bone Joint Surg Br 87:1391–1396

14. Ganz R, Gill TJ, Gautier E (2001) Surgical dislocation of the adult hip: a technique with full access to femoral head and acetabulum without the risk of avascular necrosis. J Bone Joint Surg Br 83:1119–1124

15. Tannast M, Pleus F, Bonel H, Galloway H, Siebenrock KA, Anderson SE (2010) Magnetic resonance imaging in traumatic posterior hip dislocation. J Orthop Trauma 24(12):723–731

16. Jungbluth KH, Sauer HD (1984) The internal fixation of displaced acetabular fractures: a follow study. In: Weller S, Hierholzer G, Hermichen HG (eds) Late results after osteosynthesis. Collective studies of the German section of AO/ASIF International. AO Bulletin, 63–74

17. Uchida K, Kokubo Y, Yayama T, Nakajima H, Miyazaki T, Negoro K et al (2013) Fracture of the acetabulum: a retrospective review of ninety-one patients treated at a single institution. Eur J Orthop Surg Traumatol 23:155–163

18. Mitsionis G, Lykissas M, Motsis E, Mitsiou D, Gkiatas I, Xenakis T et al (2012) Surgical management of posterior hip dislocations associated with posterior wall acetabular fracture: a study with a minimum follow-up of 15 years. J Orthop Trauma 26:460–465

19. Matta JM, Merritt PO (1988) Displaced acetabular fractures. Clin Orthop 230:83–97

18

A novel intramedullary callus distraction system for the treatment of femoral bone defects

Konstantin Horas[1] · Reinhard Schnettler[2] · Gerrit Maier[2] · Uwe Horas[3]

Abstract An intramedullary device has some advantages over external fixation in callus distraction for bone defect reconstruction. There are difficulties controlling motorized intramedullary devices and monitoring the distraction rate which may lead to poor results. The aim of this study was to design a fully implantable and non-motorized simple distraction nail for the treatment of bone defects. The fully implantable device comprises a tube-in-tube system and a wire pulling mechanism for callus distraction. For the treatment of femoral bone defects, a traction wire, attached to the device at one end, is fixed to the tibial tubercle at its other end. Flexion of the knee joint over a predetermined angle generates a traction force on the wire triggering bone segment transport. This callus distraction system was implanted into the femur of four human cadavers (total 8 femora), and bone segment transport was conducted over 60-mm defects with radiographic monitoring. All bone segments were transported reliably to the docking site. From these preliminary results, we conclude that this callus distraction system offers an alternative to the current intramedullary systems for the treatment of bone defects.

✉ Konstantin Horas
konstantin.horas@sydney.edu.au

[1] ANZAC Research Institute, Bone Research Program, University of Sydney, Gate 3 Hospital Road, Concord, NSW 2139, Australia

[2] Laboratory of Experimental Trauma Surgery, Department of Trauma Surgery, Justus-Liebig-University, Rudolf-Buchheim-Str. 7, 35392 Giessen, Germany

[3] Department of Orthopedic and Trauma Surgery, Kliniken des Main-Taunus-Kreises GmbH, Kronberger Str. 36, 65812 Bad Soden, Germany

Keywords Bone defect treatment · Callus distraction · Distraction osteogenesis · Intramedullary · Bone segment transport

Introduction

Callus distraction (distraction osteogenesis) is a process enabling the reconstruction of large bone defects and the correction of limb length discrepancies. The principle is the stimulation of new bone formation by creating strain on healing tissue between two bone segments by the application of continuous axial distraction [1]. The two bone segments are generated by a low-energy osteotomy in metaphyseal regions of long bones usually [2]. The technique of creating the osteotomy and the region of the osteotomy are important as the soft tissue envelope and vascularity have to be preserved [3]. For complete regeneration, many interrelated anatomical, biomechanical and biochemical processes must occur in a well-orchestrated manner [4].

Ilizarov described the method of distraction osteogenesis for gradual lengthening of bone using a circular ring fixator [5]. This Ilizarov apparatus is a stable yet dynamic system allowing micromotion and compressive loading at the fracture site promoting callus formation [5, 6]. However, callus distraction using external fixation is associated with problems such as frequent pin-track infections, pain, joint stiffness and axial deviation [7–10]. In an attempt to reduce complications, intramedullary callus distraction systems (IMS) have been developed. Currently, there are several intramedullary devices available [11–14], but few are suited for the treatment of large bone defects [14, 15]. Moreover, these intramedullary devices are associated still with complications such as mechanical failure or pain [16–

20]. Consequently, alternative therapeutic approaches such as bone grafting are still used commonly to bridge bone defects; Masquelet et al. [21] described a procedure of combining cancellous autografts with induced membranes that secrete growth factors for stimulating bone regeneration. Although this technique has proven suitable for reconstructing bone defects, it has disadvantages such as a limited supply of bone grafts, morbidity at the donor site (if autografts are used) and nonunion or infection (if allografts are used) [22]. The aim of this study was to design a simple non-motorized intramedullary callus distraction system for the treatment of bone defects.

Materials and methods

This novel callus distraction system (CDS) was designed for segmental bone transport in the femur but can be applied to the tibia and humerus also [23]. Distraction osteogenesis is achieved by using a fully implantable system comprising a tube-in-tube system and a wire traction mechanism (Fig. 1). There are three different components enabling a maximum distraction distance of 216 mm for the femoral version of the nail:

1. A locking intramedullary nail
2. The mechanism
3. A traction wire.

The CDS nail

The femoral version of the CDS is a 340- to 420-mm straight nail. It has an external diameter of 13 mm with additional 1-mm longitudinal wall-strengthening bulges leading to a maximum diameter of 14 mm. With an internal diameter of 10.2 mm, the wall thickness measures 1.4 mm (1.9 mm with bulge). To allow transport of a bone

segment without rotational deformity, the nail is supported by two proximal and two distal transverse interlocking holes with a diameter of 6 mm each. In addition, there is a 6-mm slit over a length of 216 mm within the nail (Fig. 2).

Mechanism

With an external diameter of 10.15 mm, the cylinder-shaped mechanical system of the CDS is fully inserted into the nail (Fig. 3). The in-line mechanics consists of a threaded rod and a threaded rod spindle on top. The connection between the bone segment and the threaded rod is produced by a spindle nut attached to the threaded rod (Figs. 4, 5). A traction wire connected to the mechanics creates a force via functional change in the length of the traction wire, occurring on active or passive movement of the knee joint. Movement of the traction wire and tensile force are converted inside the mechanism, which acts in a similar way to a mechanically driven gyroscope, into a rotational movement of the threaded rod which then transports the spindle nut and correspondingly the bone segment connected to the spindle nut. Thus, the mechanism, once set in motion inside the nail's lumen, turns the threaded rod by converting the translational movement of the traction wire.

Traction wire

A traction wire is connected to the mechanism on the one end and fixed to the tibial tubercle on the other using a screw as an anchor (Figs. 1, 6). The wire is moved by flexing the knee joint generating a traction force which then triggers the mechanism for bone segment transport. The length of the wire is adjusted at, for example, 90° flexion of the knee joint. Further flexion of the knee joint leads to force transmission as tension is put on the pulling wire (Fig. 7). Knee flexion of more than 120° generates a traction force high enough to trigger the mechanism. The system can be regarded as an all-or-none principle. Flexion of the knee joint from 90° to 119°

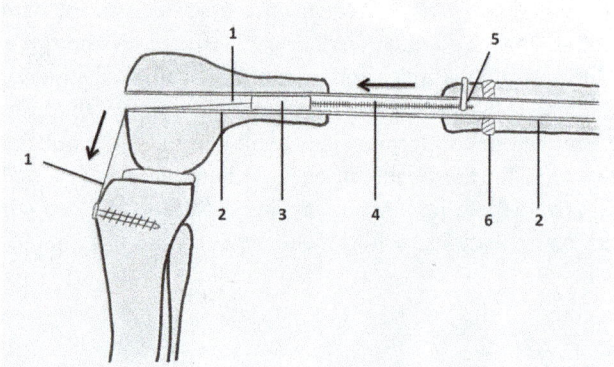

Fig. 1 Schematic of CDS implanted into the femur: *1* traction wire fixed to the tibial tubercle, *2* nail, *3* mechanics, *4* threaded rod, *5* spindle nut and connection to bone segment, *6* callus

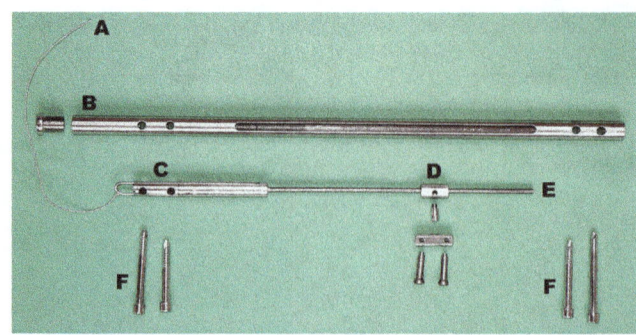

Fig. 2 Individual components of the CDS: *a* traction wire, *b* nail, *c* mechanics, *d* spindle nut, *e* threaded rod, *f* interlocking screw

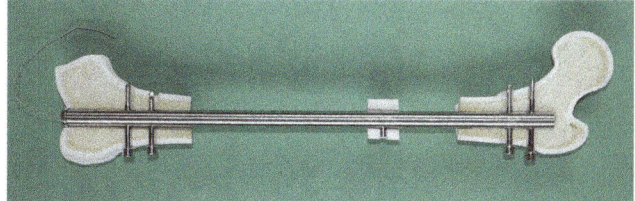

Fig. 3 CDS implanted into the femur (anteroposterior view): The traction wire is connected to the fully inserted mechanics

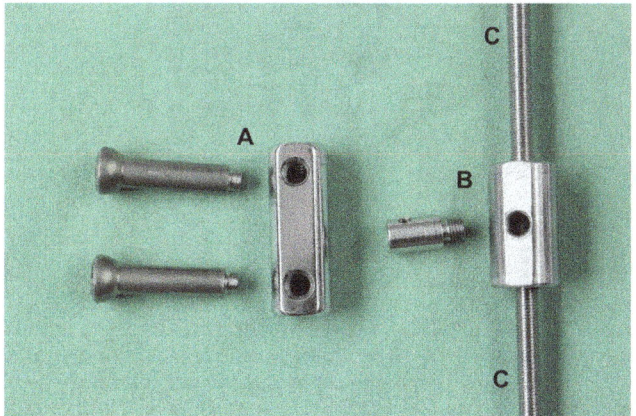

Fig. 4 Threaded rod and spindle nut: *a* spindle nut and screws for 6-mm bone segments (screws can also be applied to smaller spindle nut). *b* Spindle nut for 4-mm bone segments. *c* Threaded rod

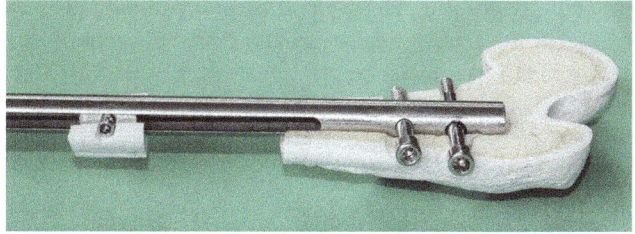

Fig. 5 CDS implanted into the femur with bone segment connected to the threaded rod via the spindle nut (lateral view)

generates an increasing traction force on the wire, but further traction force is required to release the irreversible bone segment transport. Each flexion of the knee joint over 120° results in a bone segment transport distance of 0.25 mm. It should be noted that the angle that triggers the mechanism is adjustable according to the patient's range of motion. The designated distance of bone segment transport is 1 mm per day.

Operative technique and cadaver study

In order to evaluate the implantation of the nail and the system running, a cadaver study using both femora of four human cadavers was conducted. All experiments were approved and conducted in accordance with the guidelines of the Committee of Medical Ethics. Written informed consent from the donor was obtained prior to their inclusion in this study. Each cadaver was thoroughly checked, and none of the cadavers had a history of musculoskeletal disease that could have had an impact on the experiment. All cadavers were frozen to a temperature of −18° Celsius exactly 48 h after death and defrosted for 24 h prior to the experiment. Implantation of the CDS was carried out in supine position using standard retrograde access though the knee joint. The femoral canal was reamed over a guidewire to a diameter of 15.5 mm followed by temporary insertion of the nail. After removal of the nail, a bone defect was created via a medial approach in order to avoid major damage of the surrounding soft tissues of the femur. Forty-millimeter bone segments on the right femora and 60-mm bone segments on the left femora were generated using a Gigli saw. The osteotomy was performed directly distal to the insertion of adductor brevis in such a way as to preserve as much of the periosteum as possible. The nail was then reinserted into the femoral canal across the bone segment to be transported and then locked proximally in an anteroposterior direction. Standard anteroposterior (AP) and lateral radiographs were obtained to guide the nail to the correct position. Next, a 6.5-mm lateral drill hole was generated on the bone segment followed by fixation of the bone segment on the threaded rod spindle. In order to perform distal locking of the nail, the femur had to be distracted on the side of the osteotomy as the tension force of the adherent soft tissues reduced the initial size of the bone defect. After the size of the bone defect was readjusted to a total length of 60 mm, distal locking was performed and the threaded rod was inserted into the nail. With the mechanism inserted into the nail, the traction wire was adjusted parallel to the anterior cruciate ligament (ACL) and fixed to the tibial tuberosity using a cancellous bone screw (Fig. 6). At completion, the mechanism and the system were tested by flexing the knee joint. Radiographs were taken in AP and lateral direction in order to ensure correct bone segment transport (Fig. 7). Bone transport was then conducted in all eight femora until impingement of the bone segment at the docking site. In clinical application, the screw in the tibial tuberosity will be removed at the end of segment transport and the traction wire will be cut at the distal end of the nail leading to a retraction of the wire into the nail.

Results

All eight bone segments were transported to the docking site without any complications. During continuous radiographic validation of the CDS, we did not identify any

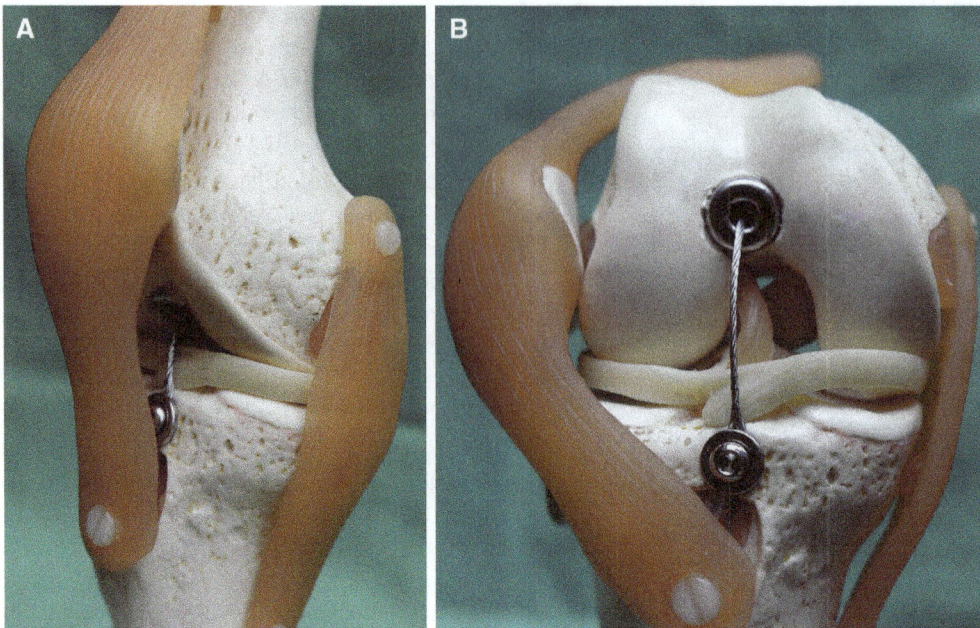

Fig. 6 Schematic model of the CDS implanted into the right femur. **a** Antero-medial view at 10° flexion of the knee joint. The traction wire is fixed to the tibial tubercle proximal to the insertion of the patellar ligament. **b** Anterior view at 90° flexion of the knee joint. The patella is laterally dislocated to fully expose the intra-articular running of the wire. The traction wire and the distal end of the nail do not impinge the menisci or impact on the ACL and the retro-patellar cartilage

mechanical obstacles of the system or axial deviation. The ratchet system ran smoothly, and no inter-locking of bone segments occurred.

Implantation

Prior to implantation, each femur was measured and the sizes of the implants were determined. The mean operative time was 75 min (without generation of bone defects). No intraoperative complications or problems occurred. There was no significant relationship, with the numbers available, between height, weight, body mass index (BMI), age of the cadaveric sample and operative time.

Use in cadavers

The anticipated transport distance of the bone segments was achieved in all eight femora. Bending of the knee joint of more than 120° reliably triggered the mechanism, whereas a knee joint movement between 0° and 119° had no impact. By stretching and flexing the knee joint every 15 s over the entire range of movement (0°–140°), bone transport of the segment over a transport distance of 0.25 mm per cycle was achieved without any difficulty. This procedure was continued until the bone segments had reached the docking site. Radiographs were obtained to evaluate the progress simultaneously showing a consistent pattern. Once the bone fragments had reached the distal

segment of the femur, no further passive flexion over 120° of knee flexion was possible. Apart from this, no other passive restrictions in knee movement in the cadavers after implantation of the CDS were noted. Additionally, we examined the intra-articular behavior of the traction wire. Radiographs (AP and lateral) were taken at 0°, 30°, 60°, 90° and 120° flexion of the knee joint (Fig. 7). By flexing the knee joint from 0° to 120°, the length of the intra-articular part of the traction wire doubled compared to its initial length. After passive extension back to the initial position of 0°, no looping of the traction wire occurred (Fig. 7). As the traction wire glided back into the distal end of the nail, no contact of the wire to the menisci or the cruciate ligaments was observed. Notably, movement of the wire occurs inside of the CDS exclusively. As there is always tension on the intra-articular part of the wire, no movement of the wire inside the joint is possible, and therefore, no interaction with the ACL or other soft tissues is to be expected (Fig. 6).

When comparing the sizes of the bone segments (60 and 40 mm) to be transported, no significant difference in implantation or distraction could be found.

Biomechanics

In order to assess the mechanical stability of the novel CDS, several static and dynamic tests were carried out comparing the novel CDS nail with the Klemm–

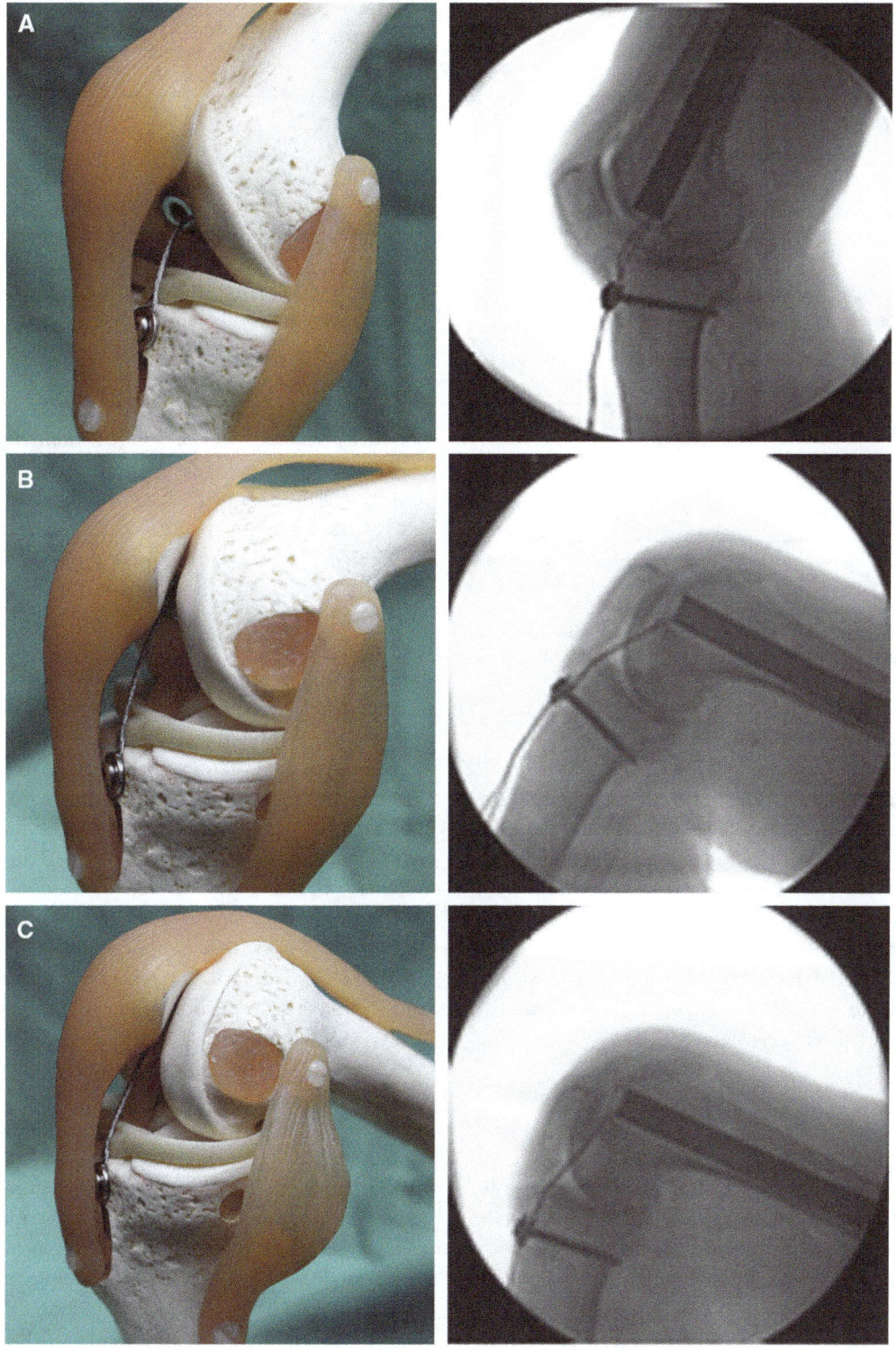

Fig. 7 Schematic model of the CDS implanted into the right femur. Antero-medial view at 30° (**a**), 90° (**b**) and 120° (**c**) flexion of the knee joint with correlating X-rays. The length of the intra-articular part of the wire doubled at 120° (**c**) compared to 30° (**a**) having constant traction on the wire

Schellmann nail [24]. For that purpose a four-point bending test, torsion tests, fatigue tests and a physical check including maximum load testing were conducted. In all tests, material properties showed satisfactory results (Tables 1, 2) and no significant difference compared to the Klemm–Schellmann nail [25–27].

Table 1 Experimental data of bending load testing

	Proportional bending moment (Nm)	Stiffness (Nm/ angular degree)	Maximal bending moment (Nm)	Bending deformity (angle)
Number of nails tested	10	10	10	10
Mean	83.2	22.1	167.1	14.1
Median	84.0	22.4	168.0	14.1
Standard deviation	5	0.7	3.8	1.3

Table 2 Experimental data of torsion stability testing (Nm/°) and prolonged swing testing

	Torsion stability (Nm/angular degree)	Prolonged swing test (load changes)
Number of nails tested	10	4
Mean	0.2930	41,850
Median	0.2965	42,000
Standard deviation	0.00761	1025

Prolonged swing testing was conducted for a period of 60 min and a force of approximately 3 kN at a frequency of 3 Hz. Prior to experiments, we set the threshold to 30.000 load changes calculated based on results by Taylor and coworkers [42, 43]. With a mean value of 41,850 load changes, the novel CDS exceeded the required threshold

Complications

Difficulties during implantation occurred such as a shortening of the generated bone defect after removal of the bone fragment due to traction forces of the adherent soft tissues. For that purpose, a spacer was inserted and fixed using two pins on subsequent experimental implantation. Nevertheless, this is a problem that only occurs in artificially generated bone defects for the use in this study and does not reflect the situation of bone defect treatment in patients that suffer from bone defects.

Discussion

The treatment of long bone defects in the lower extremity is a challenging reconstructive problem for orthopedic surgeons. For many years, bone grafting was the most common treatment to bridge segmental bone defects. Since the discovery of distraction osteogenesis, first introduced by Ilizarov, this method has become a successful alternative to bone grafting [5]. This method can be associated with several complications [9, 28]. Problems such as pin-track infection, pain, joint instability and stiffness are related mostly to the external fixator [7, 8, 29]. In an effort to reduce these complications, numerous new devices and implants have been developed [11, 12, 30]. Paley et al compared a standard Ilizarov method to a combination of external fixation with interlocking intramedullary nailing in a study on femoral lengthening. They concluded that lengthening over an intramedullary nail decreases the duration of external fixation, protects against refracture and allows earlier rehabilitation [31]. These results were supported by Kocaoglu et al. [32] in their report of external fixator-assisted bone segment transport over an intramedullary nail for reconstruction of bone defects of the lower extremity. Although several studies showed advantages in combining external with internal fixation, there is, still, the risk of pin-track infection leading to deep intramedullary infection [9, 33, 34]. With fully implantable intramedullary CDS, the potential is to overcome the problem of pin-track infection and to improve comfort during treatment [14, 28]. One of these intramedullary devices is the Albizzia nail comprising two telescopic cylinders in which lengthening is achieved by rotating movements of the limb [11]. Although clinical results were promising, patients complained about pain which made ratcheting difficult [16]. The Intramedullary Skeletal Kinetic Distractor (ISKD) is another mechanically driven device which lengthens through torsional movement of the limb [13]. Several authors published their experience with lengthening using the ISKD and described complications such as runaway nails, premature consolidation, severe pain and uncontrolled lengthening [17–20, 28]. The ISKD has, so far, been described for the use in limb lengthening but not for the treatment of bone defects. Hyodo et al. [30] have recently reported a traction cable device for bone segment transport in the canine femur using an interlocking intramedullary rod for fixation. However, this device comprises an external distraction apparatus, and local infection at the exit side of the cable and along the cable tract has been reported. To our knowledge, only three fully implantable CDS have been described for the treatment of bone defects in humans. The recent Phoenix nail is a magnetically activated drive system, and the first results for the use in bone defect treatment are promising [14]. Another recent development is the magnet-operated telescopic PRECICE nail [35]. It has both CE mark and US FDA clearance for its first- and second-generation implants, and good results for the treatment of limb length discrepancies have been reported [35]. Although the reliability of this novel system seems to be comparable to other intramedullary nails, a magnet-driven device is a novel technology and literature regarding its efficacy, reliability, complication rate and safety is sparse [36]. Baumgart et al. [15] reported a patient with a 12-cm bone defect after tumor resection who was treated successfully using an intramedullary motorized nail (Fitbone). Betz et al. [12] reported also of good clinical outcomes using the Fitbone nail in leg lengthening. These results were further supported by Singh et al. [37] and Krieg et al. [38] who published their experience with the Fitbone nail with a relatively low complication rate of 12.5 % in leg lengthening. Although these devices seem to be appropriate for the treatment of bone defects, few publications exist on their use in bone defect treatment [15]. Moreover, the Fitbone nail comprises a complex motorized mechanism that is expensive and increases the risk of technical failure which further limits its use. For that reason, our aim was to design a simple and non-motorized intramedullary CDS as a reasonable alternative to the currently existing treatment options.

In this study, we introduce a fully implantable CDS for the treatment of femoral bone defects. This novel intramedullary callus distraction system was subjected to several mechanical tests and a cadaver study with promising results. In our cadaver experiment, bone segment transport was accomplished without mechanical obstacles and the desired range of motion of the knee joint achieved. A major advantage of this CDS is that it allows physiological movement of the limb and helps prevent the frequently reported complication of knee joint contracture [9]. It is inevitable that some movement is lost, albeit temporarily, during the period of bone segment transport. However, this limitation can be minimized by adjusting the traction wire according to the patients' knee movement range. For example, if the traction wire is adjusted such that the mechanism is triggered by flexing the knee joint more than 120°, any movement between 0° and 119° is possible without any effect on the mechanism. At the end of transport, the wire and screw will be removed and further bending of the knee joint is possible without any restriction. Other mechanical devices either limit knee movement range or require frequent non-physiological and painful movement; in this novel CDS, only four cycles of knee flexion are necessary to reach the designated transport distance of 1 mm per day compared to 15 cycles of rotational movement of the femur using the Albizzia nail. An important consideration is that the data presented in this study are from an experimental setup; there are limitations on transferring the results into clinical practice. For the present time, this study confirms proof of concept that the mechanism designed for the purpose of bone segment transport within an intramedullary nail works.

There are different opinions on the adequate velocity of distraction in order to prevent premature consolidation [18, 19, 29, 39]. The velocity of distraction in this CDS has the potential to be adjusted by the patient facilitating a personalized distraction rate. Nevertheless, as with all other systems used in distraction osteogenesis, good compliance and understanding by the patient is mandatory for success. Another factor that should be taken into consideration is that the nail is designed for weight bearing (at least at an axial load of 20 kg which corresponds clinically to partial weight bearing). Axial micromotion and compressive stress at the fracture site are considered beneficial for bone healing [40, 41], and therefore, the period of time to full consolidation of the regenerated bone might be reduced in this system.

Conclusion

The findings of this study demonstrate the feasibility of bone segment transport by callus distraction using a novel CDS. Results achieved in mechanical experiments and in the cadaver study provide proof of concept that the mechanism designed is able to transport a segment of bone in the femur. These initial results have to be validated further and the novel CDS was introduced in animal experiments.

Acknowledgments We thank M. Menzel for his assistance in biomechanical experiments and C. M. Zehendner for helpful comments on the manuscript.

Informed consent Written informed consent from the donor was obtained prior to their inclusion in this study.

References

1. Claes L, Veeser A, Gockelmann M, Horvath D, Durselen L, Ignatius A (2010) A novel method for lateral callus distraction and its importance for the mechano-biology of bone formation. Bone 47(4):712–717
2. Nayagam S (2010) Femoral lengthening with a rail external fixator: tips and tricks. Strateg Trauma Limb Reconstr 5(3):137–144
3. Horas K, Schnettler R, Maier G, Schneider G, Horas U (2015) The role of soft-tissue traction forces in bone segment transport for callus distraction: a force measurement cadaver study on eight human femora using a novel intramedullary callus distraction system. Strateg Trauma Limb Reconstr 10(1):21–26
4. Marsell R, Einhorn TA (2011) The biology of fracture healing. Injury 42(6):551–555
5. Ilizarov GA (1989) The tension-stress effect on the genesis and growth of tissues. Part I. The influence of stability of fixation and soft-tissue preservation. Clin Orthop Relat Res 238:249–281
6. Gessmann J, Baecker H, Jettkant B, Muhr G, Seybold D (2011) Direct and indirect loading of the Ilizarov external fixator: the effect on the interfragmentary movements and compressive loads. Strateg Trauma Limb Reconstr 6(1):27–31

7. Mekhail AO, Abraham E, Gruber B, Gonzalez M (2004) Bone transport in the management of posttraumatic bone defects in the lower extremity. J Trauma 56(2):368–378

8. Oh CW, Song HR, Roh JY, Oh JK, Min WK, Kyung HS, Kim JW, Kim PT, Ihn JC (2008) Bone transport over an intramedullary nail for reconstruction of long bone defects in tibia. Arch Orthop Trauma Surg 128(8):801–808

9. Sun XT, Easwar TR, Manesh S, Ryu JH, Song SH, Kim SJ, Song HR (2011) Complications and outcome of tibial lengthening using the Ilizarov method with or without a supplementary intramedullary nail: a case-matched comparative study. J Bone Joint Surg Br 93(6):782–787

10. Liantis P, Mavrogenis AF, Stavropoulos NA, Kanellopoulos AD, Papagelopoulos PJ, Soucacos PN, Babis GC (2014) Risk factors for and complications of distraction osteogenesis. Eur J Orthop Surg Traumatol 5:693–698

11. Guichet JM, Deromedis B, Donnan LT, Peretti G, Lascombes P, Bado F (2003) Gradual femoral lengthening with the Albizzia intramedullary nail. J Bone Joint Surg Am 85-A(5):838–848

12. Betz A, Baumgart R, Schweiberer L (1990) First fully implantable intramedullary system for callus distraction–intramedullary nail with programmable drive for leg lengthening and segment displacement. Principles and initial clinical results. Der Chirurg; Zeitschrift fur alle Gebiete der operativen Medizien 61(8):605–609

13. Cole JD, Justin D, Kasparis T, DeVlught D, Knobloch C (2001) The intramedullary skeletal kinetic distractor (ISKD): first clinical results of a new intramedullary nail for lengthening of the femur and tibia. Injury 32(Suppl 4):SD129–SD139

14. Konofaos P, Kashyap A, Neel MD, Ver Halen JP (2012) A novel device for long bone osteodistraction: description of device and case series. Plast Reconstr Surg 130(3):418e–422e

15. Baumgart R, Betz A, Schweiberer L (1997) A fully implantable motorized intramedullary nail for limb lengthening and bone transport. Clin Orthop Relat Res 343:135–143

16. Garcia-Cimbrelo E, Curto de la Mano A, Garcia-Rey E, Cordero J, Marti-Ciruelos R (2002) The intramedullary elongation nail for femoral lengthening. J Bone Joint Surg Br 84(7):971–977

17. Schiedel FM, Pip S, Wacker S, Popping J, Tretow H, Leidinger B, Rodl R (2011) Intramedullary limb lengthening with the Intramedullary Skeletal Kinetic Distractor in the lower limb. J Bone Joint Surg Br 93(6):788–792

18. Simpson AH, Shalaby H, Keenan G (2009) Femoral lengthening with the Intramedullary Skeletal Kinetic Distractor. J Bone Joint Surg Br 91(7):955–961

19. Kenawey M, Krettek C, Liodakis E, Wiebking U, Hankemeier S (2011) Leg lengthening using intramedullay skeletal kinetic distractor: results of 57 consecutive applications. Injury 42(2):150–155

20. Burghardt RD, Herzenberg JE, Specht SC, Paley D (2011) Mechanical failure of the Intramedullary Skeletal Kinetic Distractor in limb lengthening. J Bone Joint Surg Br 93(5):639–643

21. Masquelet AC, Fitoussi F, Begue T, Muller GP (2000) Reconstruction of the long bones by the induced membrane and spongy autograft. Ann Chir Plast Esthet 45(3):346–353

22. Bieler D, Franke A, Willms A, Hentsch S, Kollig E (2014) Masquelet technique for reconstruction of osseous defects in a gunshot fracture of the proximal thigh-a case study. Mil Med 179(9):e1053–e1058

23. Horas U (2006) A novel internal callus distraction system. In: Leung KTG, Schnettler R, Alt V, Haarman HJTM (eds) Practice of Intramedullary Locked Nails. Springer, Berlin, pp 199–210

24. Contzen H (1987) Development of intramedullary nailing and the interlocking nail. Aktuelle Traumatologie 17(6):250–252

25. Menzel M (2004) Experimentelle Untersuchung zur Belastbarkeit und Funktion eines neuen Kallusdistraktionssystems unter Berücksichtigung der biologischen Rahmenbedingungen des Knochensegmenttransports. Dissertation, Justus-Liebig Universität, Giessen

26. Schandelmaier P, Krettek C, Tscherne H (1996) Biomechanical study of nine different tibia locking nails. J Orthop Trauma 10(1):37–44

27. Schandelmaier P, Farouk O, Krettek C, Reimers N, Mannss J, Tscherne H (2000) Biomechanics of femoral interlocking nails. Injury 31(6):437–443

28. Hankemeier S, Pape HC, Gosling T, Hufner T, Richter M, Krettek C (2004) Improved comfort in lower limb lengthening with the intramedullary skeletal kinetic distractor. Principles and preliminary clinical experiences. Arch Orthop Trauma Surg 124(2):129–133

29. Zhang X, Liu T, Li Z, Peng W (2007) Reconstruction with callus distraction for nonunion with bone loss and leg shortening caused by suppurative osteomyelitis of the femur. J Bone Joint Surg Br 89(11):1509–1514

30. Hyodo A, Kotschi H, Kambic H, Muschler G (1996) Bone transport using intramedullary fixation and a single flexible traction cable. Clin Orthop Relat Res 325:256–268

31. Paley D, Herzenberg JE, Paremain G, Bhave A (1997) Femoral lengthening over an intramedullary nail. A matched-case comparison with Ilizarov femoral lengthening. J Bone Joint Surg Am 79(10):1464–1480

32. Kocaoglu M, Eralp L, Bilen FE, Balci HI (2009) Fixator-assisted acute femoral deformity correction and consecutive lengthening over an intramedullary nail. J Bone Joint Surg Am 91(1):152–159

33. Brunner UH, Cordey J, Kessler S, Rahn BA, Schweiberer L, Perren SM (1993) Bone segment transport in combination with an intramedullary nail. Injury 24(Suppl 2):S29–S44

34. Liodakis E, Kenawey M, Krettek C, Wiebking U, Hankemeier S (2011) Comparison of 39 post-traumatic tibia bone transports performed with and without the use of an intramedullary rod: the long-term outcomes. Int Orthop 35(9):1397–1402

35. Paley D (2015) PRECICE intramedullary limb lengthening system. Expert Rev Med Devices 12(3):231–249

36. Kirane YM, Fragomen AT, Rozbruch SR (2014) Precision of the PRECICE internal bone lengthening nail. Clin Orthop Relat Res 472(12):3869–3878

37. Singh S, Lahiri A, Iqbal M (2006) The results of limb lengthening by callus distraction using an extending intramedullary nail (Fitbone) in non-traumatic disorders. J Bone Joint Surg Br 88(7):938–942

38. Krieg AH, Lenze U, Speth BM, Hasler CC (2011) Intramedullary leg lengthening with a motorized nail. Acta Orthop 82(3):344–350

39. Sangkaew C (2004) Distraction osteogenesis with conventional external fixator for tibial bone loss. Int Orthop 28(3):171–175

40. Claes L, Augat P, Schorlemmer S, Konrads C, Ignatius A, Ehrnthaller C (2008) Temporary distraction and compression of a diaphyseal osteotomy accelerates bone healing. J Orthop Res 26(6):772–777

41. Gessmann J, Citak M, Jettkant B, Schildhauer TA, Seybold D (2011) The influence of a weight-bearing platform on the mechanical behavior of two Ilizarov ring fixators: tensioned wires vs. half-pins. J Orthop Surg Res 6:61

42. Taylor SJ, Walker PS (2001) Forces and moments telemetered from two distal femoral replacements during various activities. J Biomech 34(7):839–848

43. Taylor SJ, Perry JS, Meswania JM, Donaldson N, Walker PS, Cannon SR (1997) Telemetry of forces from proximal femoral replacements and relevance to fixation. J Biomech 30(3):225–234

19

Distraction osteogenesis for tibial nonunion with bone loss using combined Ilizarov and Taylor spatial frames versus a conventional circular frame

Ibrahim Elsayed Abdellatif Abuomira[1,4] · Francesco Sala[2] · Yasser Elbatrawy[1] · Giovanni Lovisetti[3] · Salvatore Alati[3] · Dario Capitani[2]

Abstract This retrospective review assesses 55 tibial nonunions with bone loss to compare union achieved with combined Ilizarov and Taylor spatial frames (I–TSF) versus a conventional circular frame with the standard Ilizarov procedure. Seventeen (31 %) of the 55 nonunions were infected. Thirty patients treated with I–TSF were compared with 25 patients treated with a conventional circular frame. In the I–TSF group, an average of 7.6 cm of bone was resected and the lengthening index (treatment time in months divided by lengthening amount in centimeters) was 1.97. In the conventional circular frame group, a mean of 6.5 cm was resected and the lengthening index was 2.1. Consolidation at the docking site and at the regenerate bone occurred in 49 (89 %) of 55 cases after the first procedure. No statistically significant difference was shown between the two groups. Superiority of one modality of treatment over the other cannot be concluded from our data. Application of combined Ilizarov and Taylor spatial frames for bone transport is useful for treatment of tibial nonunion with bone loss.

Level of evidence Case series, Level III.

Keywords Bone transport · Tibial nonunion · Bone defect · Docking site · Taylor spatial frame · Ilizarov

Introduction

Treatment of segmental bone defects in the leg, especially those that are associated with soft tissue defects or an infection at the site of a nonunion, is challenging [1–4]. Treatment objectives include improvement in the quality of bone and soft tissue, correction of angulation and length, early mobilization to prevent stiff adjacent joints, promotion of union, and eradication of infection. The Ilizarov technique has improved limb reconstruction [5–8]. For small bone defects, the defect is compressed and osteotomy and lengthening are performed at the opposite end of the bone. With larger defects, lengthening and compression occur simultaneously such that the middle segment of bone is transported to fill the defect [2, 9, 10]. Once the defect has been closed, lengthening can be continued as required. The Ilizarov fixator also has been used to gradually close traumatic soft tissue defects [11]. Reconstruction is associated with longer rehabilitation time. Complications associated with bone transport and those occurring at the docking site might require additional surgical procedures and rehospitalization.

The Taylor spatial frame (TSF; Smith + Nephew, Inc., Memphis, TN USA) uses special struts and a computer program to calculate the position of imaginary "hinges" for simultaneous deformity correction in multiple planes and represents an advance in medicine and surgery. Although the TSF is more cumbersome than the standard Ilizarov frame (especially in diameter), it offers many advantages, including reliability and the ability to simultaneously correct rotation, angulation, and translation

✉ Ibrahim Elsayed Abdellatif Abuomira
ibrahim_amira2000@yahoo.com

1 Department of Orthopedic Surgery and Traumatology, Al-Azhar University Hospital, Assiut, Egypt

2 Department of Orthopedic Surgery and Traumatology, Niguarda Hospital, Piazza Ospedale Maggiore 3, 20162 Milan, Italy

3 Department of Orthopedic Surgery and Traumatology, Menaggio Hospital, Menaggio, CO, Italy

4 2 Nile Street, Sohâg, Egypt

deformities (six-axis deformity correction) without the need to apply rotational devices or to change hinge placement, as usually is necessary with the standard Ilizarov frame [12]. Primary fixation and definitive fixation with the TSF are effective. Advantages include continuity of device until union, reduced risk of infection, early mobilization, restoration of primary defect caused by bone loss, easy and accurate application, convertibility and versatility compared with a monolateral fixator, and improved union rate and range of motion for lower extremity long-bone fractures in patients with multiple traumatic injuries [13].

Our study presents outcomes of the combined Ilizarov frame and TSF (I–TSF) compared with a standard Ilizarov procedure and a conventional circular frame for correcting segmental tibial defects [9, 10]. The current study was approved by the ethical committee at our hospital.

Patients and methods

We performed a retrospective, case-matched comparison of patients who underwent tibial deformity correction with I–TSF and those who underwent correction with a conventional circular frame during tibial bone transport. Allocation of type of frame was based on medical necessity, with simpler cases of nonunion with bone loss receiving conventional circular frames and more complex cases that included rotation, angulation, and/or translation deformity receiving I–TSF. Our study group was a retrospective cohort of 55 patients with tibial nonunions and bone loss treated with bifocal and trifocal techniques during the

period from 1999 through 2011. The demographics and clinical features of the 55 patients are presented in Table 1.

Combined I–TSF was applied to 30 patients (25 male and five female patients), with a mean age of 39 years (age range 15–79 years) (group A). Local infection was present in 20 (67 %) of 30 cases. Bifocal transport was used in 10 (33 %) of the group A patients and trifocal in 20 (67 %) (Fig. 1). Refreshing procedure at the docking site with autologous bone grafting was performed in 24 (80 %) cases. Fibular osteotomy was performed in 20 (67 %) of 30 patients. Tendo-Achilles lengthening was performed in six (20 %) patients.

A conventional circular frame was used for 25 patients (19 men and six women) with a mean age of 44.5 years (age range 21–75 years) (group B). The standard Ilizarov frame (Sintea Plustek, Assago, Italy) was used in 10 patients, the TrueLok frame (Orthofix, McKinney, TX USA) in eight, the Sheffield frame (Orthofix) in five, and the full ring fixator (Synthes Gmbh, Solothurn, Switzerland) in two. The standard Ilizarov procedure was used with all four types of conventional circular frames. Local infection was present in 18 (72 %) of 25 cases. Bifocal transport was performed in 16 (64 %) patients and trifocal transport in nine (36 %). Refreshing procedure at the docking site with autologous bone grafting was performed in nine (36 %) cases. Fibular osteotomy was performed in 14 (56 %) of 25 patients.

All patients were encouraged to bear partial weight progressively with crutches on the second day after surgery. Quadriceps isometric exercises were started immediately after the operation to maintain or increase muscle strength. Range-of-motion exercises of the knee were

Table 1 Study population demographics

	Overall population ($n = 55$)	Group A ($n = 30$)	Group B ($n = 25$)
Age, year, mean ± SD (range)	41.5 ± 18 (15–79)	39 ± 20.4 (15–79)	44.5 ± 14.6 (21–75)
Sex, n (%)			
Male	44 (80)	25 (83)	19 (76)
Female	11 (20)	5 (17)	6 (24)
Local infection, n (%)	38 (69)	20 (67)	18 (72)
Bone transport, cm, mean ± SD (range)	7.1 ± 3.3 (3–17)	7.6 ± 3.5 (3–15)	6.5 ± 3 (3–17)
Treatment type, n (%)			
Trifocal	29 (53)	20 (67)	9 (36)
Bifocal	26 (47)	10 (33)	16 (64)
External fixation time, d, mean ± SD (range)	391 ± 140.5 (120–770)	418 ± 144.8 (168–770)	359 ± 130.8 (120–670)
Lengthening index, mo/cm, mean ± SD (range)	2 ± 0.8 (1.1–4)	1.97 ± 0.7 (1.1–3.4)	2.1 ± 0.9 (1.3–4)
Mean union rate after first surgery	89	90	88
Duration of follow-up, days, mean ± SD (range)	50 ± 14.7 (25–78)	48 ± 12.8 (26–78)	53 ± 16.5 (25–74)

None of the differences shown reached statistical significance

SD standard deviation

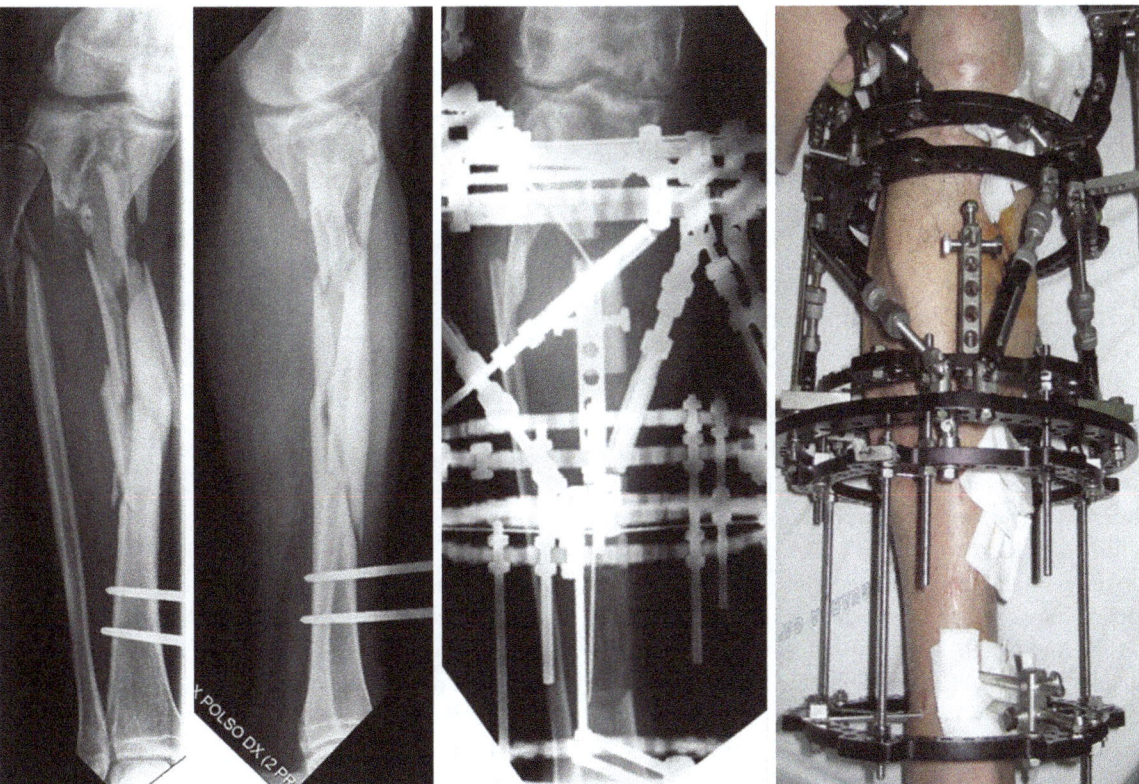

Fig. 1 43-year-old man with infected tibial nonunion treated with bony resection of all infected bone and a trifocal retrograde tibial bone transport. From *left to right*, images show radiographs of the tibial nonunion with a temporary external fixator, anteroposterior radiograph with the TSF applied, and clinical photograph after application of the TSF during tibial bone transport

initiated as soon as the comfort of the patient allowed. The TSF was removed when at least tricortical consolidation was seen on anteroposterior and lateral view radiographs before complete removal of the frame. The fixators were slowly destabilized by removing struts or bars over a period of 3 weeks. After frame removal, patients were restricted to partial weight bearing for 4–6 weeks and no brace was used. Full weight bearing was allowed between the 4th and 10th postoperative week, based on clinical and radiological evidence of healing at the nonunion site and at the site of lengthening and deformity correction.

Patients' data were collected from medical records and radiographs that were obtained every 2 weeks during the distraction phase and once a month during the consolidation phase. Complications encountered intraoperatively and during treatment were also recorded. With use of the classification system presented by Paley [14], minor complications were problems that did not require additional surgery, major complications were obstacles that resolved with additional surgery, and true complications were sequelae that remained unresolved at the end of the treatment period. Preoperative and last follow-up radiographic measurements were reviewed for all patients. External fixation time (length of time with the frame applied), lengthening index (treatment time in months divided by

lengthening amount in centimeters), amount of obtained length, and segment transfer were all calculated.

Operative technique

All nonunions were treated with radical bony resection of all necrotic bones and bone transport according to Ilizarov distraction osteogenesis principles. The TSF rings were placed on the proximal and distal fragments parallel to their respective joints, allowing adequate soft tissue clearance. The frame was mounted orthogonally to the mechanical axis of the tibia and fixed initially with two wires, one proximal and one distal. Additional wires and half-pins were then inserted, aiming for at least three points of fixation both proximally and distally. Great care must be taken to keep the master tab area of each TSF ring free for future strut applications. Six-millimeter hydroxyapatite (HA)-coated half-pins (Orthofix) were used in all patients [15].

For proximal and distal tibial nonunions, the constructs were extended to the distal femur or to the foot to increase frame stability. The total residual computer program of the TSF was used to restore the normal limb axis and to achieve lengthening if necessary. A percutaneous Gigli saw osteotomy of the tibia was made through two transverse incisions of the skin in both groups. The latency period before starting distraction osteogenesis was 12–14 days. Distraction ranged from 0.5 to 1.5 mm/day, depending on the regenerative quality and the number of sites of osteotomy. When bone capitation at the docking site was achieved, inter-fragmentary compression was continued at the rate of 0.25 mm/day for 5–7 days. Once consolidation had commenced, the rate was 0.25 mm every 2 weeks for more 2 months. Standard pin care with possible showering and application of dry gauze around the pins was recommended [13, 16]. Oral antibiotics were prescribed for patients with pin site infections.

All patients were encouraged to partially bear weight with the assistance of crutches on the 2nd day after surgery. All frames were dynamized before removal. Group A dynamization was performed by replacing the TSF struts with traditional Ilizarov rods. The HA-coated half-pins were removed with the patient under short-term sedation in the operating room. After frame removal, patients were restricted to partial weight bearing for 4–6 weeks. The final bony and functional results were classified accordingly to the criteria proposed by Paley and Maar [18].

Statistical analysis

Obtained data are presented as means ± standard deviations, ranges, numbers, and percentages. Results were analyzed by conducting one-way analysis of variance with post hoc Tukey honest significant difference test and Chi-squared test. Statistical analysis was conducted by using SPSS version 15 statistical software package (IBM Corporation, Armonk, NY). A p value < 0.05 was considered statistically significant.

Results

The mean duration of follow-up was 48 ± 12.8 months (range 26–78 months) in group A and 53 ± 16.5 months (range 25–74 months) in group B, with a nonsignificant difference in favor of group B ($p > 0.05$). Positive nonsignificant correlation was shown between presence of infection and length of duration of follow-up in both groups ($p > 0.05$). Table 2 presents the postoperative bony and functional outcomes of the study population.

In group A, tibial bone healing was achieved in all cases (100 %), with a union rate of 90 % after the first procedure. The mean external fixation time was 418 ± 144.8 days (range 168–770 days). The average distance of bone transport was 7.6 ± 3.5 cm (range 3–15 cm). The mean lengthening index was 1.97 ± 0.7 (range 1.1–3.4) (Fig. 2). At the time of the 3-year follow-up visit, the fracture sites were completely united and the

Table 2 Postoperative bony and functional outcomes

Outcomes	Overall population ($n = 55$)	Group A ($n = 30$)	Group B ($n = 25$)
Bony, n (%)			
Excellent	28 (51)	17 (47)	11 (44)
Good	18 (33)	10 (33)	8 (32)
Fair	5 (9)	2 (7)	3 (12)
Poor	4 (7)	1 (3)	3 (12)
Functional, n (%)			
Excellent	25 (45)	14 (47)	11 (44)
Good	21 (38)	12 (40)	9 (36)
Fair	5 (9)	3 (10)	2 (8)
Poor	4 (7)	1 (3)	3 (12)

None of the differences shown reached statistical significance

patients had no clinical infection, skin defect, or limb length discrepancy. Using the Association for the Study and Application of the Method of Ilizarov outcome score, the bony result was excellent and the functional result was good. Bony results were excellent in 17 cases, good in 10, fair in two, and poor in one. Functional results were excellent in 14 cases, good in 12, fair in three, and poor in one. Negative nonsignificant correlation was shown between lengthening index and both external fixation time and distance of bone transport.

In group B, tibial bone healing was achieved in 24 (96 %) of 25 cases, with a union rate of 88 % after the first surgery with a nonsignificant difference in favor of group A ($p > 0.05$). The mean external fixation time was 359 ± 130.8 days (range 120–670 days), which was nonsignificantly shorter than the external fixation time in group A ($p > 0.05$). The average distance of bone transport was 6.5 ± 3 cm (range 3–17 cm), which was shorter than the average distance reported in group A, but the difference did not reach statistical significance ($p > 0.05$). The mean lengthening index was 2.1 ± 0.9 (range 1.3–4.0) and was nonsignificantly higher than the index reported for group A ($p > 0.05$). Bony results were excellent in 11 patients, good in eight, fair in three, and poor in three. Functional results were excellent in 11 patients, good in nine, fair in two, and poor in three. Bony and functional results were nonsignificantly lower in group B compared with group A ($p > 0.05$). A negative nonsignificant correlation was shown between lengthening index and both external fixation time and distance of bone transport ($p > 0.05$).

In both groups, negative nonsignificant correlation was shown between lengthening index and external fixation time ($p > 0.05$). Likewise, in both groups, negative nonsignificant correlation was shown between lengthening index and distance of bone transport ($p > 0.05$).

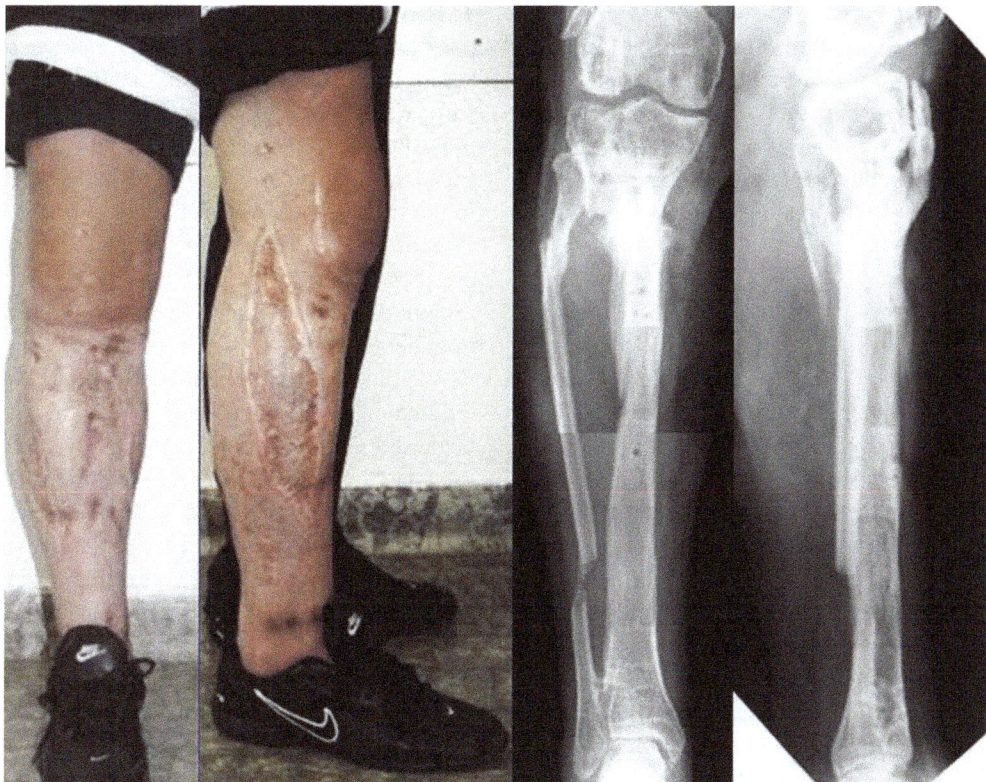

Fig. 2 Clinical and radiographic follow-up images obtained 3 years after tibial frame removal. Treatment time, 16 months; lengthening amount, 140 mm; lengthening index (months/cm), 1.14. Mechanical axis deviation was 8 mm medial to the center of the knee joint line. Patient resumed full weight bearing without support and with no discomfort

Complications

No intraoperative complications were caused by insertion of the pins or use of the Gigli saw. No compartment syndrome occurred in association with tibial osteotomy. In both groups, pain was the most common complaint during the distraction period, particularly in patients requiring lengthening in excess of 4 cm. Pain was relieved by orally administered analgesics. The most frequently occurring complication in our study was pin tract infection, which occurred in 31 patients in both groups (56 %).

Other minor complications occurred in group A: 1) half-pin breakage occurred in three patients and half-pin loosening, requiring early removal, in two; 2) residual limb length discrepancies measuring 1.5 cm occurred in two patients and 2.0 cm in one (treated with internal shoe lifts, no functional problems); 3) minimal (<5°) regenerate bending occurred in three patients.

Seven major complications occurred in group A: 1) osteitis occurred in the distal tibia of one patient 3 months after fixator removal (healed with arthrodesis of the ankle after two repeated bifocal bone transports); 2) bending of regenerate bone occurred in two patients (both recovered after additional surgical procedures: reapplication of fixator for 3 months in one and plate fixation in the other; 3)

uncommon delayed peroneal artery pseudoaneurysm occurred in one patient after surgical procedure at the docking site (supported by angiography, embolization with coil treatment was successful) [17]; 4) equinus ankle contractures occurred in three patients with large bone defects (trifocal bone transports: two retrograde and one antegrade). Correction was obtained with Achilles tendon lengthening and was maintained with extension of the frame to the foot.

Minor complications occurred in group B: 1) three pins fractured in three patients; 2) five pins were added during the course of treatment of three patients to provide additional function; 3) minimal (<5°) regenerate bending occurred in four patients; 4) limb length discrepancies measuring 1.5 and 2.0 cm occurred in two patients without causing functional problems.

Four major complications occurred in group B: 1) refracture of previously consolidated docking sites occurred in two patients at 318 and 121 days because of recurrent sepsis (both treated with second bifocal treatment with simple compression at docking site: one healed with optimal bony and functional results, the other, a 61-year-old man who was diabetic and a heavy smoker with an initial septic nonunion of the leg, was still receiving treatment at the time of this writing; 2) nonunion of the regenerate bone in an immunosuppressed patient who was a heavy smoker and who otherwise achieved consolidation of the docking site (further treatment was refused); 3) equinus ankle contracture occurred in one patient (correction obtained with Achilles tendon lengthening and extension of the frame to the foot); 4) misalignment of the transported distal fragment before docking in one patient (required additional correction surgery).

Discussion

The bifocal and trifocal bone transport using the I–TSF technique in group A produced excellent and good bony and functional results, respectively, in 27 and 26 cases, respectively, versus 19 cases in group B. In three (10 %) cases in group A, previous treatment had failed compared with three (12 %) cases in group B. The treatment times with the bifocal and trifocal techniques were long in both groups. Considering the intrinsically long treatment times, careful patient selection is necessary.

In a recent review of our experience [10], we assessed and compared I–TSF trifocal and bifocal techniques for the treatment of seven segmental tibial bone defects, achieving union without malalignment of the mechanical axis [19]. With this report, we updated our series with 18 new cases, introducing a second group of 25 cases in which a bone transport procedure was performed with a conventional circular frame. These results represent the early experience with use of the TSF with this technique. As time has progressed, the technique has been refined and results have become more reliable. In the present study, no case developed malalignment or bony deformity in either group.

Bone transport is inherently more complicated than compression–distraction, with respectively longer treatment times and further operative procedures being necessary. Because the defect is closed gradually, a time delay exists before bony contact and compression occur at the docking site, thus prolonging treatment time. As noted by Paley and Maar [18], the bone healing index gradually decreases the longer the lengthening time and/or the larger bone transport gap is. The transported segment of bone can be deviated as it passes through the soft tissues, leading to translation at the docking site.

In the three-dimensional space, six different directions of displacement are possible between an upper and a lower ring: the six degrees of freedom. The TSF allowed the necessary ring displacements in all cases without time-consuming preoperative planning of joint or slider positions using the software mode of the total residual program [20].

Treatment of rotation deformities with respect to the vertical axis is known to be especially difficult. With the TSF, rotation with respect to any axis in space can be performed, and translations attributable rotations can be taken into account mathematically [21]. In bifocal and trifocal transports, strut bars of TSF can interfere with half-pins during bone transfer or axial and rotational corrections. Strut bars allow precise docking of the bone transport to the target point, with accurate axis alignment and, when resections are correctly performed, circumferential compression of the docking site [18]. At times, partial remounting of the fixator is required during the course of treatment.

We did not treat bone loss with acute shortening and re-lengthening for immediate contact of the resected ends because infection was present in 38 (69 %) of 55 cases and the bone defects were larger than 3 cm in all patients. Bone grafting at the docking site was required in 33 (60 %) of 55 cases of bone transport [22, 23]. Consolidation of the regenerate bone without further complications was achieved in 28 (93 %) of 30 patients in group A and 24 (96 %) of 25 patients in group B. Consolidation of the docking site without further complications was achieved in 29 (97 %) of 30 patients in group A and 23 (92 %) of 25 patients in group B. Percentages of healing were therefore similar. Group B patients, however, had shorter transports (6.5 versus 7.6), and this factor could be a bias affecting the results of group A, as has been observed in terms of total external fixation time in different groups. In addition, the lengthening index seems to be superior in group B (2.10 versus 1.97 in group A), but the difference is largely because of a higher number of trifocal procedures. Several complications occurred in our study; however, the rate was reasonable considering the complexity of the cases.

One limitation of our study was the variety of fixators used in group B. Four types of conventional circular frames were included. However, the standard Ilizarov procedure was used with all four types. Also, cases that were allocated to receive I–TSF were more complex cases than those receiving only conventional circular frames, which might have introduced selection bias. Further limitations of our study include the small sample size and retrospective design. Further comparative studies are needed to prove the efficacy of bone transport with a TSF in combination with an Ilizarov frame compared with a conventional circular frame only.

Conclusion

When it is necessary to perform bone transport, to optimize conditions for healing, the necrotic or infected bone ends should be resected and fashioned in such a way as to enhance docking. The frame should be carefully mounted to be parallel in both planes to prevent translation. Bone grafting of the docking site, if necessary, should be performed early. Our results are promising in terms of achieved union rates, axis alignment of the lower extremity, and eradication of infections. Although the superiority of one treatment modality over the other cannot be concluded based on our data, the study shows that the combined use of the TSF and Ilizarov frame for bone transport is useful for treatment of tibial nonunion with bone loss.

Acknowledgments No financial support was received for this study. The authors thank Dori Kelly, MA, for professional manuscript editing.

Human participants and animals rights This article does not contain any studies with human participants or animals performed by any of the authors.

Informed consent Informed consent was obtained from all individual participants included in the study.

References

1. Brownlow HC, Reed A, Simpson AH (2002) The vascularity of atrophic non-unions. Injury 33(2):145
2. Cierny G III, Zorn KE (1994) Segmental tibial defects: comparing conventional and Ilizarov methodologies. Clin Orthop Relat Res 301:118
3. Lavini F, Dall'Oca C, Bartolozzi P (2010) Bone transport and compression-distraction in the treatment of bone loss of the lower limbs. Injury 41(11):1191
4. Taylor JC (1992) Delayed union and nonunion of fractures. In: Crenshaw AH (ed) Campbell's operative orthopaedics. Mosby, St. Louis, pp 1287–1313
5. Dendrinos GK, Kontos S, Lyritsis E (1995) Use of the Ilizarov technique for treatment of non-union of the tibia associated with infection. J Bone Joint Surg Am 77(6):835
6. Ilizarov GA (1992) The apparatus: components and biomechanical principles of application. Transosseous osteosynthesis. Springer, Berlin, pp 63–120
7. Ilizarov GA, Ledyaev VI (1992) The replacement of long tubular bone defects by lengthening distraction osteotomy of one of the fragments. Clin Orthop Relat Res 280:7
8. Song HR, Cho SH, Koo KH, Jeong ST, Park YJ, Ko JH (1998) Tibial bone defects treated by internal bone transport using the Ilizarov method. Int Orthop 22(5):293
9. Rozbruch SR, Pugsley JS, Fragomen AT, Ilizarov S (2008) Repair of tibial nonunions and bone defects with the Taylor spatial frame. J Orthop Trauma 22(2):88
10. Sala F, Thabet AM, Castelli F, Miller AN, Capitani D, Lovisetti G, Talamonti T, Singh S (2011) Bone transport for post infectious segmental tibial bone defects with a combined Ilizarov/Taylor spatial frame technique. J Orthop Trauma 25(3):162
11. Rozbruch SR, Weitzman AM, Watson JT, Freudigman P, Katz HV, Ilizarov S (2006) Simultaneous treatment of tibial bone and soft-tissue defects with the Ilizarov method. J Orthop Trauma 20(3):197
12. Elbatrawy Y, Fayed M (2009) Deformity correction with an external fixator: ease of use and accuracy? Orthopedics 32(2):82
13. Sala F, Elbatrawy Y, Thabet AM, Zayed M, Capitani D (2013) Taylor spatial frame fixation in patients with multiple traumatic injuries: study of 57 long-bone fractures. J Orthop Trauma 27(8):442
14. Sala F, Salerno CF, Albisetti W (2013) Pseudoaneurysm of the peroneal artery: an unusual complication of open docking site procedure in bone transport with Taylor spatial frame. Musculoskelet Surg 97(2):183
15. Paley D (1990) Problems, obstacles, and complications of limb lengthening by the Ilizarov technique. Clin Orthop Relat Res 250:81
16. Moroni A, Vannini F, Mosca M, Giannini S (2002) Techniques to avoid pin loosening and infection in external fixation. J Orthop Trauma 16(3):189
17. Shirai T, Shimizu T, Ohtani K, Zen Y, Takaya M, Tsuchiya H (2011) Antibacterial iodine-supported titanium implants. Acta Biomater 7(4):1928
18. Paley D, Maar DC (2000) Ilizarov bone transport treatment for tibial defects. J Orthop Trauma 14(2):76
19. Lovisetti G, Sala F, Thabet AM, Catagni MA, Singh S (2011) Osteocutaneous thermal necrosis of the leg salvaged by TSF/Ilizarov reconstruction: report of 7 patients. Int Orthop 35(1):121
20. Feldman DS, Shin SS, Madan S, Koval KJ (2003) Correction of tibial malunion and nonunion with six-axis analysis deformity correction using the Taylor spatial frame. J Orthop Trauma 17(8):549
21. Seide K, Wolter D, Kortmann HR (1999) Fracture reduction and deformity correction with the hexapod Ilizarov fixator. Clin Orthop Relat Res 363:186
22. Giotakis N, Narayan B, Nayagam S (2007) Distraction osteogenesis and nonunion of the docking site: is there an ideal treatment option? Injury 38(Suppl 1):S100
23. Lovisetti G, Sala F, Miller AN, Thabet AM, Zottola V, Capitani D (2012) Clinical reliability of closed techniques and comparison with open strategies to achieve union at the docking site. Int Orthop 36(4):817

20

Distal femoral valgus osteotomy: bone healing time in single plane and biplanar technique

J. A. D. van der Woude[1] · S. Spruijt[1] · B. T. J. van Ginneken[1] · R. J. van Heerwaarden[2]

Abstract Varus deformity can be localized in the tibia, in the femur or in both. If varus deformity is localized within the femur, it is mandatory to correct it in the femur. This report presents the technique and results of a consecutive case series of lateral uniplanar and biplanar closed-wedge valgus osteotomy of the distal femur for the treatment of varus deformity of the knee. Retrospectively, fifteen patients (sixteen knees) were identified. Indications for surgery varied from unloading an osteoarthritic medial compartment to reduction to symmetrical varus leg alignment. Pre- and post-operative X-rays, including a full leg radiograph, were assessed as well as bone healing time at follow-up intervals. Clinical outcome was assessed using different questionnaires. There were nine male and six female patients with a median age at surgery of 45 (±14) years. The mLDFA changed from 95.9° (±2.7°) preoperatively to 89.3° (±2.9°) post-operatively. Preoperative planning and the use of angle stable implants resulted in accurate corrections according to preoperative aims in all but one patient. At follow-up (mean, 40 months), the mean VAS score was 2.5 (±2.4) and the WOMAC score averaged 80 (±20). The mean bone healing time of biplanar osteotomies (4 ± 3 months) was shorter than in the uniplanar osteotomies (6 ± 3 months). Distal lateral closed-wedge valgus osteotomy of the femur for the treatment of femoral varus deformities resulted in clinical improvement and accurate corrections in patients with different aims for correction. A biplanar osteotomy technique shortens bone healing time.

Keywords Distal femoral osteotomy · Valgus producing · Closed-wedge · Limb alignment · Biplanar · Uniplanar

Introduction

Varus malalignment of the knee is associated with the development and progression of knee osteoarthritis [1]. In a biomechanical study, it was demonstrated that the cartilage of the medial compartment of the knee is loaded predominantly in a varus knee; a neutral mechanical axis loads the medial slightly more than the lateral compartment; and in valgus alignment the main load is through the lateral compartment [2].

The rationale for osteotomies around the knee in symptomatic osteoarthritic joints is to offload the affected compartment by shifting the weight-bearing axis to the more normal compartment and achieve a more even distribution of pressure and accomplish pain relief. In addition, osteotomies are indicated to correct deformity or to obtain alignment symmetrical to the contralateral side. Traditionally, a high tibial osteotomy (HTO) is used to correct varus deformity and distal femoral osteotomy (DFO) to correct a valgus deformity. However, the source of a varus deformity can be localized in the tibia, in the femur (Fig. 1) or in both. The same is true for a valgus deformity. If a varus deformity that is localized in the femur is corrected using a valgus-producing HTO, the end results will be a re-aligned limb axis at the cost of an excessively oblique joint line [3, 4]. Joint-line obliquity of

✉ R. J. van Heerwaarden
vanheerwaarden@yahoo.com

[1] Limb Deformity Reconstruction Unit, Department of Orthopaedic Surgery, Maartenskliniek Woerden, Polanerbaan 2, 3447 GN Woerden, The Netherlands

[2] Centre for Deformity Correction and Joint Preserving Surgery, Kliniek ViaSana, Hoogveldseweg 1, 5451 AA Mill, The Netherlands

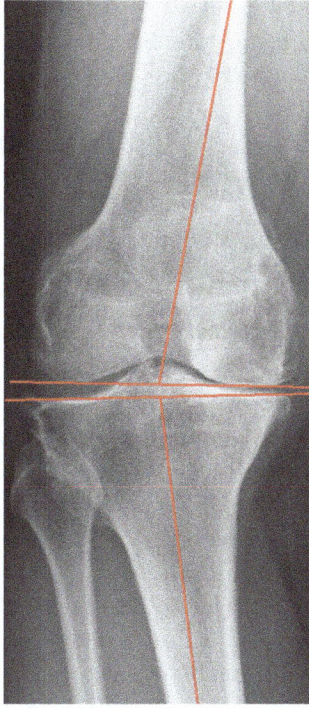

Fig. 1 Example of varus deformity in the distal femur (mLDFA 100°, MPTA 86°)

the knee is not tolerated well because of increased shear stresses [3] and may lead to technical difficulties when performing a total knee arthroplasty [5].

Distal femoral osteotomy techniques for lateral OA from femoral deformities have evolved to more accurate corrections, decreased bone healing problems and improved clinical scores [6–9]. Whilst the literature on varus osteotomies on the distal femur is increasing, reports on valgus distal femoral osteotomies are scant. This retrospective review presents the technique and results of a consecutive series of lateral closed-wedge valgus osteotomies of the distal femur for the treatment of symptomatic varus deformity.

Materials and methods

Sample

We identified fifteen patients (sixteen knees) who underwent a closed-wedge valgus-producing osteotomy of the femur for the treatment of varus deformity in our department in the past decade. The osteotomies were performed between 2005 and 2012, in two centres in the Netherlands (Maartenskliniek Woerden and Sint Maartenskliniek Nijmegen). Two experienced surgeons (RJvH and SS) performed all osteotomies using the techniques described below. The objectives of surgery differed: indications included medial compartment offloading in medial

osteoarthritis; a decrease in varus alignment to normal; and a restoration of leg alignment symmetrical to the contralateral leg.

Radiograph measurements

All patients underwent preoperative and post-operative plain X-rays of the knee in 3 planes (AP weight-bearing view, lateral view, PA 45° weight-bearing tunnel view and patella skyline view) and a standing full leg AP radiograph. The standing full leg antero-posterior radiographs were obtained using a standardized protocol; patients stood on both feet with the knees in full extension and with the X-ray beam centred on the knee [10]. The degree of osteoarthritis was scored using Kellgren and Lawrence scale [11]. In addition, the degree of varus deformity was assessed by measuring the mechanical tibiofemoral angle, the medial proximal tibia angle (MPTA), the mechanical lateral distal femoral angle (mLDFA) and the knee joint-line convergence angle (JLCA) preoperatively and post-operatively [4]. The mechanical axis of the femur is defined as the line between the centre of the femoral head (identified using Mose circles) and the apex of the inter-condylar notch of the femur. The mechanical axis of the tibia runs from the mid-point between the tibial spines to the mid-width of the distal tibia. The mechanical tibiofemoral angle is the angle between the mechanical axis of the femur and tibia [4] and was expressed as a deviation from 180° (positive values indicate varus, negative values valgus). The MPTA is the angle measured medially between the mechanical tibial axis and the tibial joint line (defined as a line tangential to the flat or concave aspect of the subchondral line of the two tibial plateaus) [4]. The mLDFA is the angle measured laterally between the femoral mechanical axis and the femoral joint line (a line tangential to the most distal points on the convexity of the two femoral condyles) [4]. MPTA and mLDFA values between 85° and 90° are considered normal. A MPTA less than 85**°** indicates that the varus deformity is located in the tibia. When there is a mLDFA higher than 90**°**, the femur contributes to the varus deformity. The JLCA was defined as the angle between the femoral and tibial knee joint lines in the frontal plane. A medially converging joint line greater than 3° is abnormal and indicates either ligamentous laxity or loss of cartilage thickness as source of varus malalignment [4]. All measurements were performed by two of the authors (SS and JTW). There were no cases of joint contractures to influence radiographic measurements.

Clinical outcome

The range of motion of the knee was measured preoperatively and during post-operative visits. Knee joint function and quality of life (QoI) were evaluated post-operatively using the validated Dutch knee injury and osteoarthritis outcome score (KOOS) [12] and the Western Ontario and McMaster Universities Osteoarthritis Index (WOMAC) [13], both normalized to a 100 % scale, 100 being the maximum score. The VAS pain score (0–100 mm; "0" meaning no pain) was used to evaluate pain. The Lysholm knee score provided information on instability and functional limitations [14], and the Tegner knee function score (range 0–10) was used to determine the level of activity in work and sports [15]. Questionnaires were sent by postal mail to all patients.

Operative technique

Surgery is performed in supine position with the knee in full extension, and a tourniquet is placed at the root of the thigh to create a bloodless field. A single dose of antibiotic is used preoperatively. Fluoroscopic visualization of the hip, knee and ankle joint is used during surgery.

A 10–15 cm straight lateral incision is made, starting 3 cm proximal to the knee joint line and extending proximally. With the fascia lata split longitudinally, a lateral subvastus approach is started by palpation of the natural opening under the distal part of the vastus lateralis muscle belly at the level of the supratrochlear area. A retractor is used to lift the muscles anteriorly. The dorsal part of the lateral vastus muscle is freed from the intermuscular septum by blunt and sharp dissection. Special care is taken to visualize and ligate the perforating vessels present whilst creating enough room proximally for plate fixation. A blunt Hohmann retractor is placed posteriorly in contact with the bone to protect the popliteal neurovascular bundle.

The starting point for the distal osteotomy on the lateral femur is determined through preoperative digital planning and an intraoperative fluoroscopy check using temporary plate application to locate osteotomy level to optimal plate position (Fig. 2) The desired level of the osteotomy is marked. Under fluoroscopic control, two K-wires are inserted for an oblique down-sloping wedge with the wedge base length at the lateral cortex corresponding to the preoperative planning. The K-wires converge just proximal to the medial femoral condyle, ending 0.5–1 cm short of the medial cortex, and may be inserted freehand or with an osteotomy guide.

A uniplanar closing-wedge osteotomy was performed between 2005 and 2008 by making two transverse cuts with an oscillating saw within the two K-wires. After 2009, we used a biplanar osteotomy technique [16]. In the biplanar technique, the dorsal three-fourth is used for the two transverse osteotomy cuts, whereas a proximally directed frontal plane saw cut is made in the ventral one-fourth of the distal femur. The dorsal cortex is used as a reference for directing the frontal plane cut across the ventral surface; this is performed with a thinner saw blade (Fig. 3).

After wedge removal, the resected wedge is inspected for completeness as remaining bone fragments may cause incomplete closure and fracture of the medial cortical hinge during closure. If this is found, additional bone removal and weakening of the hinge (with help of a special bone impaction instrument—a blunt chisel) are then indicated. Closure of the wedge must be performed gradually and with a gentle valgus force. It may take several minutes to enable plastic deformation of the medial cortex to close the osteotomy gap. It should be noted that the medial cortex of the distal femur in general is weaker and the hinge point of the osteotomy will fracture more often as compared to the lateral cortex hinge point in a medial closing-wedge osteotomy. An intact medial cortex after osteotomy closure provides for higher axial and rotational stability.

Limb alignment is evaluated fluoroscopically using a long rigid alignment rod between the centre of the femoral head and the centre of the ankle. The rod, representing the weight-bearing line, should pass through the knee joint at the preoperatively defined position for the mechanical axis. If adequate correction has been achieved, the osteotomy is stabilized with either a TomoFix (Depuy/Synthes) Lateral Distal Femur plate (LDF) (ipsilateral version) or with a TomoFix Medial Distal Femur Plate (MDF) (contralateral version). The decision is based on personal choice of the surgeon. However, the MDF plate is less pronounced after insertion and therefore more suitable in shorter and smaller femurs.

The plate is mounted with drill guides and is, with a spacer to protect the periosteum, distally placed on the lateral femur condyle and proximally in line with the femur shaft in the frontal and sagittal plane. Temporary fixation distal to the osteotomy is performed with a K-wire drilled through a guiding sleeve. Plate position is checked fluoroscopically. As the TomoFix is an internal fixator, precise fit to the femur is not necessary. After drilling, at least four self-tapping locking screws are inserted distally. Next, a bicortical self-tapping lag screw is inserted eccentrically in the dynamic part of the combi-hole directly superior to the osteotomy putting the osteotomy under axial compression. Three self-tapping monocortical or bicortical (depending on bone quality and patient's stature) screws are inserted in the remaining holes proximal of the lag screw. Finally, the lag screw is changed for a self-tapping bicortical locking screw inserted in the locking part of the combi-hole. After a final check with the image intensifier, the wound is closed over a non-suction drain. Care is taken to meticulously close the fascia lata before subcutaneous closure. The skin is closed subcuticularly.

Fig. 2 The starting point for the distal osteotomy at the lateral femur is defined by preoperative digital planning (**a**) and intraoperative fluoroscopy check using temporary plate application (**b**) to relate osteotomy height to optimal plate position

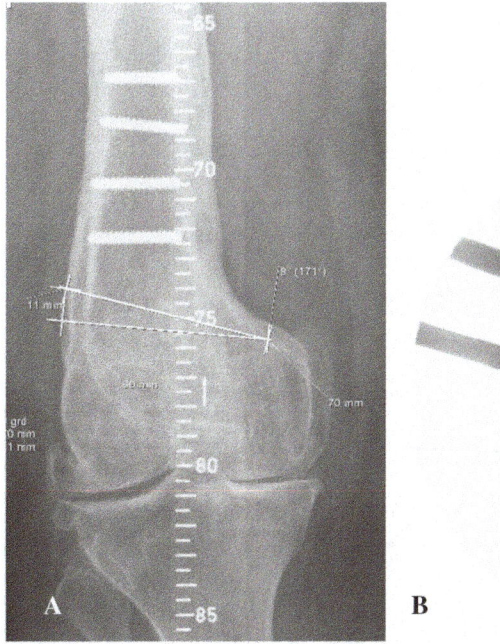

Fig. 3 Example of the biplanar technique in a left distal femur intraoperatively (**a**) and in a sawbone (**b**). The two transverse cuts are made in the dorsal three-fourth, whereas the proximal directed frontal plane saw cut is made in the ventral one-fourth of the distal femur

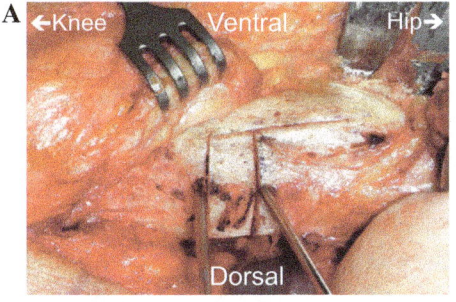
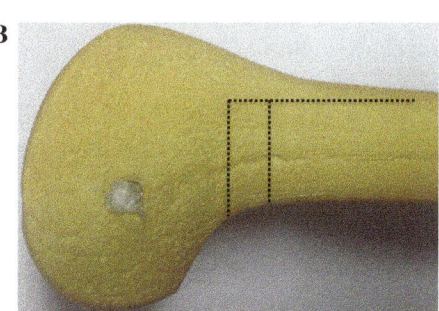

Post-operative care

A sterile compressive bandage is applied after surgery. In the first 24 h during rest, the knee is positioned in a 60–90° flexion position to prevent adhesions of the vastus lateralis muscle to the femur [17, 18]. Full range of active and passive movement of the knee is started as soon as tolerated by the patient with the help of a physiotherapist. During the first 6 weeks partial (no more than 15–20 kg) weight-bearing is allowed between crutches. Clinical and radiographic proof of bone healing at 6 weeks enables progressive weight-to-full-weight bearing.

Comparison of bone healing time

Bone healing at 6 weeks, 3 months, 6 months, 9 months and 12 months post-surgery was evaluated on standard coronal and sagittal radiographs. Full bone healing was defined as full reformation, though osteotomy recognizable, as described by van Hemert et al. [19] Bone healing time at different

follow-up times for biplanar and uniplanar osteotomies was scored and compared using standard *T* test for comparison.

Results

Of the fifteen patients (sixteen knees) who underwent an isolated valgus-producing closing-wedge distal femoral osteotomy (DFO), one patient had a total knee arthroplasty within 2 years. There were nine male and six female patients with a median age at surgery of 45 (±14) years. Preoperatively, 63 % of the cases had a Kellgren and Lawrence grade of III. Table 1 shows the sample characteristics. One patient had a bilateral closed-wedge valgus DFO. The causes of varus deformity were: femoral malunion in five knees; overcorrection of a valgus deformity (previous osteotomy) in four knees; secondary to an (hemi)-epiphysiodesis in two knees; and idiopathic in five knees with osteochondritis dissecans of the medial femoral condyle in two knees. Five osteotomies were preceded by

Table 1 Characteristics of the study population

Number of patients (n)	15
Number of osteotomies (n)	16
Mean age at surgery [years (±SD)]	45 ± 14
Gender ratio (M:F)	9:6
Mean body length at surgery [cm (±SD)]	180 ± 11
Mean weight at surgery [kg (±SD)]	86 ± 20
Mean body mass index at surgery [kg/m² (±SD)]	26 ± 4
Side (left:right)	6:10
Kellgren and Lawrence grade	
Grade 1 [n (%)]	2 (12.5 %)
Grade 2 [n (%)]	3 (18.8 %)
Grade 3 [n (%)]	10 (62.5 %)
Grade 4 [n (%)]	1 (6.3 %)
Mean follow-up [months (±SD)]	40 ± 30

an arthroscopy; one had a partial lateral meniscectomy and four a partial medial meniscectomy.

Operative data

There were no intraoperative complications. The mean duration of the surgery was 89 min (range 50–135 min). In six knees, the DFO was uniplanar and in ten biplanar. An angular stable LDF plate was used in twelve knees, an angular stable MDF plate (contralateral) in three and in one knee, because of non-availability of other plates at time of surgery, a LISS plate. In two knees, additional fixation was used: in one knee a staple at the fractured medial hinge and in one other knee an antero-posterior lag screw through the anterior flange of the biplane osteotomy. A fracture of the hinge without dislocation was observed in eight knees.

No systemic complications, wound infections, or nerve palsies occurred. Due to tenderness, seven patients required plate removal. In one patient, an ACL-reconstruction as well as an open-wedge valgus high tibial osteotomy was performed several years after the index surgery for progressive symptomatic medial osteoarthritis causing tibial varus deformity and instability. In two patients, an arthroscopy was necessary (amongst them the patient who underwent the total knee arthroplasty).

Radiographic measurement results

The mean preoperative mechanical tibiofemoral axis was 10.0° (±2.6°) of varus which reduced to 3.1° (±2.6°) varus after surgery. The mLDFA changed from 95.9° (±2.7°) preoperatively to 89.3° (±2.9°) post-operatively. The mean MPTA did not substantially contribute to varus in this group of patients, being 87.8° (±2.3°) preoperatively.

Figure 4 shows pre- and post-operative leg alignment in two cases. All pre- and post-operative radiographic measurements are in Table 2 and Fig. 5. The preoperative indication and aim of correction of each case are displayed in Table 3.

Clinical results

As one patient had a total knee arthroplasty, fourteen (fifteen knees) of the included fifteen patients (sixteen knees) could be evaluated clinically (Table 3). The clinical results were assessed at a mean of 40 months (±30) post-operatively. At follow-up, the mean VAS score was 2.5 (±2.4). The subjective result according to the Lysholm score was excellent in one patient, good in three patients, fair in six patients and poor in four patients. All the patients who scored good or excellent on the Lysholm scale had grade I or II of osteoarthritis according to the scale of Kellgren and Lawrence. On the Tegner activity scale, the mean level was 3 (±1.7). At follow-up, the WOMAC score averaged 80 (±20). The mean score at follow-up of the individual components of the WOMAC index (pain, stiffness and function) were 80 (±18), 75 (±26) and 81 (±21), respectively. The range of flexion and extension did not change between preoperative and post-operative measurements (118° ± 14° preoperative versus 117° ± 15° post-operative). The mean length of hospital stay was 3 (±1) days.

Bone healing time results

All but 3 patients in the biplane DFO group showed union at the 3 months follow-up radiographs. The remaining patients showed union at, respectively, 6, 7 and 9 months of follow-up. In the single plane DFO group, two patients showed union at the 3 months follow-up radiographs, one at 5 months, one at 7 months, one at 8 months and one at 10 months. Comparison of the mean time to union between the biplane osteotomy group (3.9 ± 2.5 months) and the single plane group (6.1 ± 2.7 months) did not show a significant difference (p = 0.118).

Discussion

This retrospective cohort study is a report on the short- to mid-term results of the distal lateral closed-wedge valgus osteotomy of the femur. Carefully planned single plane and biplane osteotomies have produced significant symptom relief in most patients although clinical scores in two patients indicated persistent functional impairments.

Deformities around the knee should be subject to a systematic deformity analysis using standardized full leg standing radiographs [20]. In this sample, a femoral

Fig. 4 Leg alignment preoperative (**a–c**) and 3 months post-operative in two cases (**b–d**)

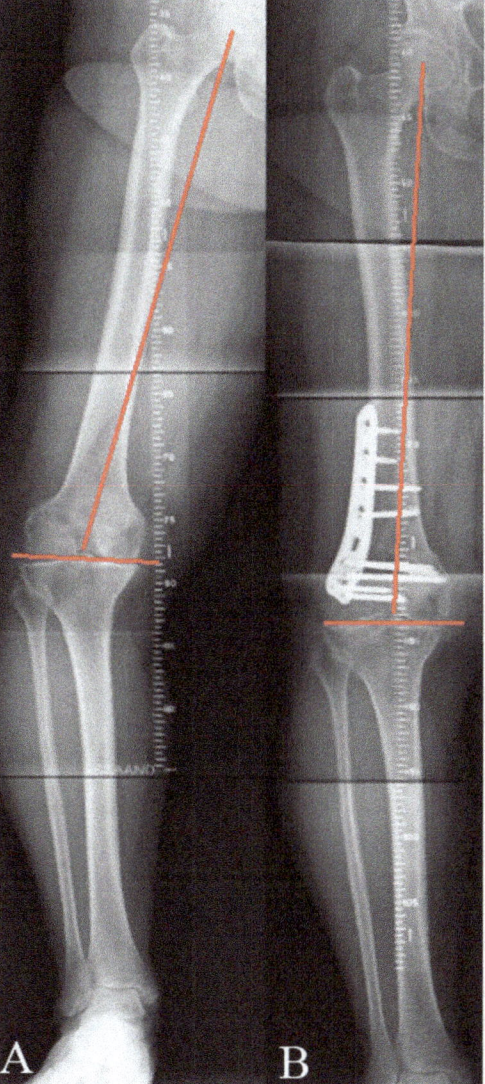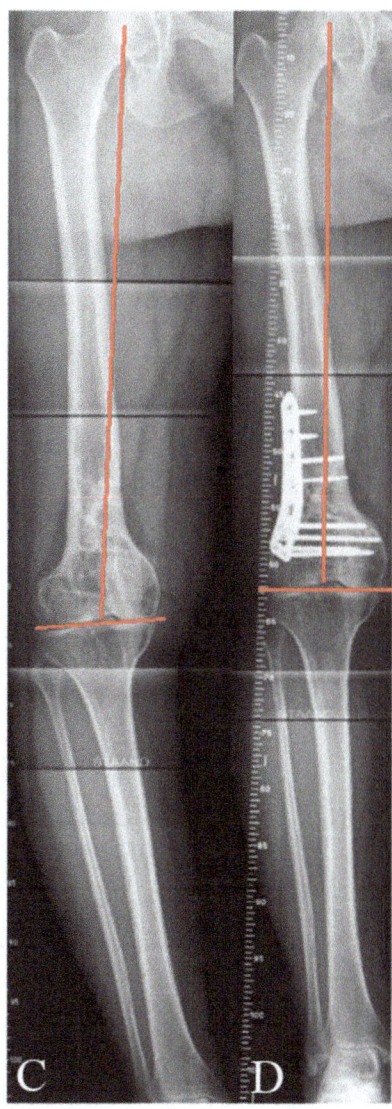

deformity was identified as the origin of the varus of the leg. Each deformity should be corrected at its source otherwise joint-line obliquity will be the result [5, 21]. Accordingly, valgus osteotomies are performed at the tibial level, femoral level or both levels simultaneously depending on the source of the deformity (i.e. a tailored approach) [3]. Joint-line obliquity is to be avoided as it results in increased shear stresses at the cartilage joint surface (even tibiofemoral subluxation) and may hamper subsequent joint replacement surgery.

The influence of joint-line obliquity and varus orientation of the distal femur on the results of osteotomies around the knee has been reported. Terauchi et al. [22] found that the presence of a preoperative varus deformity of the distal femur was associated with recurrence of varus deformity and poor results after HTO. Van Raaij et al. [23] did not find a significant correlation between distal femoral joint-line orientation and failure of HTO. This can be explained by the fact that the mean preoperative distal femur alignment in their patients was mild valgus (mean mLDFA 89.1 ± 2.1°), whereas our patients had a clear varus malalignment of the distal femur with a mean mLDFA of 95.9° (±2.7°). Babis et al. [5] looked at obliquity of the joint line as a prognostic factor. In a series of patients with large varus deformities and medial compartment osteoarthritis, treated with a double level osteotomy, normal knee joint-line orientation was preserved and they showed in a computer model that the tension of stabilizing ligaments (i.e. collateral ligaments) remained normal after correction.

The leg alignment after deformity correction ranged from 1.3° valgus to 7.1° varus; the aims for correction differed from unloading in case of medial compartment osteoarthritis, decrease in varus to normal varus or restoration of limb symmetry (see also Table 3). In four patients, the valgus osteotomies were performed for a varus that had arisen from a previous overcorrection of a valgus

Table 2 Preoperative and post-operative radiographic measurements

	Preoperative					Post-operative					
Case	K&L	TFA	MPTA	mLDFA	JLCA	K&L	TFA	mLDFA	JLCA	HF	BHT
1	3	10	90	99	2	4	2.5	90.7	1.4	Yes	9
2	4	5.5	92	95	3.5	4	4.0	89	2.5	No	3.8
3	3	14	86	95	5	3	3.5	85	5.5	Yes	4.8
4	1	10.5	86.5	95	3	1	1.5	85.5	3.5	No	3.5
5	2	10	87.5	96.5	2	2	2.5	88	2	Yes	3
6	3	8.5	93	102	0.5	3	1.5	95.5	2 Lat	Yes	3
7	2	8.5	89	95.5	3	2	0.2	90.5	0.5 Lat	No	5.5
8	3	10.5	88	95	4	3	6	91	5	Yes	10
9	3	7	88	93	2	3	−1	87	1.5	No	2.3
10	3	16	86	100	2.5	3	5.5	91	1 Lat	Yes	2.3
11	2	13	86	98	0.5	2	7.1	93.9	1.4	Yes	7
12	3	9	88.5	95	3	3	4.5	90	3	No	1.5
13	3	9	86	93	2	3	3	86	3	Yes	8
14	3	9.5	87	91	5	3	7	88	5	No	7
15	3	11	85	95	1.5	3	3.5	90	0	No	4
16	1	8.5	86	95.5	0.5 Lat	1	−1.3	87.5	1 Lat	No	1.5

K&L scale of Kellgren and Lawrence, grade 0 normal, grade 1 min osteophytes, grade 2 definite osteo-phyte, grade 3 moderate joint-space reduction, grade 4 severe joint-space narrowing with sclerosis and osteophytes, TFA mechanical tibiofemoral angle (degree, positive values indicate varus alignment, nega-tive values indicate valgus alignment), MPTA medial proximal tibial angle (degree)

mLDFA mechanical lateral distal femoral angle (degree), *JLCA* joint-line convergence angle (degree), *Lat* lateral convergence, *HF* hinge fracture, *BHT* bone healing time (months)

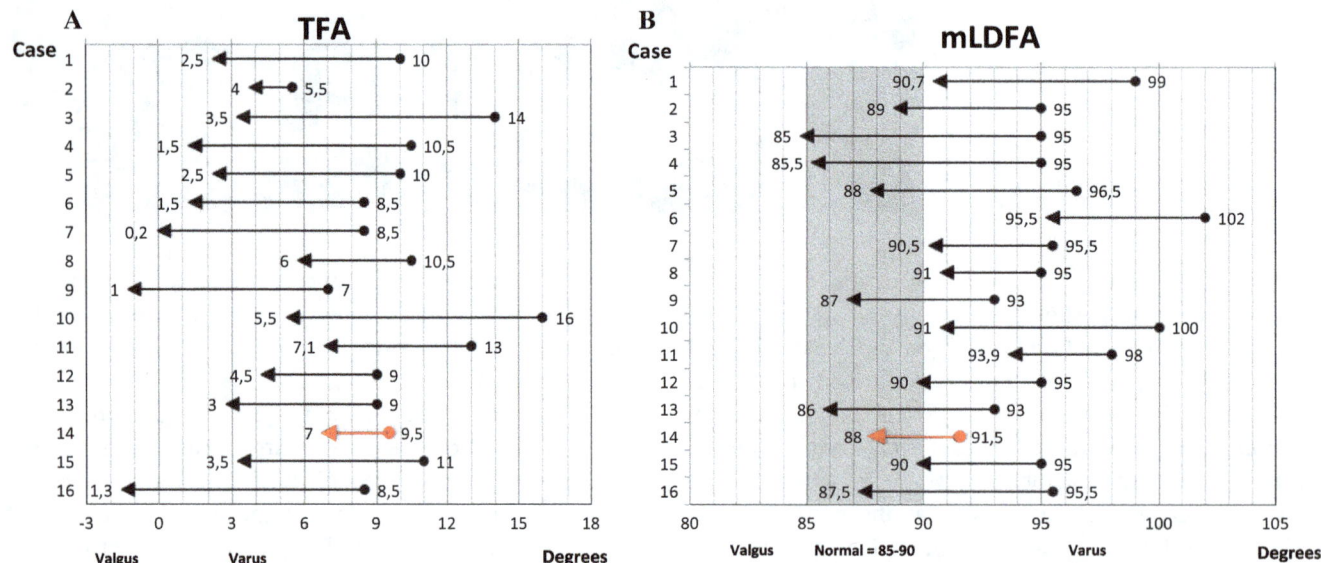

Fig. 5 Change of mechanical tibiofemoral angle (TFA) per patient (**a**) and the change of mechanical lateral distal femoral angle (mLDFA) per patient (**b**). The preoperative deformities are represented by the *circles* and the post-operative values are represented by the *arrowheads*. The *red line* represents the failure (i.e. total knee arthroplasty) (color figure online)

deformity. In most of these cases, a neutral mechanical axis was intended. One osteotomy had resulted in an under correction. Performing a closed-wedge osteotomy is known to be difficult technically because the surgeon has to rely on the accuracy of the bone resection. Careful preoperative planning and the use of oblique osteotomy cuts of equal length in an isosceles triangle prevent cortical overlap after gap closure [6, 16]. Our final range of tibiofemoral angles were within a similar range to that published for distal femoral varus osteotomies (6° varus to 10° valgus) [24].

Table 3 Indication, aim of correction, clinical scores and plate complaints

Preoperative			Post-operative				
Case	Ind.	Aim	VAS	WOMAC	Lys	Teg	PC
1	PO	B	1	81	73	2	No
2	ID	A	5	74	63	5	No
3	PE	C	1	93	82	2	No
4	PT	B	2	99	92	7	Yes
5	PT	B	0	100	85	3	Yes
6	PO	B	0	92	80	2	No
7	ID	A	7	21	32	0	Yes
8	OCD/ID	A	2	75	58	3	Yes
9	OCD/ID	A	2	75	58	3	Yes
10	PE	C	3	57	78	2	No
11	PT	B	1	98	97	5	No
12	PO	B	7	76	67	2	No
13	ID	A	–	84	60	2	No
14	PT	A	–	–	–	–	Yes
15	PT	B	4	81	75	3	Yes
16	PO	A	2	94	90	3	No

Ind. indication, *PT* post-traumatic (femoral malunion), *PE* previous epiphysiodesis, *ID* idiopathic, *PO* previous osteotomy, *OCD* osteochondritis dissecans, Aim: A unloading, B correction to normal varus, C correction to symmetrical leg alignment, Lys Lysholm, Teg Tegner, PC plate complaints resulting in plate removal. Case 14 represents the failure (i.e. total knee arthroplasty)

Our rate of hinge fractures (50 %) (Table 2) is high compared with the 10–20 % reported after closing-wedge HTO [25]. One of the main reasons for this difference may lie in the correction. For example, in six of the sixteen osteotomies the correction angle was greater than 8°; the risk of a hinge fracture gets higher when the correction angle increases due to the limited plasticity of the cortical (supracondylar) bone [26]. None of the fractured hinges displaced and, by using a temporary bicortical lag screw compression over the osteotomy, including the hinge, stability was restored. In those patients who had more developed leg muscles (and were thought to expose the osteotomy to more axial and torsional loading), a medially placed staple was used or an antero-posterior lag screw through the anterior flange of the biplane osteotomy.

The highest clinical scores were found in patients with post-traumatic deformities that according to aim had been corrected to normal varus alignment (Tables 2, 3). Patients with a failed previous femoral osteotomy had high clinical scores also, whereas lower scores were found in patients presenting with grade III osteoarthritis following osteochondritis dissecans (cases 8 and 9). In our sample, eleven osteotomies were performed in patients with moderate and

severe (stage III and IV) osteoarthritis according to the scale of Kellgren and Lawrence. As observed by other authors a significant association exists between preoperative Kellgren and Lawrence grade and HTO failure [27]. There were moderate results in these patients with an average WOMAC score of 80 and only one patient requiring a total knee arthroplasty. It should be noted that in a femoral realignment osteotomy, axis restoration is planned and accomplished for the extended knee (i.e. walking). In 90° of flexion, the contact point of the loaded posterior condyles on the tibia remains unchanged [6].

One case (6.3 %) required a total knee arthroplasty and was classified as a failure. This is in line with failure rates of HTO (3.4 % before 24 months to 7.8 % between 24 and 47 months [25]) and double level osteotomy (3.7 %) [5]. In hindsight, this patient might not have been the ideal candidate for a closed-wedge valgus DFO. In this case, the aim was to correct the femoral deformity with unloading the OA. The preoperative Kellgren and Lawrence grade was III, the mLDFA was not that abnormal (91.5°) preoperatively and the post-operative mechanical tibiofemoral axis was 7° of varus. In seven cases (44 %), the fixation implant was removed. Jacobi et al. [28] reported that fixation of an osteotomy on the lateral side of the distal femur leads to irritation of the iliotibial band. Nevertheless, our rate of 44 % is lower than the 86 % of Jacobi et al. [28]. The lower rate of plate irritation in our sample may be due to the use of the less prominent MDF plate for fixation. None of the three patients with a MDF plate needed removal.

After the introduction of a biplanar technique in medial closing-wedge distal femur osteotomies [8] in our group, a biplanar osteotomy technique was used for lateral closing-wedge osteotomies. Clinical observations and demonstrations in sawbone models would suggest that a biplane medial closing-wedge osteotomy has better bone healing potential over a uniplanar technique [29]. In clinical studies, rapid and uncomplicated bone healing has been found using biplanar osteotomies in medial closing-wedge osteotomies [9] as well as for lateral opening-wedge [30] osteotomies. Bone healing time of the uniplanar osteotomies in the present study was 6.1 ± 2.7 months, whereas the bone healing time of the patients operated with a biplanar technique averaged 3.9 ± 2.5 months. Bone healing was complete in 7 of 10 patients operated on with the biplanar technique at the 3-month follow-up; this is comparable to the bone healing times reported for uniplanar [7, 8] and biplanar medial closing-wedge distal femoral techniques [9] and to those for the lateral open-wedge biplanar osteotomy results of Bagherifard et al. [30]. Of the remaining 3 patients with longer bone healing times in the biplanar osteotomy group, 2 had medial hinge fractures. Increased bone healing time from hinge fractures causing instability in closing-wedge osteotomies has been reported for DFO and HTO [31, 32]. In our population, the mean bone healing time in patients with hinge fractures was 5.8 ± 2.8 months.

Our study has limitations. It was a retrospective study with a small sample. Due to this limited number of patients, the correlation of different variables was not possible. The next step would be a prospective study comparing patients preoperatively and post-operatively after a distal lateral closed-wedge valgus osteotomy of the femur. Nevertheless, the results in our series are encouraging for selected knees. Regarding bone healing time evaluation, the intervals of follow-up hampers an accurate registration of bone healing time. A monthly follow-up would have given us more accurate information on bone healing time.

Based on the results of this study, a biplane distal lateral closed-wedge valgus osteotomy of the femur for the treatment of varus deformity of the knee is a valuable procedure when the deformity is localized in the femur with clinical benefit in most of the patients.

Informed consent Informed consent was obtained from all individual participants included in this study.

References

1. Brouwer GM, van Tol AW, Bergink AP et al (2007) Association between valgus and varus alignment and the development and progression of radiographic osteoarthritis of the knee. Arthritis Rheum 56(4):1204–1211
2. Agneskirchner JD, Hurschler C, Wrann CD et al (2007) The effects of valgus medial opening wedge high tibial osteotomy on articular cartilage pressure of the knee: a biomechanical study. Arthroscopy 23(8):852–861
3. Hofmann S, Lobenhoffer P, Staubli A, Van Heerwaarden R (2009) Osteotomies of the knee joint in patients with mono-compartmental arthritis. Orthopade 38(8):755–769
4. Paley D (2003) Normal lower limb alignment and joint orientation. In: Paley D, Herzenberg JE (eds) Principles of deformity correction, 2nd edn. Springer, New York, pp 1–18
5. Babis GC, An K, Chao EYS et al (2002) Double level osteotomy of the knee: a method to retain joint line obliquity. J Bone Joint Surg Am 84:1380–1388
6. Brinkman JM, Freiling D, Lobenhoffer P, Staubli AE, van Heerwaarden RJ (2014) Supracondylar femur osteotomies around the knee. Patient selection, planning, operative techniques, stability of fixation and bone healing. Orthopade 43(11):988–999
7. Van Heerwaarden R, Wymenga A, Freiling D, Lobenhoffer P (2007) Distal medial closed wedge varus femur osteotomy stabilized with TomoFix plate fixator. Oper Tech Orthop 17(1):12–21
8. Van Heerwaarden RJ, Wymenga AB, Freiling D, Staubli AE (2008) Supracondylar varization osteotomy of the femur with plate fixation. In: Lobenhoffer P, van Heerwaarden RJ, Staubli AE, Jakob RP (eds) Osteotomies around the knee. Georg Thieme Verlag, Stuttgart, pp 147–166
9. Freiling D, van Heerwaarden R, Staubli A et al (2010) Medial closed-wedge osteotomy of the distal femur for the treatment of unicompartmental lateral osteoarthritis of the knee. Oper Orthop Traumatol 22:317–334
10. Paley D (2003) Radiographic assessment of lower limb deformities. In: Paley D, Herzenberg JE (eds) Principles of deformity correction, 2nd edn. Springer, New York, pp 31–60
11. Kellgren JH, Lawrence JS (1957) Radiological assessment of osteoarthritis. Ann Rheum Dis 16:494–502
12. De Groot IB, Favejee MM, Reijman M et al (2008) The Dutch version of the knee injury and osteoarthritis outcome score: a validation study. Health Qual Life Outcomes 16(6):1–11
13. Bellamy N (1995) Outcome measurement in osteoarthritis clinical trials. J Rheumatol Suppl 43:49–51
14. Lysholm J, Gillquist J (1982) Evaluation of knee ligament surgery results with special emphasis on use of a scoring scale. Am J Sports Med 10(3):150–154
15. Tegner Y, Lysholm J (1985) Rating systems in the evaluation of knee ligament injuries. Clin Orthop 198:43–49
16. Van Heerwaarden R, Spruijt S (2014) Die suprakondyläre varisierende und valgisierende Femurosteotomie mit Plattenfixateur. In: Lobenhoffer P, van Heerwaarden R, Agneskirchner JD (eds) Kniegelenknahe Osteotomien. Indikation—Planung—Operationstechniken mit Plattenfixateuren. Georg Thieme Verlag Stuttgart, New York, pp 180–198
17. Müller ME (1977) Suprakondyläre Osteotomien. In: Müller ME, Allgöwer M, Schneider R, Willenegger H (eds) Manual der osteosynthese, 2nd edn. Springer, Berlin, pp 376–377
18. Schatzker J (2005) Postoperative care—supracondylar fractures of the femur. In: Schatzker J, Tile M (eds) The rationale of operative fracture care, 3rd edn. Springer, Berlin, p 437
19. Van Hemert WLW, Willems K, Anderson PG, van Heerwarden RJ, Wymenga AB (2004) Tricalcium phosphate granules or rigid wedge preforms in open wedge high tibial osteotomy: a radiologic study with a new evaluation system. Knee 11(6):451–456
20. Paley D, Herzenberg JE, Tetsworth K et al (1994) A deformity planning for frontal and sagittal plane corrective osteotomies. Orthop Clin North Am 25(3):425–465
21. Saragaglia D, Mercier N, Colle PE (2010) Computer-assisted osteotomies for genu varum deformity: which osteotomy for which varus? Int Orthop 34(2):185–190
22. Terauchi M, Shirakura K, Katayama M et al (2002) Varus inclination of the distal femur and high tibial osteotomy. J Bone Joint Surg Br 84(2):223–226
23. Van Raaij TM, Takacs I, Reijman M, Verhaar JA (2009) Varus inclination of the proximal tibia or the distal femur does not influence high tibial osteotomy outcome. Knee Surg Sports Traumatol Arthrosc 17(4):390–395
24. Saithna A, Kundra R, Modi CS et al (2012) Distal femoral varus osteotomy for lateral compartment osteoarthritis in the valgus knee. A systematic review of the literature. Open Orthop J 6:313–319
25. Virolainen P, Aro HT (2004) High tibial osteotomy for the treatment of osteoarthritis of the knee: a review of the literature and a meta-analysis of follow-up studies. Arch Orthop Trauma Surg 124(4):258–261
26. Vena G, D'amio S, Amendola A (2013) Complications of osteotomies about the knee. Sports Med Arthrosc 21(2):113–120
27. Efe T, Ahmed G, Heyse TJ et al (2011) Closing-wedge high tibial osteotomy: survival and risk factor analysis at long-term follow up. BMC Musculoskelet Disord 12:46
28. Jacobi M, Wahl P, Bouaicha S et al (2011) Distal femoral varus osteotomy: problems associated with the lateral open-wedge technique. Arch Orthop Trauma Surg 131(6):725–728
29. Van Heerwaarden R, Najfeld M, Brinkman M et al (2013) Wedge volume and osteotomy surface depend on surgical technique for distal femoral osteotomy. Knee Surg Sports Tramatol Arthrosc 21(1):206–212
30. Bagherifard A, Jabalameli M, Ali Hadi H et al (2015) The results of biplanar distal femoral osteotomy; a case series study. Arch Bone Jt Surg 3(1):35–38

21

Bone transport for the management of severely comminuted fractures without bone loss

Mootaz F. Thakeb[1] · Mahmoud A. Mahran[1] · El-Hussein M. El-Motassem[1]

Abstract This study aims to provide a new method for treatment of severely comminuted fractures without bone loss using the well-known technique of bone transport. Sixteen patients suffering from severely comminuted fractures with closed soft tissue injury were prospectively treated using bone transport by Ilizarov circular fixator. There were 14 male and 2 female patients. The mean age was 36.5 years (27–45). There were 13 proximal tibial metaphyseal fractures, one tibial diaphyseal fracture and two femoral distal metaphyseal fractures. All patients had closed soft tissue. The mean length of the comminution gap was 50.3 mm (40–64). Fracture healing occurred in 15 patients. The mean healing time was 23.4 weeks (14–30). No bone stimulating procedures were needed for either the fracture or distraction site. Using the IOWA knee and ankle score for assessment of the 15 patients who completed treatment: the functional outcome for the knee was excellent in 11 patients, good in three and fair in one. The ankle score was excellent in 12 patients, good in two and fair in one. According to Paley and Maar's, bone results were excellent in 14 patients, good in one patient and poor in the patient who had failure of the procedure. The results achieved in this work are encouraging to keep on applying this technique to treat fractures that meet the following criteria: metaphyseal, with total circumferential comminution involving more than 4 cm of the bone length.

Keywords Bone transport · Comminuted fractures · Ilizarov technique · Contained bone defect · Internal bone loss

Introduction

Bone transport for the management of traumatic bone loss is a well-known technique [1–4]. Bone loss may occur from extrusion of fragments at the time of injury or during debridement of an open fracture when devitalized segments of bone are removed. This creates a segmental defect or gap between the remaining bone ends.

A severely comminuted fracture with intact soft tissue envelope, having circumferentially widely separated fragments that involve more than 2 cm of the bone length, should be considered as a fracture with "contained defect" or "internal bone loss." Open fractures with segmental defects more than 2 cm are unlikely to heal spontaneously following bone stabilization alone. Fractures with 50 % or more of circumferential bone loss require bone graft to restore normal volume and strength [5–8].

Comminuted fractures with contained bone defects present difficulties in management because of the high potential of reduced fragments' viability, soft tissue compromise and problems with stabilization. Various surgical methods have been proposed for treating such complex fractures including: internal fixation by plates and screws, intramedullary nailing and external fixation [5, 9, 10].

Circular external fixator provides multilevel stabilization of the fractured limb segments with minimal disruption of the soft tissue envelope. It is particularly useful where bone gaps need reconstruction by distraction osteogenesis.

✉ Mootaz F. Thakeb
m.thakeb@med.asu.edu.eg

[1] The Department of Orthopedic Surgery, Ain Shams University, Cairo, Egypt

This is a report of using bone transport technique to manage closed comminuted fractures with "contained bone defects" to bridge the gap and achieve healing in a reasonable time.

Patients and methods

Between June 2005 and January 2011, 16 patients suffering from severely comminuted fractures with closed soft tissue injury were treated using bone transport by Ilizarov circular fixator.

There were 14 males and 2 females. The mean age was 36.5 years (range 27–45). There were 14 tibial fractures (13 proximal metaphyseal and one diaphyseal), and two femoral distal metaphyseal fractures. According to AO/OTA system [11], ten fractures were classified as 41.A3, three as 41.C2, one as 42.C3, one as 33.A3.3 and one fracture as 33.C2.3.

All patients had closed soft tissue injuries that were graded according to Tscherene and Gotsen method [12]. Eight were grade I, five were grade II and three were grade III. Nine patients had their fractures as isolated injury while seven had other fractures (Table 1). The mechanism of injury was road traffic accident in 11 patients, trauma from

a heavy object in three patients and falls from a height in two patients.

The length of the segmental comminution gap was measured between two points of circumferentially intact bone at the proximal and distal main bone segments (Fig. 1). The mean length of this gap was 50.3 mm (range 40–64).

Four patients had their fracture initially immobilized with a mono-lateral spanning external fixator. Twelve patients had their fractures immobilized in plaster back slab until definitive stabilization. The mean time to definitive surgery was 8.8 days (range 1–28). The operative delay in some patients was due to late referral from primary centers.

Four patients (three type 41-C2 proximal tibia and one type 33-C2.3 distal femur) had their articular fragments reduced and fixed percutaneously with one or two cannulated 6.5 screws and washers. Tibial fractures were stabilized with an Ilizarov frame; each segment of bone was fixed either by two rings or a single ring with a drop wire or half pin on either side. Each ring was fixed by at least two tensioned 1.8-mm wires and a 6-mm predrilled half pin. The femoral frames comprised two femoral arches proximally and two distal rings. Three or four 6-mm half pins fixed each arch. Two tensioned wires and half pins were fixed to the rings.

Table 1 Patients data

Case	Age	Gender	Grade of soft tissue injury	AO classification	Comminution gap (mm)	Associated injuries	Primary treatment	Time to frame (days)
1	27	M	2	41-A3	64	Contralateral fracture distal humerus	Back Slab	7
2	45	M	1	41-A3	52	–	Back Slab	1
3	36	M	3	41-C2	58	–	Temporary fixator	28
4	40	M	1	33-C2.3	45	Ipsilateral fracture distal radius	Back Slab	1
5	38	M	2	41-A3	42	–	Back Slab	10
6	28	M	1	33-A3.3	40	Contralateral fracture tibia	Back Slab	1
7	32	F	1	41-A3	55	–	Back Slab	1
8	43	M	1	41-A3	52	–	Back Slab	1
9	35	M	2	42-C3	40	–	Back Slab	7
10	33	M	3	41-A3	60	Contralateral fracture Posterior wall acetabulum	Temporary fixator	25
11	44	M	2	41-C2	50	–	Temporary fixator	18
12	28	M	1	41-A3	40	Contralateral fracture femur	Back Slab	1
13	34	F	1	41-A3	44	–	Back Slab	1
14	36	M	3	41-C2	50	–	Temporary fixator	28
15	45	M	2	41-A3	58	Ipsilateral fracture humerus	Back Slab	10
16	40	M	1	41-A3	55	Ipsilateral fracture calcaneus	Back Slab	1

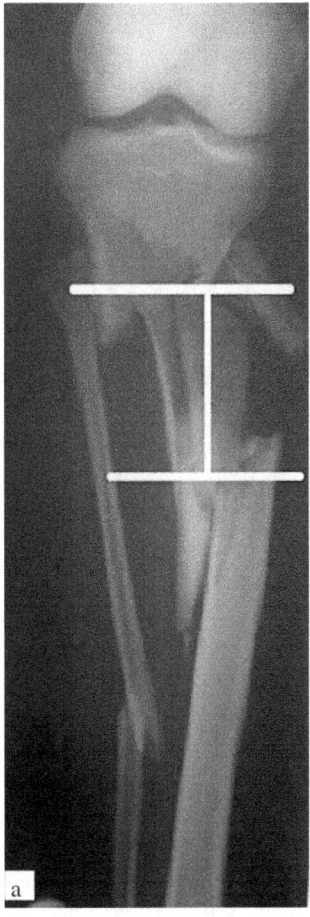

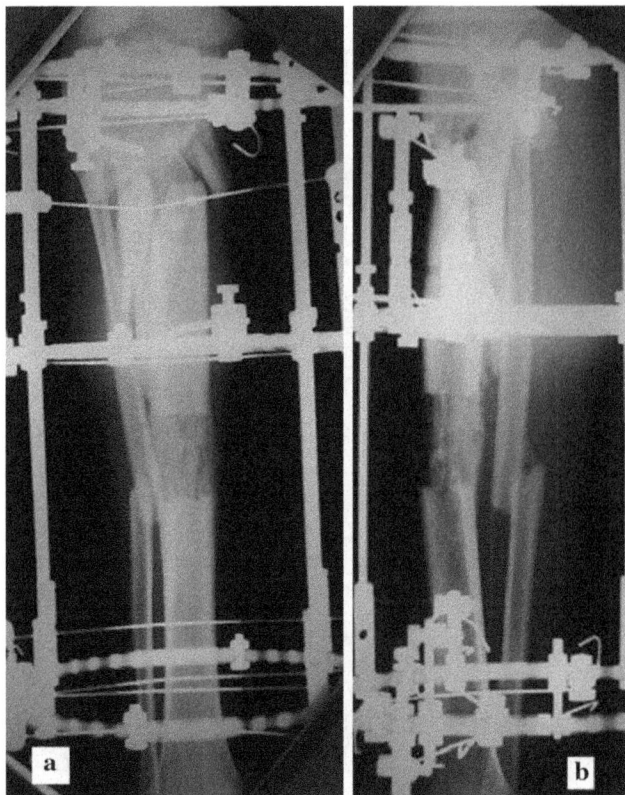

Fig. 2 **a**, **b** Antero-posterior and lateral radiographs showing the distracted segment bridging the comminution gap, with good consolidation

Fig. 1 Antero-posterior radiograph showing comminuted fracture proximal tibia, 41-A3, with a segmental comminution gap of 64 mm

The two femoral fractures and the tibial diaphyseal fracture had proximal to distal bone transport. The 13 proximal tibial fractures had distal to proximal bone transport. Corticotomies were done using predrilling technique.

Postoperatively, patients were allowed partial weight bearing unless contraindicated by the presence of other injuries. Knee and ankle range of motion exercises started on the first postoperative day or as tolerated by the patient. Distraction started after a latent period of 7 days at a rate of 0.25 mm/6 h. This continued till the comminuted fragments resisted transport. Thus, the amount of distraction was not necessarily equal to the preoperative measured length of contained defect (Fig. 2).

Pin site care included daily removal of crusts with normal saline and application of compressive dressing. Alcoholic chlorhexidine antiseptic solution was used only if pin site inflammation occurs.

Patients were followed up weekly during the distraction period and then every 2 weeks till frame removal. All frames were dynamized 2 weeks before removal.

Healing was determined radiologically and clinically: radiologically, callus bridging the fracture site and the appearance of three cortices bridging the distraction corticotomy on antero-posterior and lateral radiographs indicated healing. Clinical fracture healing was determined when the patient was able to bear weight freely without supporting aids after frame dynamization.

The final follow-up was done after 12 months using the IOWA [13] knee and ankle functional score and Paley and Maar's bone results [4].

Results

Fifteen fractures healed uneventfully (Fig. 3). The mean healing time was 23.4 weeks (range 14–30). The mean consolidation time for the distraction site was 19 weeks (range 10–24). No bone healing stimulating procedures were needed for either the fracture or distraction site (Table 2). The mean length gained (the transported distance) was 39.4 (range 20–50) mm.

Pin site infection was the most common problem encountered in almost all patients and treated with oral

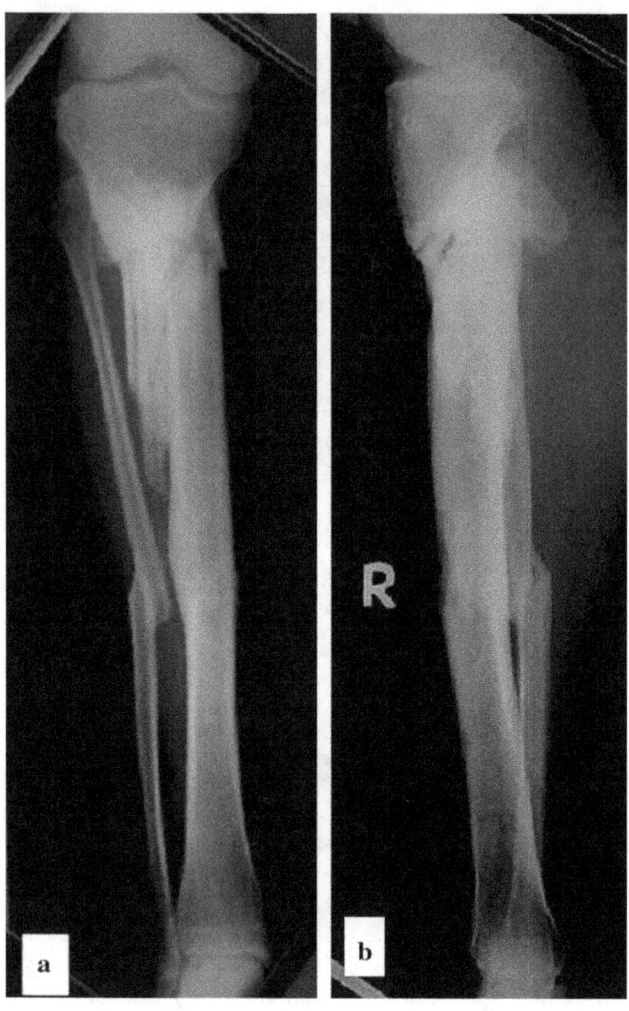

Fig. 3 a, b Antero-posterior and lateral radiographs at final follow-up showing fully consolidated fracture and distraction sites with 10 mm medial translation of the mechanical axis

assessment and was considered as a failure of the procedure.

According to Paley and Maar's scoring system, bone results for all 16 patients were excellent in 14 patients, good in one patient and poor in the patient who had failure of the procedure.

Discussion

High-energy fractures have soft tissue compromise and a potentially reduced viability of bone ends which can alter the normal healing process with considerable delay in union expected. The method chosen for treatment of these fractures has a substantial effect on the local mechanical and biological environment. The treatment strategy for these fractures focuses on fixation stability while respecting the biological reserve.

Restoration of limb length and alignment together with preservation of function are the main goals in treatment of these injuries. Severely comminuted metaphyseal fractures challenge the ability of standard implants to provide adequate stability. Fixation by plates and screws pose an additional surgical injury to an already compromised soft tissue envelope, even with minimally invasive plate designs. Furthermore, the presence of a segmental gap or defect will compromise the stability of plate fixation; when prolonged bone healing time is expected, failure may occur by cantilever loading [5, 14].

The use of intramedullary nails in comminuted fractures with contained metaphyseal defects is not suitable. Short metaphyseal proximal tibial or distal femoral segments are difficult to control and malalignment can be difficult to avoid, even with the use of nails with multidirectional locking screws [5, 15].

The Ilizarov external fixator can be applied with minimal soft tissue disruption. Moreover, it offers the mechanical advantage of resisting all prevailing loads except the axial ones that are beneficial for osteogenesis. The multidirectional fixation can adequately stabilize short metaphyseal segments allowing early weight bearing and rehabilitation; additionally, it has the versatility for correcting any residual postreduction deformities.

A severely comminuted fracture forms a "contained defect" comprised of fracture fragments with reduced viability. In this series, the bone transport technique was used knowing corticotomy increases blood flow to the limb [16] and the transported bone segment is able to bridge the area of the contained defect and avoid need for bone graft.

Pin site infections encountered in all patients were successfully controlled with oral antibiotics. This is considered a problem of external fixation used in limb reconstruction as opposed to an obstacle or true complication as

antibiotics. None progressed to deep infection or required exchange of wires or half pins.

One patient (with 42-C3 diaphyseal fracture) was not able to tolerate the procedure; the frame was removed prematurely. A back slab was applied temporarily for 4 weeks until consolidation of the distraction gap. Revision of fixation was performed with an unreamed interlocking nail and iliac crest bone graft used. This patient was excluded from the final functional assessment and was rated as a poor bony result due to failure of the bone transport procedure alone to achieve healing.

The IOWA knee and ankle score was used for assessment of the 15 patients who completed treatment. The functional outcome for the knee was excellent in 11 patients, good in three and fair in one. The ankle score was excellent in 12 patients, good in two and fair in one. The patient who did not complete treatment with bone transport was not included in this final functional

Table 2 Results

Case	Time to healing		Amount of distraction (mm)	Comminution gap (mm)	Residual deformity	IOWA score		Bone results
	Distraction site (weeks)	Fracture site (weeks)				Knee	Ankle	
1	22	24	45	64	Medial translation 10 mm	96	94	Excellent
2	20	22	42	52	–	98	100	Excellent
3	24	24	45	58	5° Varus, 1 cm shortening	90	96	Excellent
4	15	20	35	45	–	86	100	Excellent
5	12	16	30	42	1 cm shortening	94	98	Excellent
6	10	15	25	40	–	90	96	Excellent
7	24	28	50	55	5° Varus, 1 cm shortening	96	100	Excellent
8	20	26	40	52	–	100	100	Excellent
9	–	–	20	40	–	–	–	Poor
10	22	28	50	60	1.5 cm shortening	84	79	Excellent
11	18	24	44	50	–	92	94	Excellent
12	12	14	25	40	5° Varus	94	98	Excellent
13	18	24	40	44	10° varus	89	92	Good
14	22	28	42	50	1.5 cm shortening	74	89	Excellent
15	24	30	50	58	5° Valgus	98	100	Excellent
16	22	28	48	55	1 cm shortening	92	83	Excellent

described by Paley [17]. The only true complication was the non-union encountered with one patient with the diaphyseal fracture who did not tolerate the procedure.

The functional outcome in this series indicates the limited knee and ankle range of motion that can be encountered in some patients treated by Ilizarov method is temporary and can be resolved after frame removal. Early postoperative knee and ankle range of motion exercises are imperative to avoid this problem.

The mean time to bone healing was 23.4 weeks which the authors consider as a reasonable time for such fractures. This is comparable to the healing time reported for complex and segmental fractures stabilized by circular fixators [9, 10, 18].

Conclusion

We describe a technique of bone transport to stimulate and overcome the comminution in high-energy fractures of the tibia and femur using the Ilizarov fixator as an alternative to other methods of stabilization with or without bone graft. The results presented confirm the suitability of the strategy for this cohort of patients who have metaphyseal fractures with total circumferential comminution involving more than 4 cm of the bone length.

Informed consent Informed consent was obtained from all individual participants included in the study.

References

1. Ilizarov GA, Ledyaev VI (1992) The replacement of long tubular bone defects by lengthening distraction osteotomy of one of the fragments. Clin Orthop Relat Res 280:7–10
2. Green SA, Jackson JM, Wall DM, Marinow H, Ishkanian J (1992) Management of segmental defects by the Ilizarov intercalary bone transport method. Clin Orthop Relat Res 280:136–142
3. Song HR, Cho SH, Koo KH, Jeong ST, Park YJ, Ko JH (1998) Tibial bone defects treated by internal bone transport using the Ilizarov method. Int Orthop 22(5):293–297
4. Paley D, Maar DC (2000) Ilizarov bone transport treatment for tibial defects. J Orthop Trauma 14(2):76–85
5. Keating JF, Simpson AH, Robinson CM (2005) The management of fractures with bone loss. J Bone Joint Surg Br 87(2):142–150
6. Blick SS, Brumback RJ, Lakatos R, Poka A, Burgess AR (1989) Early prophylactic bone grafting of high-energy tibial fractures. Clin Orthop Relat Res 240:21–41
7. Court-Brown CM, McQueen MM, Quaba AA, Christie J (1991) Locked intramedullary nailing of open tibial fractures. J Bone Joint Surg Br 73(6):959–964
8. Sledge SL, Johnson KD, Henley MB, Watson JT (1989) Intramedullary nailing with reaming to treat non-union of the tibia. J Bone Joint Surg Am 71(7):1004–1019
9. Giotakis N, Panchani SK, Narayan B, Larkin JJ, Al Maskari S, Nayagam S (2010) Segmental fractures of the tibia treated by circular external fixation. J Bone Joint Surg Br 92(5):687–692

10. Foster PA, Barton SB, Jones SC, Morrison RJ, Britten S (2012) The treatment of complex tibial shaft fractures by the Ilizarov method. J Bone Joint Surg Br 94(12):1678–1683

11. Marsh JL, Slongo TF, Agel J, Broderick JS, Creevey W, DeCoster TA, Prokuski L, Sirkin MS, Ziran B, Henley B, Audigé L (2007) Fracture and dislocation compedium - 2007: orthopedic trauma association classification, database and outcomes committee. J Orthop Trauma 21(10 suppl):S1–S133

12. Tscherne H, Gotzen L (eds) (1984) Fractures with soft tissue injuries (German). Telger TC (trans). Springer, Berlin, pp 1–9

13. Merchant TC, Dietz FR (1989) Long-term follow-up after fractures of the tibial and fibular shafts. J Bone Joint Surg Am 71(4):599–606

14. Fulkerson E, Egol KA, Kubiak EN, Liporace F, Kummer FJ, Koval KJ (2006) Fixation of diaphyseal fractures with a segmental defect: a biomechanical comparison of locked and conventional plating techniques. J Trauma 60(4):830–835

15. Lindvall E, Sanders R, Dipasquale T, Herscovici D, Haidukewych G, Sagi C (2009) Intramedullary nailing versus percutaneous locked plating of extra-articular proximal tibial fractures: comparison of 56 cases. J Orthop Trauma 23(7):485–492

16. Aronson J (1994) Temporal and spatial increases in blood flow during distraction osteogenesis. Clin Orthop Relat Res 301:124–131

17. Paley D (1990) Problems, obstacles, and complications of limb lengthening by the Ilizarov technique. Clin Orthop Relat Res 250:81–104

18. Ozturkmen Y, Karamehmetoglu M, Karadeniz H, Azboy I, Caniklioglu M (2009) Acute treatment of segmental tibial fractures with the Ilizarov method. Injury 40(3):321–326

22

Patterns of healing: a comparison of two proximal tibial osteotomy techniques

Anna C. Peek[1] · Anna Timms[1] · Kuen F. Chin[1] · Peter Calder[1] · David Goodier[1]

Abstract Several low-energy osteotomy techniques are described in the literature, but there is limited evidence comparing them. Our study evaluates the patterns of regenerate formation using two different osteotomy techniques. Two cohorts of patients underwent osteotomy of the tibia using a Gigli saw ($n = 15$) or De Bastiani corticotomy ($n = 12$) technique. The patient radiographs were assessed by the two senior authors who were blinded to the osteotomy type. Regenerate quality was assessed along the anterior, posterior, medial and lateral cortices, graded 1–5 from absent to full consolidation over time. The time to 3 cortices healed/regenerate length was calculated. The time to consolidation of the anterior, posterior, medial and lateral cortices was compared. The mean 3 cortices index in the Gigli group was 2.0 months/cm and in the De Bastiani group 1.8 months/cm. This was not a significant difference. In both groups, anterior bone formation was slower, and anterior cortical deficiency with a scalloped appearance was seen in 25 % of cases overall with no statistically significant difference between the two groups. Both Gigli saw and De Bastiani corticotomy techniques result in good bone formation following distraction osteogenesis. The anterior tibial cortex consolidates more slowly than the other cortices in both groups. This is likely due to deficient soft tissue cover and direct periosteal damage at time of osteotomy.

Keywords Regenerate · Osteotomy · Healing

✉ Anna C. Peek
anna.peek@rnoh.nhs.uk

[1] Royal National Orthopaedic Hospital, Stanmore, UK

Introduction

Limb lengthening and segmental bone transport are techniques based upon the principles of 'Callus Distraction Osteogenesis' discovered by Ilizarov in the 1950s. Ilizarov pioneered the use of a low impact division of the cortex of bone, attempting to preserve the medullary blood supply ('corticotomy') followed by a latent period of 5–7 days to allow callus to start forming, then gradual distraction in increments totalling 1 mm per day [1].

This corticotomy technique has been adapted by various authors, notably De Bastiani [2] and Patkiss and Gross [3] who described the 'Afghan Percutaneous Osteotomy' using a Gigli saw. The De Bastiani technique purports to keep the medullary blood supply intact; the Gigli saw technique divides it. On the other hand, the usual approach for the De Bastiani corticotomy is an anterior incision over the tibial crest, whereas the incisions to pass a Gigli saw tend to be smaller but require more periosteal elevation.

We had observed in our limb reconstruction practice that the subcutaneous border of the tibia (shown on AP and lateral radiographs as the most anterior cortex on lateral projection and most medial cortex on AP) was the slowest to 'fill in' after corticotomy. Our study was to evaluate whether there was a difference in formation of bone in this area between these two techniques.

Method

We conducted a retrospective review of patients undergoing limb reconstruction surgery identified using a prospectively collected database. Indications for surgery included tibial lengthening or bone transport for defect reconstruction with a minimal distraction of 2 cm

Table 1 Indications for frame, number of patients

Group	Lengthening or deformity correction	Aseptic nonunion or malunion	Infected nonunion
GS	2	11	2
DB	6	5	1

(Table 1). There was no significant difference in indication between the 2 groups (Chi-square, p value NS). Children and patients with metabolic bone disorders were excluded. The osteotomy for bone distraction was performed in the proximal tibia with a Gigli saw in 15 patients (GS group) and by the De Bastiani technique in 12 patients (DB group). The mean age was similar in both groups (DB 36 years, GS 41 years p value NS).

Surgical technique [4]

- Gigli saw

  Two transverse incisions are made and via subperiosteal dissection a suture is passed from the posteromedial to anterolateral using a right-angled and curved clamp. The Gigli saw is tied to the suture and is pulled from posterior to anterior. Elevators are inserted, and the posterior and lateral cortices divided. The medial periosteum is then elevated, and the cortex divided. The saw is cut with a wire cutter and removed.

- De Bastiani

  A small 1-cm incision is made over the anterolateral aspect of the tibia. The periosteum is elevated along the anterior and lateral cortices. The tibia is predrilled from anterior to posteromedial and posterolateral, 3–5 drill holes. An osteotome is then passed along the anterior and lateral cortices. The osteotomy is completed by rotation of the osteotome.

The osteotomy technique was based on the surgeon's choice. Following osteotomy, a latent period of 6 days was followed by lengthening of 1 mm per day in four quarterly turns with Ilizarov frames and 1 mm per day in a single correction using Taylor Spatial Frames. The type of frame was also the surgeon's choice. Follow-up including radiographs was every 2 weeks during the lengthening period and every 4–6 weeks during regenerate consolidation.

The patient radiographs during lengthening and consolidation periods were anonymised, and the regenerate assessed by the two senior authors, in an attempt to blind the assessors to the type of osteotomy performed.

The bone quality of the regenerate was recorded along the anterior, posterior, medial and lateral cortices. This was graded 1–5, from absent to full consolidation over time in

Table 2 Cortex grading

Grade of cortex	Appearance of cortex
1	No visible callus
2	Concave callus
3	Straight callus
4	Convex callus
5	Consolidated

frame. Each cortex was graded independently (Table 2; Fig. 1).

A modified healing index was used as the time for a minimum of 3 cortices to consolidate [5]. This measure was used rather than the healing index to frame removal, as some patients spent a considerable length of time in frame undergoing bifocal treatment. The proximal regenerate had consolidated, but there was considerable delay in waiting for the transport docking site to unite.

The time to consolidation of the anterior, posterior, medial and lateral cortices was compared between the two osteotomy techniques.

Statistical analysis was performed using SPSS software version 22. The Chi-square test and paired T test were used, and significance level was set at $p < 0.05$.

Results

The overall time to 3 cortices grade 4 was similar: 2.2 months per cm in the GS group and 1.8 months per cm in the DB group (Chi-square, p value NS).

The anterior cortex was slower to heal than the posterior (Chi-square, $p < 0.05$) and lateral cortices in both groups (Chi-square, $p < 0.05$); although there was no statistically significant difference between the two groups, the trend seemed more marked in the anterior cortex relative to the other cortices in the DB group (Figs. 2, 3). Although the absolute scores were lower in the GS group in comparison with the DB group, this was not statistically significant (paired t test, p value NS).

Anterior cortical deficiency with a scalloped appearance was seen in 25 % of cases overall at some point during treatment, with no statistically significant difference between the two groups (13 % GS vs. 41 % DB, Chi-square $p = 0.09$).

Discussion

Experimental and clinical studies examining the factors influencing regenerate formation have been described [6, 7]. These include the site, the age of the patient and the

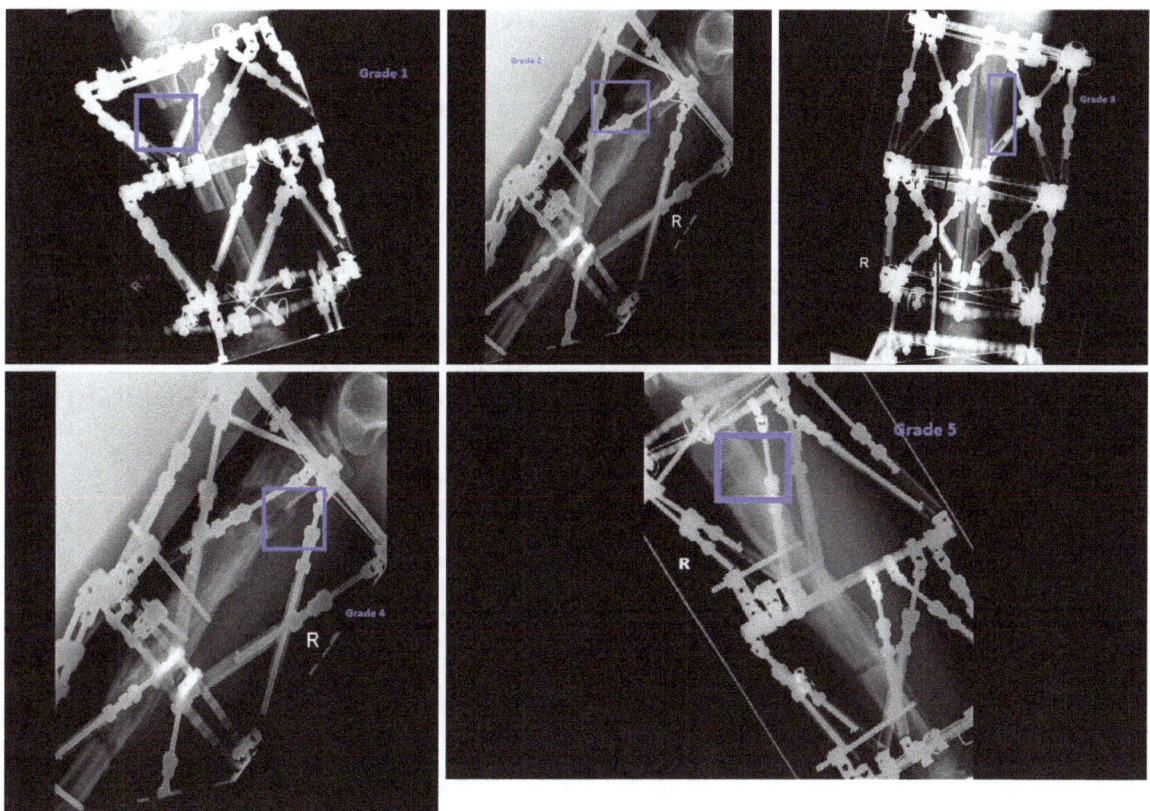

Fig. 1 Illustrations of the scoring system

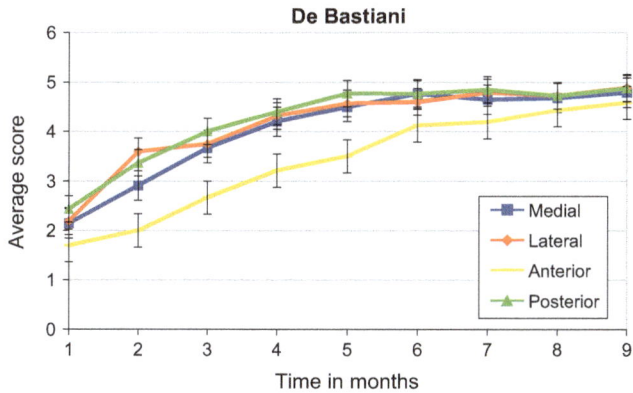

Fig. 2 Average score of each cortex vs time since corticotomy in the De Bastiani group

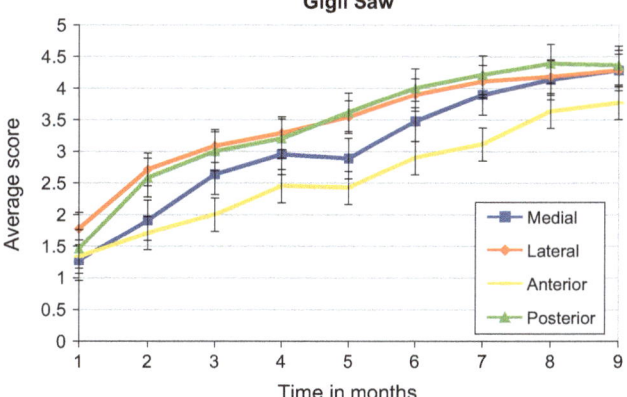

Fig. 3 Average score of each cortex vs time since corticotomy in the Gigli saw group

amount of distraction applied. In a canine model, tibial osteotomies made with a mallet and hammer, drill holes and an osteotome, or an oscillating saw were compared. In this study, fewer bone divisions made using the oscillating saw were consolidated at 10 weeks [8]. In a direct comparison in 41 patients between a Gigli saw Afghan osteotomy and an osteotomy made with drill holes and an osteotome, the Gigli saw method was found to result in a

shorter healing index [9]. The authors concluded the Gigli saw-type osteotomy caused less periosteal disruption.

We note proximal tibial osteotomies demonstrate a distinct pattern of healing with the anterior cortex in particular lagging behind the other cortices. Although it is more apparent in the De Bastiani group, there is no statistically demonstrable difference between the two, concluding that this pattern of healing relates primarily to the soft tissue attachments in this region of the tibia rather than any periosteal striping or thermal damage provoked at the time of the osteotomy. One might assume that, due to the triangular shape of the tibia at this level, posterior healing conveys more stability to the regenerate, but this was not tested in this study.

We have not demonstrated any significant difference in the healing index between the two methods in this study.

The limitations of this study are its retrospective nature and the small numbers studied with a potential for a type 2 error. Additionally, use of an unvalidated scoring system for the grading of the cortical appearance will introduce bias. The two groups were treated by different surgeons, and there may be unknown confounding factors related to this.

Acknowledgments No financial support was received for this study.

References

1. Ilizarov GA (1990) Clinical application of the tension-stress effect for limb lengthening. Clin Orthop 250:8–26
2. De Bastiani G, Aldegheri R, Renzi-Brivio L, Trivella G (1987) Limb lengthening by callus distraction (callotasis). J Pediatr Orthop 7:129–134
3. Paktiss AS, Gross RH (1993) Afghan percutaneous osteotomy. J Pediatr Orthop 13:531–533
4. Paley D (2005) Principles of deformity correction. Springer, Berlin
5. Paley D, Herzenberg JE, Paremain G, Bhave A (1997) Femoral lengthening over an intramedullary nail. A matched-case comparison with Ilizarov femoral lengthening. J Bone Joint Surg Am 79:1464–1480
6. Koczewski P, Shadi M (2013) Factors influencing bone regenerate healing in distraction osteogenesis. Ortop Traumatol Rehabil 15:591–599. doi:10.5604/15093492.1091515
7. Fischgrund J, Paley D, Suter C (1994) Variables affecting time to bone healing during limb lengthening. Clin Orthop 301:31–37
8. Frierson M, Ibrahim K, Boles M et al (1994) Distraction osteogenesis. A comparison of corticotomy techniques. Clin Orthop 301:19–24
9. Eralp L, Kocaoglu M, Ozkan K, Turker M (2004) A comparison of two osteotomy techniques for tibial lengthening. Arch Orthop Trauma Surg 124:298–300. doi:10.1007/s00402-004-0646-9

23

External fixation reconstruction of the residual problems of benign bone tumours

Levent Eralp[1] · F. Erkal Bilen[2]⊙ · S. Robert Rozbruch[3] · Mehmet Kocaoglu[2] ·
Ahmed I. Hammoudi[4]

Abstract The mechanical features of and biologic response to using distraction osteogenesis with the circular external fixator are the unique aspects of Ilizarov's contribution that allows deformity correction and reconstruction of bone defects. We present a retrospective study of 20 patients who suffered from a variety of benign tumours for which external fixators (EF) were used to treat deformity, bone loss, and limb-length discrepancy. A total of 26 bony segments in twenty patients (10 males, 10 females; mean age 17 years; range 7–58 years) were treated with EF for residual problems from the tumour itself (primary treatment) in 8 patients and for complications related to the primary surgery (secondary treatment) in 12 patients. Histological diagnoses were Ollier's disease ($n = 4$), Fibrous Dysplasia ($n = 5$), Congenital multiple exostosis ($n = 5$), giant cell tumour ($n = 2$) and one case for chondromyxoid fibroma, desmoid fibroma, chondroma and unicameral bone cyst. Various types of external fixators used to treat these problems. These were Ilizarov, unilateral fixator, multiaxial correction frame (Biomet, Parsippany, NJ), Taylor spatial frame (Memphis, TN) and smart correction multiaxial frame. The mean follow-up time was 69.5 months (range 35–108 months). The mean external fixation time was 159.5 days (range 27–300 days). The mean external fixation index was 67.4 days/cm (12–610) in 26 limbs who underwent distraction osteogenesis. The mean length of distraction was 4.9 cm (range 0.2–14 cm). At final follow-up, all patients had returned to normal activities. Complications were in the form of knee arthrodesis in one patient, pin tract infection in six and residual shortening in eight patients. The use of EF and the principles of distraction osteogenesis, in the management of problems associated with benign bone tumours and related surgery yields successful results especially in young patients. With this approach, the risk for recurrence of shortening and deformity may be minimized with over-correction or over-lengthening as dictated by preoperative planning.

Keywords Benign bone tumours · External fixation · Limb reconstruction · Distraction osteogenesis · Shortening · Bone deformity

✉ F. Erkal Bilen
bilenfe@gmail.com

[1] Department of Orthopaedics and Traumatology, Istanbul Faculty of Medicine, Istanbul University, 34390 Topkapi, Istanbul, Turkey

[2] Department of Orthopaedics and Traumatology, Memorial Health Group, 34385 Okmeydani, Istanbul, Turkey

[3] Hospital for Special Surgery, Limb Lengthening and Complex Reconstruction Service (LLCRS), Weill Cornell Medical College, Cornell University, 535 East 70th Street, New York, NY 10021, USA

[4] Orthopedic Department, Faculty of Medicine, Al-Azhar University Hospitals, Nasr City, Cairo 11884, Egypt

Introduction

The management of limb deformity, shortening and bone defects in the treatment of benign tumours is a major challenge [1, 2]. The radical and aggressive nature of surgical therapy has to be balanced with the treatment-related morbidity, i.e. complications, the need for reconstructive stabilization and potential functional deficit. The decision is a challenge for the orthopaedic surgeon [3]. Conventional methods of correcting deformity and limb-length inequality, such as shortening, single or multiple osteotomies or epiphysiodesis are limited in their scope and

often unpredictable or unsatisfactory. Alternative methods of treating bone defects include free autograft, vascularized bone graft, allograft, artificial bone substitutes and prostheses [4]. However, these methods have disadvantages and a high incidence of complications. Long-term results can be unsatisfactory especially after resection of extensive or juxta-articular tumours [2, 5–7].

Ilizarov introduced the concept of induction of local bone formation with a minimally invasive procedure, the process he called distraction osteogenesis (DO) [8]. DO has been used widely to treat traumatic bone loss, nonunion, osteomyelitis, malunion, limb-length discrepancy and to correct deformity [9–12]. The method embraces biomechanical stability, minimally invasive surgery, regeneration of new bone with gradual lengthening of the soft tissues [5]. There are few studies of its use in the treatment of benign bone tumours [13, 14]. In this study we describe our experience of the use of external fixators to correct deformity, limb-length discrepancy, contractures and similar problems related to the primary treatment of benign bone tumours or for the secondary complications of other primary treatment.

Materials and methods

Informed consent to participate in this study was obtained from all patients and the Institutional Review Board approved this study. External fixation techniques with or without intramedullary nailing (IMN) were used in 26 bony segments in 20 patients (10 males and 10 females) who had been treated for benign bone tumours and subsequently developed shortening, deformity or other complications. The reconstruction procedures were performed in two centres. The mean age at surgery was 17 years (7–58 years). Physical examination of the affected limb was complemented by plain radiography, computerized tomography and magnetic resonance imaging as necessary. The treatment was related to residual problems from the tumour itself (primary treatment) in 8 patients and for complications related to the primary surgery (secondary treatment) in 12 patients. All problems were either deformity or shortening, or both, or osteomyelitis.

Histological diagnoses included Ollier's disease (OD) in 6 segments (four patients) (Figs. 1, 2, 3, 4, 5), fibrous dysplasia (FD) in 8 (five patients) (Figs. 6, 7, 8, 9, 10, 11, 12), congenital multiple exostosis (CME) in 6 (five patients) (Figs. 13, 14, 15, 16, 17, 18a, b), giant cell tumour (GCT) in 2 (two patients), desmoid fibroma (DF) in 1 (one patient), chondromyxoid fibroma (CMF) in 1 (one patient), chondroma in 1 (one patient) and unicameral bone cyst (UBC) in 1 (one patient) (Table 1).

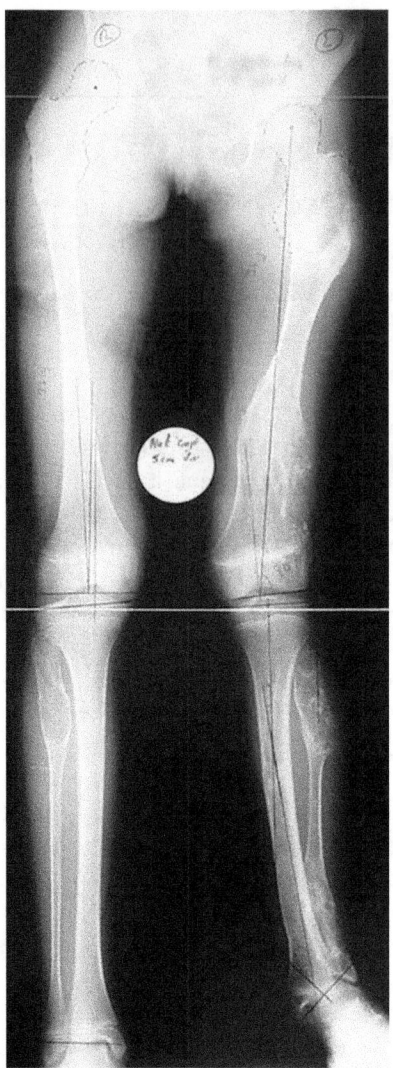

Fig. 1 An eight-year-old girl with Ollier's disease Lt. femur and tibia who developed valgus deformity and shortening following initial surgery of excision. Preoperative orthoroentgenogram denoting the LLD and the valgus deformity

A variety of fixation and reconstructive devices were used to accomplish the objectives of surgery. Limb lengthening was performed in three segments (one femur was treated using the Ilizarov fixator, one tibia was treated using the Ilizarov fixator with IM nailing and one tibia using the Ilizarov fixator combined with ipsilateral femoral IMN, both to compensate for limb discrepancy resulting after primary tumour excision). Combined limb lengthening with deformity correction was performed in 22 segments (22/26). We used the Taylor Spatial Frame (TSF) (Smith & Nephew, Memphis, TN, USA) to treat three femurs and five tibias, and Smart correction (computer assisted circular fixator system, Response Ortho, USA) to treat four femurs. A unilateral fixator was applied to treat one femur, one radius and four ulnas; Steinman pins were used as intramedullary devices for two ulnar cases. EBI

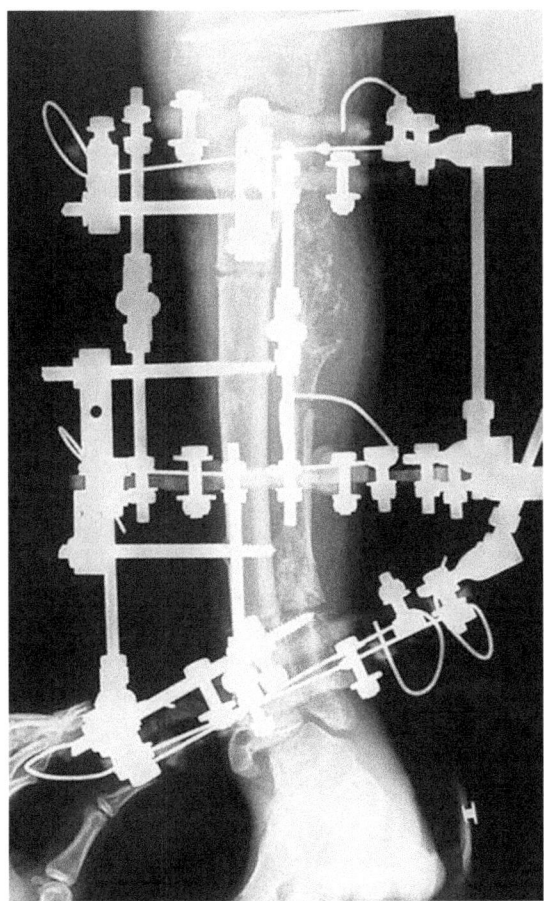

Fig. 2 Tibial Ilizarov with proximal osteotomy for gradual lengthening and distal osteotomy for gradual correction of valgus

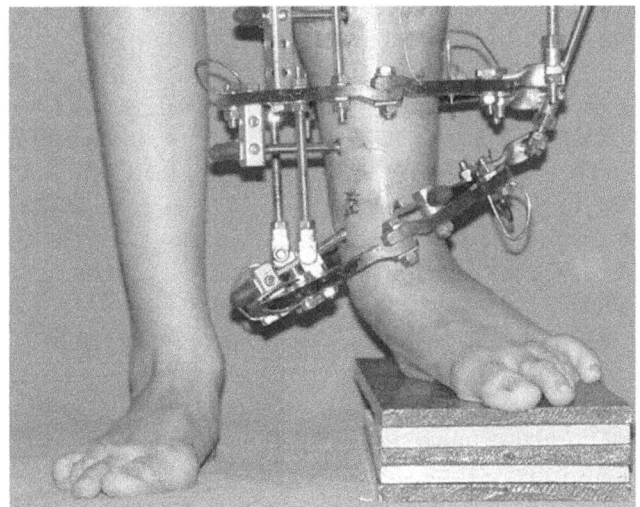

Fig. 3 Clinical photo of the Ilizarov frame

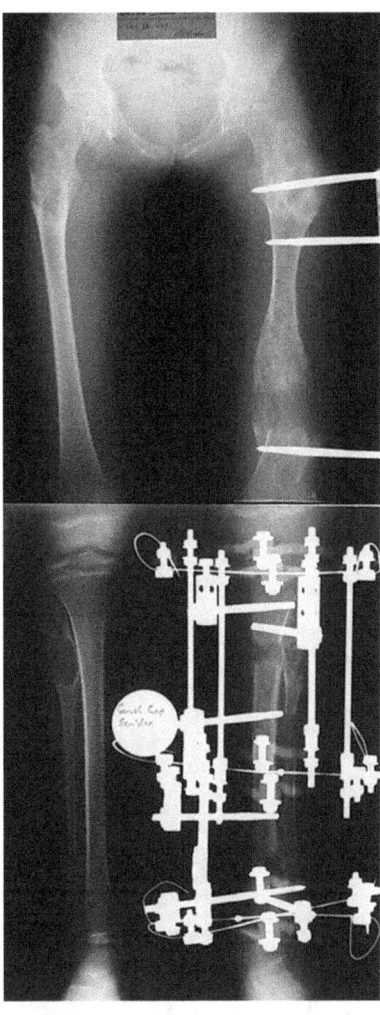

Fig. 4 Femoral unilateral fixator for acute deformity correction and gradual lengthening, note the consolidation of the regenerates with corrected deformity

external fixators (Dynafix; EBI, Parsippany, NJ, USA) were used to treat one fibula and one humerus, the Ilizarov fixator to treat one femur and a Multi-Axial Correction (MAC) monolateral external fixator (Biomet, Parsippany, NJ, USA) for one femur. Bone transport was performed in one limb (the Ilizarov device was used to treat tibia by bifocal compression distraction) (Table 1).

Prophylactic antibiotics were given to all patients for 2 days post-operatively. Distraction at the osteotomy site was often started 7 days post-operatively, at a rate of 0.25 mm every 6 h, with radiographs every 2 weeks. A rehabilitation programme of muscle and joint exercises was initiated immediately after surgery.

The mean follow-up time was 69.5 months (range 35–108 months). A functional assessment was done using criteria described by Paley et al. [15]. They are substantial limp, equinus rigidity of the ankle, soft tissue dystrophy (skin hypersensitivity, insensitivity of the sole, or decubitus ulcer), pain and inactivity (unemployment because of the leg injury or an inability to return to daily activities because of the leg injury). The results were considered

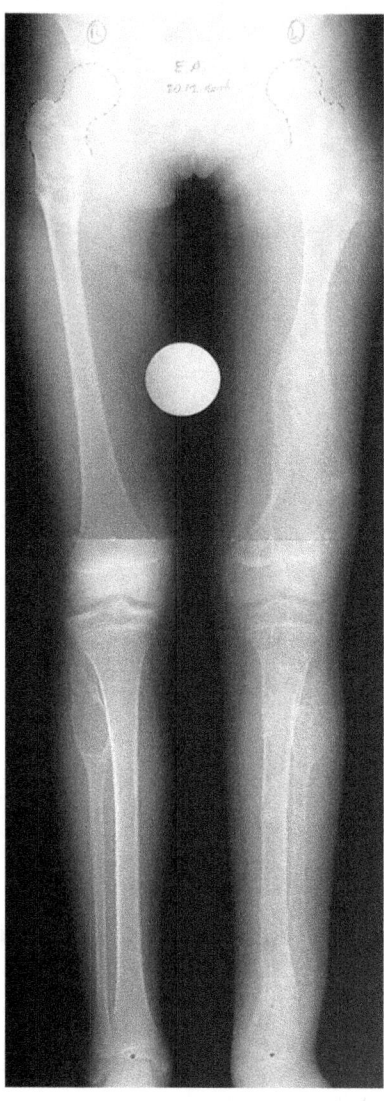

Fig. 5 After removal of the fixators, restored length with deformity correction

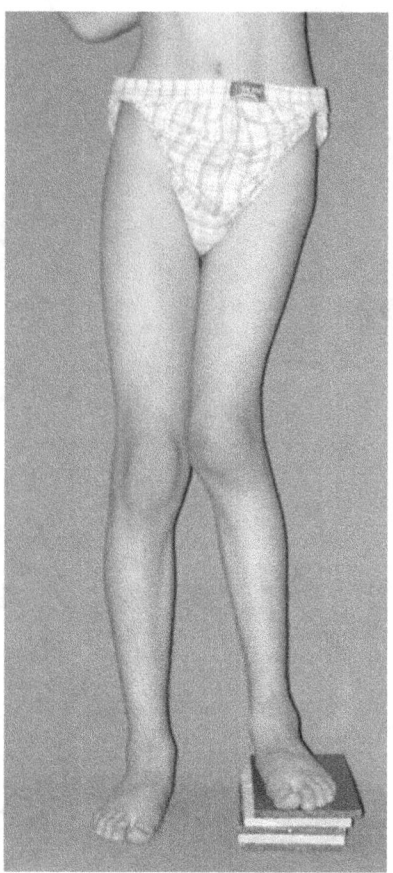

Fig. 6 A thirteen-year-old boy with Fibrous dysplasia Lt. distal femur treated initially by excision. Clinically, block test denoting 5 cm shortening

excellent when the patient was active and had none of the other four criteria, good when the patient was active and had one or two of the other four criteria, fair when the patient was active and had three or four of the other criteria or had had an amputation, and poor when the patient is inactive or had five criteria.

Results

The mean external fixation time was 159.5 days (range 27–300 days): 168 days in the OD group (129–210); 123.8 days in the FD group (51–152); 201 days in the CME group (105–300); 148.5 days in the GCT group (117–180); 90 days in the DF patient; 270 days in the CMF patient; 210 days in the chondroma patient; 27 days in the

UBC patient. The mean length of distraction was 4.9 cm (range 0.2–14 cm) (Tables 2, 3, 4, 5). This gave a mean external fixation index of 67.4 days/cm (12–610) in 26 limbs that underwent distraction osteogenesis. This was 31.8 days/cm in the OD group (12–55), 140.4 days/cm in the FD group (14–610), 62.2 days/cm in the CME group (43–108), 28.5 days/cm in the GCT group (24–33), 26 days in the DF patient, 60 days in the CMF patient, 25 days in the chondroma patient and 39 days in the UBC patient.

All 20 patients returned to normal daily activities without pain at final follow-up. Only one patient with the proximal tibial GCT had a knee arthrodesis due to sepsis and prosthesis failure following initial surgery.

All patients were evaluated as excellent (using Paley's functional criteria) except one with DF who developed a foot drop from sciatic nerve injury after initial surgery of tumour excision; this was treated by pantalar arthrodesis. Complications encountered included pin track infections in 6 patients which was treated by oral antibiotics, residual shortening in 8 patients and diminished joint motion due to knee arthrodesis in one patient.

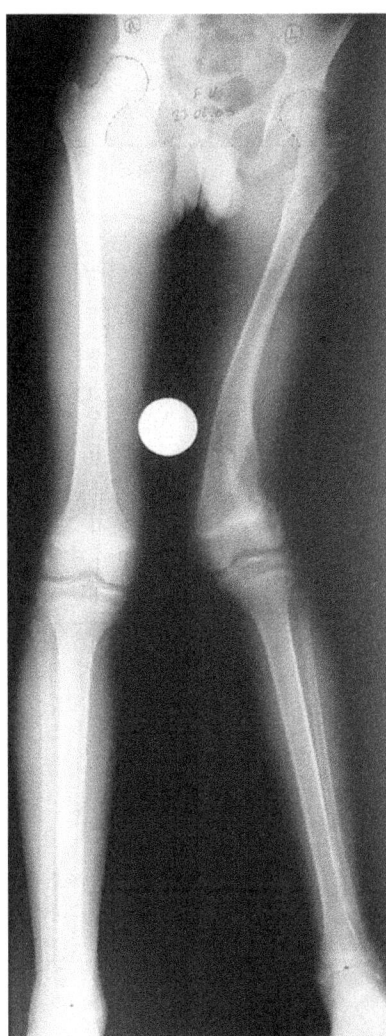

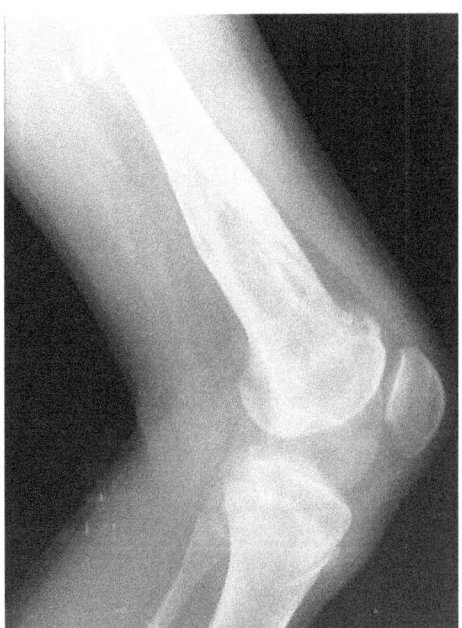

Fig. 8 Lateral X-ray of the same patient

Fig. 7 AP orthoroentgenogram, denoting valgus deformity with the CORA at the site of previous initial treatment

Discussion

Benign bone tumours are diagnosed in the juvenile age group usually with the deformity and shortening encountered progressive. Correction of the deformity but ignoring the limb shortening does not provide for a fully functional extremity at maturity [16].

A number of surgical treatments are proposed for correction of deformity, limb-length equalization and reconstruction in patients with bone tumours [16]. In this series of patients with benign bone tumours, we were able to treat most problems using external fixators. The aim was to achieve normal physiological alignment at maturity, and this may prompt a need for overcorrection and or overlengthening with distraction osteogenesis and the Ilizarov method. Currently, whilst different devices are used for this objective, the underlying principles are unchanged [16].

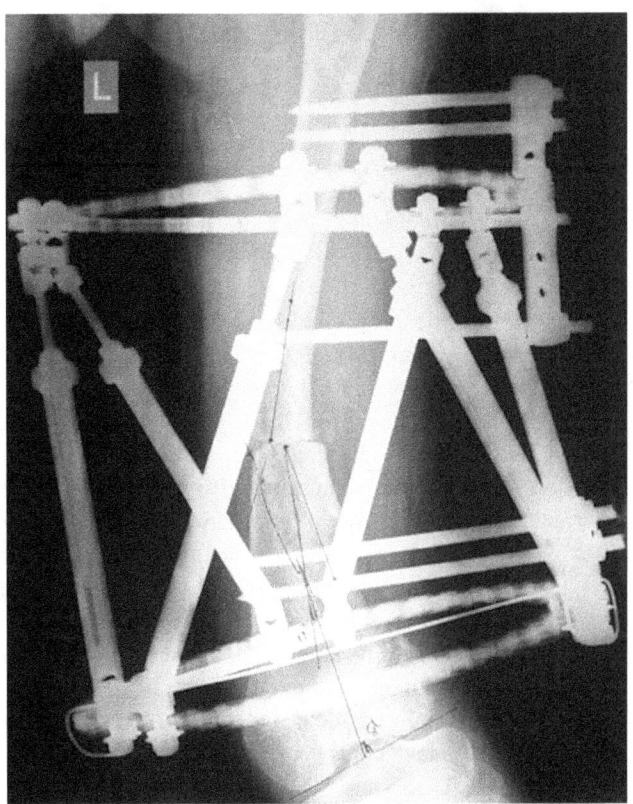

Fig. 9 Immediately after the operation, with Smart correction multiaxial frame and distal femoral osteotomy

Multiple enchondromatosis (Ollier's disease) is a common intraosseous benign cartilaginous tumour that develops in close proximity to the growth plate. It can cause

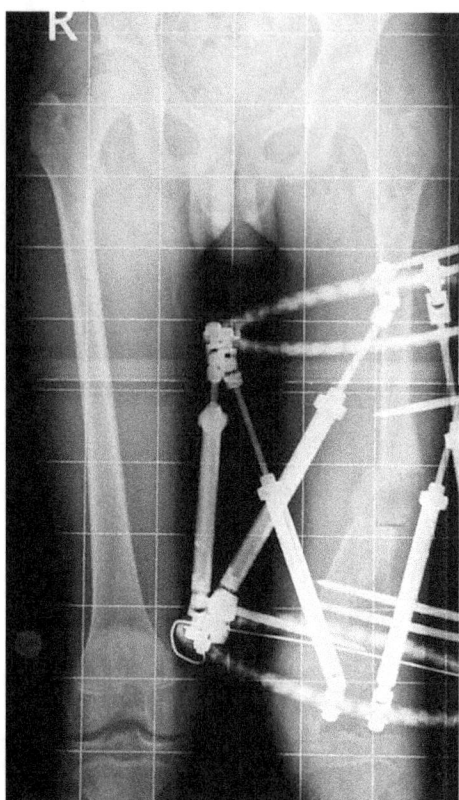

Fig. 10 After correction and lengthening with good regenerate (note the amount of translation as the osteotomy site is not at the CORA)

deformity and limb-length discrepancy and carries a risk of malignant change to chondrosarcoma [17]. Conventional treatment is curettage and bone grafting which may result in severe deformities requiring repeated osteotomies. It is often difficult to obtain adequate stabilization and normal bone growth by autogenous bone grafting. Jesus-Garcia et al. [18] reported the use of the Ilizarov method in ten patients with Ollier's disease. They reported excellent results and claimed the technique led to conversion of the abnormal cartilage to histologically mature bone in all their patients [18]. In this series all cases had accurate deformity correction with stable and mature bony regenerate. Three of the four cases had residual shortening (0.5 cm) that was not significant. One developed a knee contracture that resolved with physiotherapy. In spite of lengthening, which for some cases was over 9 cm and up to 14 cm, all four patients had excellent bony healing illustrated by the low EFI values (12, 23, 37 and 55 days/cm).

In fibrous dysplasia, curettage of the lesion and bone grafting may be effective for monostotic lesions but not for polyostotic fibrous dysplasia [19–21]. If the fibrous material is curetted and replaced by autogenous bone chips, these chips are often resorbed [22]. Curettage and bone grafting is not suitable in patients with deformity and pathological fracture. Corrective osteotomy with plate and

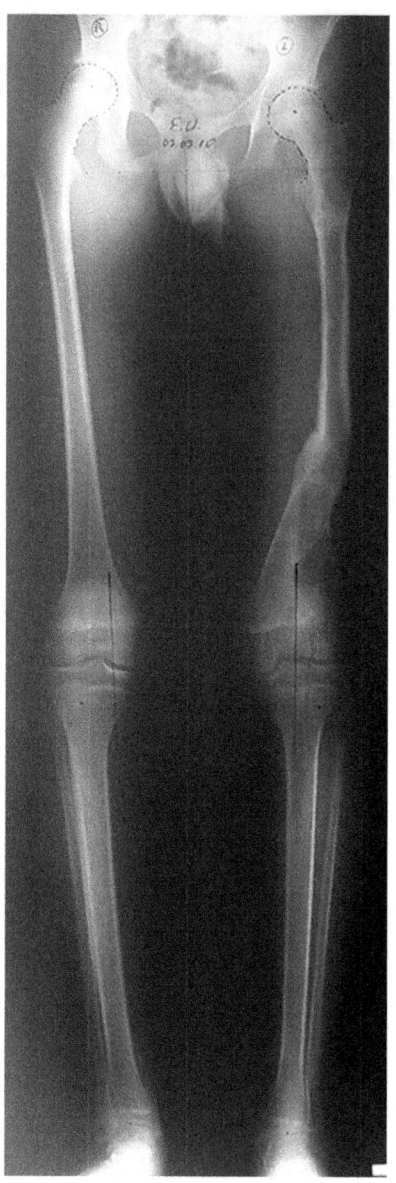

Fig. 11 Orthoroentgenogram after removal of the frame with healed regenerate and fully corrected limb

screw fixation is relatively simple, but it can be difficult to achieve sufficient stability in fixation with screws in weakened bone; additionally, a fracture may occur because of stress shielding at the distal end of the plate [23]. Radical excisional surgery of the dysplastic bone will result in deformity frequently and lead to functional losses that can be of greater damage to the patient than the disease itself. [24] In this series, surgical lengthening and alignment of the mechanical axis was effective in preventing recurrent deformity and fracture. Of the five patients, four had residual shortening (Fig. 12). Three cases developed pin track infection during treatment which resolved completely using oral antibiotic therapy. The EFI in the FD group is high (140.4 days/cm). The external fixation time

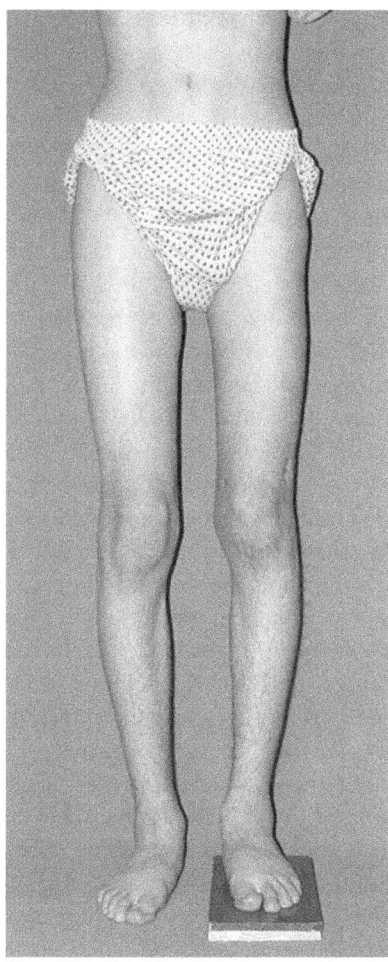

Fig. 12 Clinically straight limb with the block test denoting residual shortening

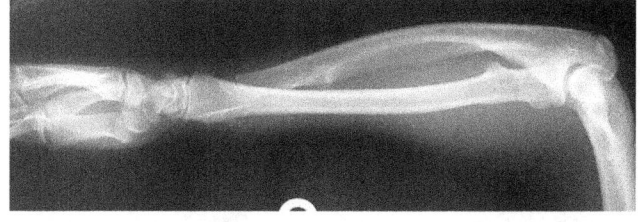

Fig. 13 A fourteen-year-old boy with Congenital Multiple Exostosis Rt. Ulna treated initially by excision. X-ray showing type 1 deformity in which there is ulnar deviation of the hand and deformity of the radius

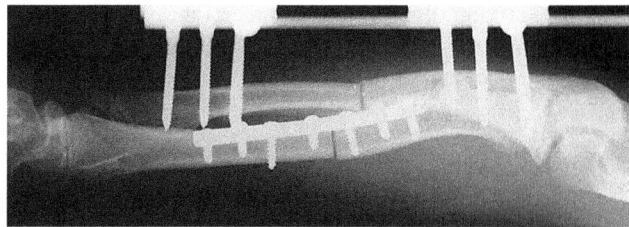

Fig. 14 Acutely corrected radius by plate and screws. Also unilateral fixator in the ulna for gradual lengthening

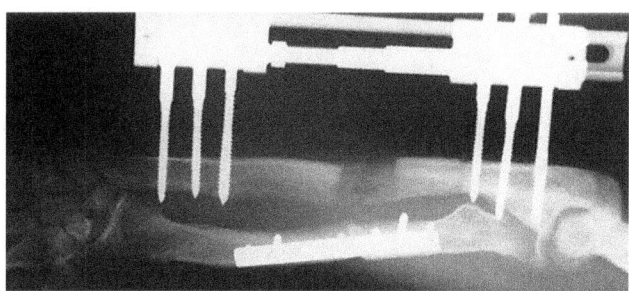

Fig. 15 X-ray at the end of lengthening

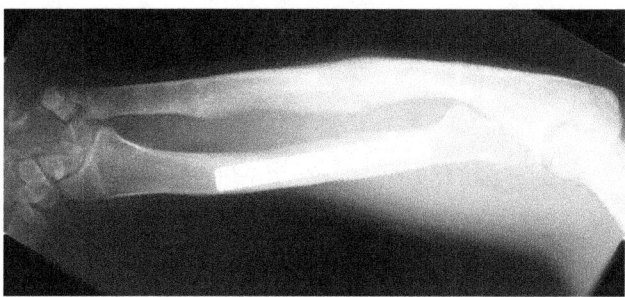

Fig. 16 X-ray after removal of the external fixator, fully corrected deformity with excellent regenerate (note the 0.5 over-lengthening to avoid complications of recurrence and to improve the function

and index can be decreased using a combined technique such as an intramedullary nail and external fixator, but the consistency of the fibrous lesions in this condition may lead to technical difficulties in reaming and inserting an intramedullary nail into a long bone.

Congenital multiple exostosis (CMO) is characterized by growths of multiple osteochondromas (benign cartilage-capped bone tumours that grow outward from the metaphyses of long bones). Osteochondromas can be associated with an inhibition of skeletal growth, development of bony deformities, restricted joint motion, shortened stature, premature osteoarthrosis, and compression of peripheral nerves. Most individuals with CMO have at least one operative procedure and many have multiple procedures [25]. Femoral or tibial involvement often requires surgical deformity correction and lengthening. Early surgical treatment of tibio-talar tilt may prevent or decrease the incidence of late deterioration of ankle function, but long-term follow-up studies are needed to confirm [26]. Surgery for forearm deformity may involve excision of the osteochondromas, corrective osteotomies, and or ulnar lengthening procedures that may improve pronation, supination, and forearm alignment [27]. Radial hemiepi-physeal stapling, used alone or with ulnar lengthening, has been effective but causes unacceptable shortening of the forearm and the final result unpredictable [28]. In this series, the main problems in the three cases included ulnar deviation of the hand and deformity of the radius. After prior resection of the osteochondroma, ulnar lengthening

was carried out with an external unilateral fixator concomitant with a corrective osteotomy of the radius with plate and screw fixation; there were satisfactory results and complete restoration of length of the ulna. We opted to perform over-lengthening by 0.5 cm in all the three cases to avoid recurrence of the ulna-radial length mismatch and to maintain improved function for longer (Fig. 16). One of these patients developed a recurrent radial deformity. The last two patients in this group had, in addition, femoral deformity and shortening which were treated successfully with using the Smart correction multiaxial fixator. One centimetre of residual shortening resulted in both cases.

The approach to treating giant cell tumours (GCT) has remained unchanged partly due to the lack of randomized clinical trials [29]. Surgery is the treatment of choice if the tumour is determined to be resectable. A number of strategies have been advocated including: curettage and grafting with autogenous bone graft; allograft or synthetic bone substitutes; either graft alone or combined with adjuvant therapy such as cryotherapy or the application of phenol after curettage [30–34]. Curettage is the commonly used technique [35], but it has reported recurrence rates of 27–55 % [36]. This high rate of recurrence is likely from an inadequate tumour resection rather than the use of adjuvant therapy [38]. Nonetheless, the high risk of recurrence led several surgeons to replace bone graft packing of the lesion with Poly Methyl Methacrylate (PMMA). The PMMA technique, compared with bone grafting, offers the advantages of lack of donor-site morbidity, an unlimited supply, immediate structural stability,

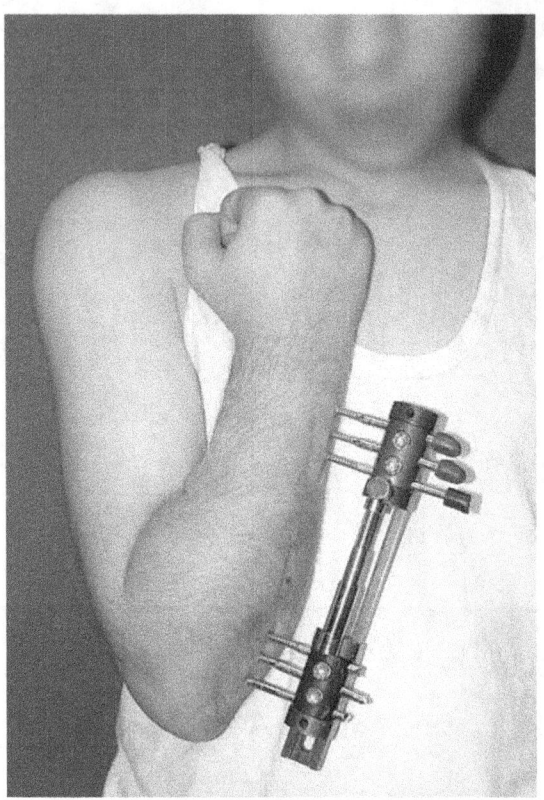

Fig. 17 Photographic documentation during external fixation period

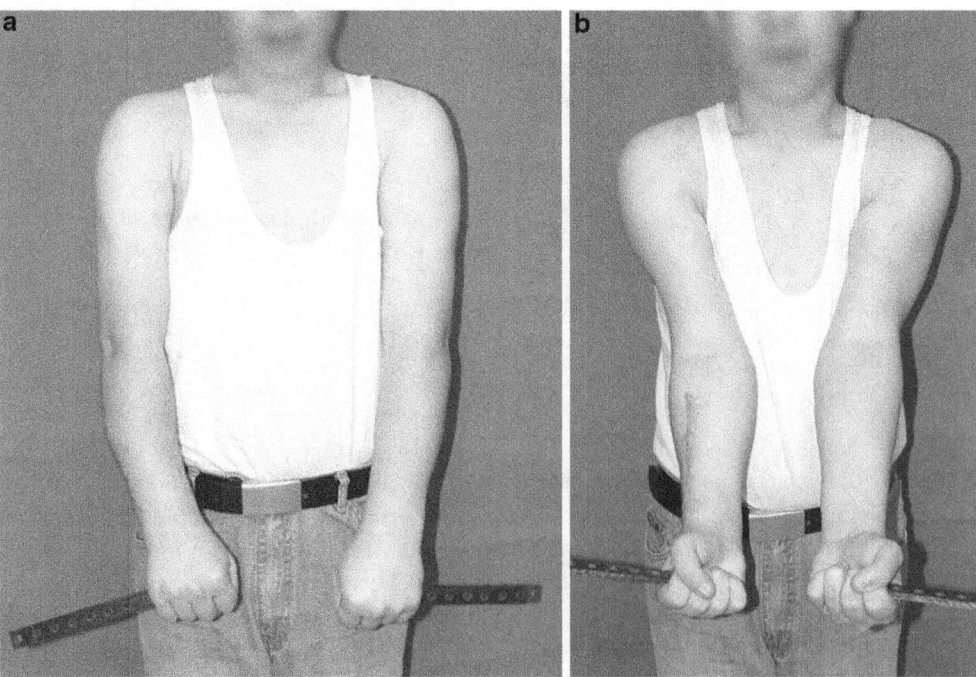

Fig. 18 a, b Photographic documentation denoting fully corrected deformity and functional limb

Table 1 Patient demographic data

Patient groups (according to histological diagnosis)	Number of limbs	Mean age (range, years)	Location	Number of external fixators	External fixation time in days (mean, range)	Lengthening	Deformity correction plus lengthening	Bone transport
Ollier's Disease	6	9.5 (7–14)	Femur 3 Tibia 2 Humerus 1	Ilizarov 1 Unilateral Fixator 1 MAC 1 EBI 1 TSF 1 Smart 1	168 (129–210)		5	1
Fibrous dysplasia	8	26.8 (11–58)	Femur 4 Tibia 4	TSF 7 Smart 1	123.8 (51–152)		8	
Congenital multiple exostosis	6	12 (10–14)	Femur 2 Ulna 4	Unilateral Fixator 4 Smart 2	201 (105–300)		6	
Giant cell tumour	2	22.5 (15–30)	Tibia 1 Radius 1	Ilizarov 1 Unilateral Fixator 1	148.5 (117–180)	1	1	
Desmoid fibroma	1	21	Tibia 1 + Gluteal region	Ilizarov & IM nail 1	90	1		
Chondromyxoid fibroma	1	22	Acetabulum 1	Ilizarov 1	270	1		
Chondroma	1	13	Femur 1	Ilizarov 1	210		1	
Unicameral bone cyst	1	14	Fibula 1	EBI 1	27		1	

MAC Multi-Axial Correction monolateral external fixation system (Biomet, Parsippany, NJ, USA), *EBI* External fixators (Dynafix; EBI, Parsippany, NJ, USA), *TSF* Taylor Spatial Frame (Smith & Nephew, Memphis, TN, USA) Smart Correction Multiaxial Frame: computer assisted circular fixator system (Response Ortho, USA)

low cost and ease of use. In addition, the barium contained in the methylmethacrylate results in a radiopaque substance that sharply contrasts with the surrounding bone. Local recurrences are more readily apparent than in cases in which bone graft is used [35]. However, there has disadvantages such as a thermal effect on articular cartilage, degenerative arthritis and that PMMA is not a biological substrate [37]. In this series there were two patients with GCT. One lesion located in the proximal tibia was managed initially by resection and prosthetic replacement. This became infected and was removed and followed by a course of antibiotics. The limb was then salvaged and the bone defect treated by knee arthrodesis, tibial Ilizarov and femoral lengthening over nail (LON). The second lesion was located in the distal radius. The patient developed a recurrence and osteomyelitis in the fibular graft used in the primary treatment. This was treated with further resection and distraction osteogenesis until both length and deformity were corrected.

Meary et al. in their nineteen cases of desmoid fibroma of the limbs noticed a large number of recurrences after surgical excision [39]. They concluded that treatment based on surgical excision should be as extensive as possible which leads usually to deformity and shortening. There was one patient with a desmoid fibroma affecting gluteal region and the tibia. After initial tumour excision, the patient developed shortening and a sciatic nerve palsy. This complication was addressed using the Ilizarov fixator and an IM nail for tibial lengthening and a pantalar arthrodesis to correct the foot drop. A residual shortening of 2 cm was the end result.

Chondromyxoid fibroma (CMF) is one of the rarest of bone tumours, accounting for less than 1 % of all bone tumours. The tumour is more common in males and located mostly in the metaphyseal areas of the lower extremity [40]. The most common method of treating CMF is with curettage followed by autograft or allograft. Occasionally, additional chemicals, such as phenol or liquid nitrogen, are placed inside the bone cavity to try to reduce the risk of recurrence. Lersundi et al., in their thirty cases of CMF, concluded that tumours treated with curettage alone did less well than those that were packed with allograft bone or polymethylmethacrylate and those treated by excision did not recur [40]. There was one patient with CMF in the

Table 2 Patients with Ollier's disease

Patient and age (years)	Site	(a) Initial treatment (b) Complication	Final treatment	EFT (days)	(a) Shortening (b) Lengthening (cm)	EFI (days/cm)	End result
F8	L Tibia and femur	(a) Excision (b) Shortness and deformity	Tibia bifocal compression distraction (Ilizarov), Femur deformity correction and lengthening (Unilateral fixator)	210	(a) 9.5 (b) 9	23	Def. corrected Res. shortening
F 14	R Femur and tibia	(a) Osteotomy distal femur and tibia (b) Deformity	MAC Frame for Femur TSF for Tibia	129	(a) 3.9 (b) 3.5	37	Def. corrected Res. shortening Knee joint contracture (resolved with PT)
F9	R Humerus	(a) Corrective osteotomy (b) Deformity	EBI frame	168	(a) 14 (b) 14	12	Def. corrected
F7	R Femur	(a) Biopsy (b) Pathologic fracture, shortening and deformity	Deformity correction and lengthening (Smart Correction multiaxial fixator)	165	(a) 4 (b) 3	55	Def. corrected Res. shortening

EFT External Fixation Time (in days), *EFI* External Fixation Index (in days/cm), *PT* Physiotherapy

Table 3 Patients with Fibrous dysplasia

Patient and age (years)	Site	(a) Initial treatment (b) Complication	Final treatment	EFT (days)	(a) Shortening (b) Lengthening (cm)	EFI (days/cm)	End result
M11	L Distal tibia	(a) Excision for recurrence, bone grafting, 8 mm fibular resection (b) Nonunion, recurrence and pin track inf	TSF	152	(a) 8.5 (b) 6.2	25	Def. corrected Res. shortening
F23	R&L Femur and tibia	(a) Bilateral femur and tibia osteotomy (b) Deformity	TSF	122	(a) 1.2 (b) 0.2	610	Def. corrected Res. shortening
F58	R Tibia	(a) Valgus osteotomy (b) Deformity and shortening	TSF	144	(a) 14.7 (b) 8.6	17	Def. corrected Res. shortening
M29	L Proximal femur	(a) Excision (b) Ankle equinus-treated with PT	TSF	51	(a) 3.7 (b) 3.7	14	Def. corrected
M13	L Femur	(a) Excision (b) Deformity and shortening	Smart correction multiaxial fixator	150	(a) 5 (b) 4.2	36	Def. corrected Res. shortening

EFT External Fixation Time (in days), *EFI* External Fixation Index (in days/cm)

acetabulum in this series. Initial treatment of resection led to shortening which was treated by femoral lengthening using the Ilizarov fixator.

The chondroma is a self-limiting lesion that, in most of cases, heals spontaneously with no treatment required for asymptomatic lesions. However, if a pathological fracture

Table 4 Patients with congenital multiple exostosis

Patient and age (years)	Site	(a) Initial treatment (b) Complication	Final treatment	EFT (days)	(a) Shortening (b) Lengthening (cm)	EFI (days/cm)	End result
M 14	L Ulna	(a) Excision (b) Ulnar club hand	Corrective osteotomy of radius, ulnar lengthening (Unilateral fixator)	270	(a) 2 (b) 2.5	108	Def. corrected
M 14	R Ulna	(a) Excision (b) Ulnar club hand	Corrective osteotomy of radius, ulnar lengthening (Unilateral fixator)	120	(a) 2 (b) 2.5	48	Def. corrected
F 10	R&L Ulna	(a) Excision (b) Bilateral ulnar club hand	Ulnar lengthening over Steinman pins (Unilateral fixator)	210	(a) 3 (b) 3.5	60	Def. corrected
M 10	R Femur	(a) Excision (b) Pathologic fracture, genu varum, 10 cm shortening	Deformity correction and lengthening (Smart correction multiaxial fixator)	300	(a) 8 (b) 7	43	Def. corrected Res. shortening
M 12	L Femur	(a) Excision (b) Deformity and knee contracture	Deformity correction and lengthening (Smart correction multiaxial fixator)	105	(a) 3 (b) 2	52	Def. corrected Res. shortening

EFT External Fixation Time (in days), *EFI* External Fixation Index (in days/cm)

Table 5 All other patients

Diagnosis	Patient and age (years)	Site	(a) Initial treatment (b) Complication	Final treatment	EFT (days)	(a) Shortening (b) Lengthening (cm)	EFI (days/cm)	End result
GCT	M 30	L Tibia	(a) Excision and tumour prosthesis (b) Septic prosthesis failure	Implant removal Femur LON, Tibia Ilizarov	180	(a) 7.5 (b) 7.5	24	Knee arthrodesis
	F15	L Radius	(a) Wide resection and non vascularized fibula graft (b) Recurrence, osteomyelitis	Lengthening and deformity correction (Unilateral External Fixator)	117	(a) 3.5 (b) 3.5	33	Def. corrected
DF	M 21	Tibia and gluteal region	(a) Wide resection (b) Shortening and sciatic nerve palsy	Pantalar arthrodesis (Ilizarov and IM nail)	90	(a) 5.5 (b) 3.5	26	Res. shortening
CMF	M 22	L Acet.	(a) Wide resection (b) Shortening	Femur lengthening (Ilizarov)	270	(a) 6 (b) 4.5	60	Res. shortening
Chondroma	F 13	R Distal Femur	(a) Wide resection (b) Shortening and deformity	Lengthening and deformity correction (Ilizarov)	210	(a) 9 (b) 8.5	25	Def. corrected Res. shortening
UBC	F 14	R Distal Fibula	(a) Curettage and bone grafting (b) Deformity	EBI frame	27	(a) 0.7 (b) 0.7	39	Def. corrected

EFT External Fixation Time (in days), *EFI* External Fixation Index (in days/cm), *LON* Lengthening over nail

occurs it is treated with curettage and bone grafting [41]. The patient from this series was treated initially by wide resection for a distal femoral chondroma. The Ilizarov fixator was applied for deformity correction and lengthening; a residual 0.5 cm shortening was the outcome.

Despite an extensive literature on the unicameral bone cyst (UBC), there remains an uncertainty regarding optimal treatment. Bensahel et al. [42] have stated the solitary bone cyst has not revealed all its secrets. Surgical therapy of a UBC may be divided into open and percutaneous procedures. Success is quite varied and the very definition of success has also varied amongst authors [43]. The initial treatment of the patient with UBC of the distal fibula in this series was of curettage and bone grafting, after which shortening and deformity occurred. We applied EBI monolateral fixator for lengthening and deformity correction.

There is a concern regarding the risk for malignant degeneration in patients when an osteotomy is performed in bone with a coexisting benign tumour [5]. Similarly, there are concerns over the quality of new bone formation during distraction osteogenesis in what is 'diseased' bone [5]. Despite these concerns, we did not encounter these problems during a mean follow-up of 69.5 months.

Conclusion

There are advantages of using distraction osteogenesis in the treatment of problems and sequelae after primary treatment for benign bone tumours. The risks for recurrence of shortening and deformity in young patients may be minimized with overcorrection or over-lengthening. There appears to be no increased risk of malignant degeneration from osteotomy through diseased bone or there being low-quality regenerate bone at the distraction site. We believe that external fixation is an effective technique for treating defects, problems and complications related to benign bone tumours or the effects arising from wide excision of the primary lesion. It offers a good alternative to other conventional methods of management. There are some disadvantages to this technique such as pin track infection, the bulk and encumbrance of the fixator and the prolonged treatment period. The choice of external fixator is dictated by the complexity of problem and the anatomical location but, in general, the circular fixators are more suitable than the unilateral fixators for the simultaneous treatment of deformity and limb-length discrepancy.

Acknowledgments No financial support was received for this study.

Informed consent Informed consent was obtained from all individual participants included in this study.

References

1. Donati D, Giacomini S, Gozzi E, Mercuri M (2002) Proximal femur reconstruction by an allograft prosthesis composite. Clin Orthop 394:192–200
2. Eckardt JJ, Kabo JM, Kelley CM et al (2000) Expandable endoprosthesis reconstruction in skeletally immature patients with tumors. Clin Orthop 373:51–61
3. Schaser KD, Bail HJ, Haas NP, Melcher I (2002) Treatment concepts of benign bone tumors and tumor-like bone lesions. Chirurg 73(12):1181–1190
4. Tsuchiya H, Tomita K, Shinokawa Y et al (1996) The Ilizarov method in the management of giant-cell tumors of the proximal tibia. J Bone Joint Surg [Br] 78:264–269
5. Tsuchiya H, Tomita K, Minematsu K et al (1996) Limb salvage using distraction osteogenesis: a classification of the technique. J Bone Joint Surg [Br] 78:403–411
6. Enneking WF, Campanacci DA (2001) Retrieved human allografts: a clinico-pathological study. J Bone Joint Surg [Am] 83:971–986
7. Shih LY, Chen TS, Lo WH (1993) Limb salvage surgery for locally aggressive and malignant bone tumors. J Surg Oncol 53:154–160
8. Aronson James (1997) Current concepts review—limb-lengthening, skeletal reconstruction, and bone transport with the Ilizarov method. J Bone Joint Surg [Am] 79(8):1243–1258
9. Atesalp AS, Basbozkurt M, Erler K et al (1998) Treatment of tibial bone defects with the Ilizarov circular external fixator in high-velocity gunshot wounds. Int Orthop 22:343–347
10. Green SA (1991) Osteomyelitis: the Ilizarov perspective. Orthop Clin North Am 22:515–521
11. Rozbruch SR, Herzenberg JE, Tetsworth K, Tuten HR, Paley D (2002) Distraction osteogenesis for nonunion after high tibial osteotomy. Clin Orthop 394:227–235
12. Koseoglu E, Yildiz C, Atesalp AS, Basbozkurt M, Gur E (2000) Treatment of posttraumatic lower limb deformities with the Ilizarov method. Acta Orthop Traumatol Turc 34:480–487
13. Canadell J, San-Julian M, Cara J, Forriol F (1998) External fixation in tumor pathology. Int Orthop 22:126–130
14. Millett PJ, Lane JM, Paletta GA Jr (2000) Limb salvage using distraction osteogenesis. Am J Orthop 29:628–632
15. Paley D, Catagni MA, Argnani F, Villa A, Benedetti GB, Cattaneo R (1989) Ilizarov treatment of tibial nonunions with bone loss. Clin Orthop 241:146–165
16. Tsuchiya H, Morsy AF, Matsubara H, Watanabe K, Abdel-Wanis ME, Tomita K (2007) Treatment of benign bone tumours using external fixation. J Bone Joint Surg [Br] 89(8):1077–1083
17. Erol B, Tetik C, Sirin E, Kocaoglu B, Bezer M (2006) Surgical treatment of hand deformities in multiple enchondromatosis: a case report. Acta Orthop Traumatol Turc 40:89–93
18. Jesus-Garcia R, Bongiovanni JC, Korukian M et al (2001) Use of the Ilizarov external fixator in the treatment of patients with Ollier's disease. Clin Orthop 382:82–86
19. Freeman BH, Bray EW 3rd, Meyer LC (1987) Multiple osteotomies with Zickel nail fixation for polyostotic fibrous dysplasia involving the proximal part of the femur. J Bone Joint Surg [Am] 69:691–698
20. Funk F Jr, Well RE (1973) Hip problems in fibrous dysplasia. Clin Orthop 90:77–82

21. Ozaki T, Sugihara M, Nakatsuka Y, Kawai A, Inoue H (1996) Polyostotic fibrous dysplasia: a long-term follow up of 8 patients. Int Orthop 20:227–232

22. Edgerton MT, Persing JA, Jane JA (1985) The surgical treatment of fibrous dysplasia. With emphasis on recent contributions from cranio-maxillo-facial surgery. Ann Surg 202(4):459–479

23. Guille JT, Kumar SJ, MacEwen GD (1998) Fibrous dysplasia of the proximal part of the femur: long-term results of curettage and bone-grafting and mechanical realignment. J Bone Joint Surg [Am] 80:648–658

24. Jaffe HL (1958) Fibrous dysplasia. In: Tumors and tumorous conditions of the bones and joints. Lea and Febiger, Philadelphia, pp 117–142, 244–255

25. Porter DE, Lonie L, Fraser M, Dobson-Stone C, Porter JR, Monaco AP, Simpson AH (2004) Severity of disease and risk of malignant change in hereditary multiple exostoses. A genotype–phenotype study. J Bone Joint Surg [Br] 86:1041–1046

26. Noonan KJ, Feinberg JR, Levenda A, Snead J, Wurtz LD (2002) Natural history of multiple hereditary osteochondromatosis of the lower extremity and ankle. J Pediatr Orthop 22:120–124

27. Watts AC, Ballantyne JA, Fraser M, Simpson AH, Porter DE (2007) The association between ulnar length and forearm movement in patients with multiple osteochondromas. J Hand Surg [Am] 32:667–673

28. Pritchett JW (1986) Lengthening the ulna in patients with hereditary multiple exostoses. J Bone Joint Surg [Br] 68:561–565

29. Thomas DM, Skubitz T (2009) Giant-cell tumor of bone. Curr Opin Oncol 21:338–344

30. Dahlin DC, Cupps RE, Johnson EW Jr (1970) Giant-cell tumor: a study of 195 cases. Cancer 25:1061–1070

31. Campanacci M, Cervellati C, Donati U (1985) Autogenous patella as replacement for a resected femoral or tibial condyle: a report on 19 cases. J Bone Joint Surg [Br] 67:557–563

32. Cappana R, Fabbri N, Bettelli G (1990) Curettage of giant cell tumor of bone: the effect of surgical technique and adjuvants on local recurrence rate. Chir Organi Mov 75(Suppl 1):206

33. Clohisy DR, Mankin HJ (1994) Osteoarticular allografts for reconstruction after resection of a musculoskeletal tumor in the proximal end of the tibia. J Bone Joint Surg [Am] 76:549–554

34. Trieb K, Bitzan P, Lang S, Dominkus M, Kotz R (2001) Recurrence of curetted and bone grafted giant-cell tumors with and without adjuvant phenol therapy. Eur J Surg Oncol 27:200–202

35. Balke M, Schremper L, Gebert C, Ahrens H, Streitbuerger A, Koehler G et al (2008) Giant cell tumor of bone: treatment and outcome of 214 cases. J Cancer Res Clin Oncol 134(9):969–978

36. Gitelis S, Mallin BA, Piasecki P (1993) Intralesional excision compared with en bloc resection for giant-cell tumors of bone. J Bone Joint Surg [Am] 75(11):1648–1655

37. Camargo OP, Croci AT, Oliveira CR, Baptista AM, Caiero MT (2005) Functional and radiographic evaluation of 214 aggressive benign bone lesions treated with curettage, cauterization, and cementation: 24 years of follow up. Clinics 60:439–444

38. Blackley HR, Wunder JS, Davis AM et al (1999) Treatment of giant-cell tumors of long bones with curettage and bone-grafting. J Bone Joint Surg [Am] 81-A:811–820

39. Méary R, Danan JP, Tomeno B, Forest M, Cirotteau Y (1978) Desmoid fibroma of the limbs. Rev Chir Orthop Reparatrice Appar Mot 64(3):195–204

40. Lersundi A, Mankin HJ, Mourikis A, Hornicek FJ (2005) Chondromyxoid fibroma: a rarely encountered and puzzling tumor. Clin Orthop 439:171–175

41. Vanni R (2003) Bone: chondroma. Atlas Genet Cytogenet Oncol Haematol 7(3):191–193

42. Bensahel H, Jehanno P, Desgrippes Y, Pennecot GF (1998) Solitary bone cyst: controversies and treatment. J Pediatr Orthop B 7(4):257–261

43. Wright JG, Yandow S, Donaldson S, Marley L (2008) A randomized clinical trial comparing intralesional bone marrow and steroid injections for simple bone cysts. J Bone Joint Surg [Am] 90(4):722–730

24

Internal bone transport using a cannulated screw as a mounting device in the treatment of a post-infective ulnar defect

Konstantinos Tsitskaris[1] · Heledd Havard[1] · Paulien Bijlsma[2] · Robert A. Hill[1]

Abstract Bone transport techniques can be used to address the segmental bone loss occurring after debridement for infection. Secure fixation of the bone transport construct to the bone transport segment can be challenging, particularly if the bone is small and osteopenic. We report a case of a segmental ulnar bone defect in a young child treated with internal bone transport using a cannulated screw as the mounting device. We found this technique particularly useful in the treatment of bone loss secondary to infection, where previous treatment and prolonged immobilisation had led to osteopenia. This technique has not been previously reported.

Keywords Internal bone transport · Ulnar segmental bone defect · Cannulated screw · PVL *S. aureus*

Segmental bone loss can occur as a consequence of fractures, after tumour resection and following extensive debridement for bone infection [1]. Treatment methods used to address large bone defects include traditional bone grafting, vascularised bone grafts, the induced membrane technique and bone transport techniques [2]. Secure fixation of the bone transport construct to the bone transport

segment can be challenging, particularly if the bone is small and osteopenic. We report a case of a segmental ulnar bone defect in a young child treated with internal bone transport using a cannulated screw as the mounting device. This technique has not been previously reported.

Case report

A 2-year-old girl presented to her local hospital with pain and swelling in the left forearm and elevated inflammatory markers. Plain radiographs and a magnetic resonance imaging scan confirmed the clinical diagnosis of osteomyelitis of the left ulna. She was started on broad-spectrum antibiotics and transferred to our unit where she underwent surgical debridement. Tissue samples were positive for infection with Panton–Valentine leukocidin (PVL) *Staphylococcus aureus* (*S. aureus*), sensitive to flucloxacillin and clindamycin. She underwent two further surgical debridements and received a six-week course of intravenous antibiotics. The inflammatory markers returned to normal levels, and the debridement wounds healed with no local sequelae.

During the following 3 months, a segment of the ulna became osteolytic and after minor trauma, a midshaft fracture occurred which was treated in a cast (Fig. 1). Substantial dissolution of the ulnar shaft took place, leaving the distal ulna and its growth plate radiographically intact. During this period, the patient was assessed at frequent intervals and no clinical or biochemical evidence of an active infection was identified. The ulnar bone defect measured approximately 3.5 cm and showed no evidence of recovery. After the osteolytic process had reached a plateau on sequential radiographs, ulnar reconstruction was undertaken.

✉ Konstantinos Tsitskaris
tsitskaris@yahoo.com

[1] Department of Orthopaedics, Great Ormond Street Hospital for Children, London WC1N 3JH, UK

[2] Department of Orthopaedics, St Mary's Hospital and Hillingdon Hospital, London, UK

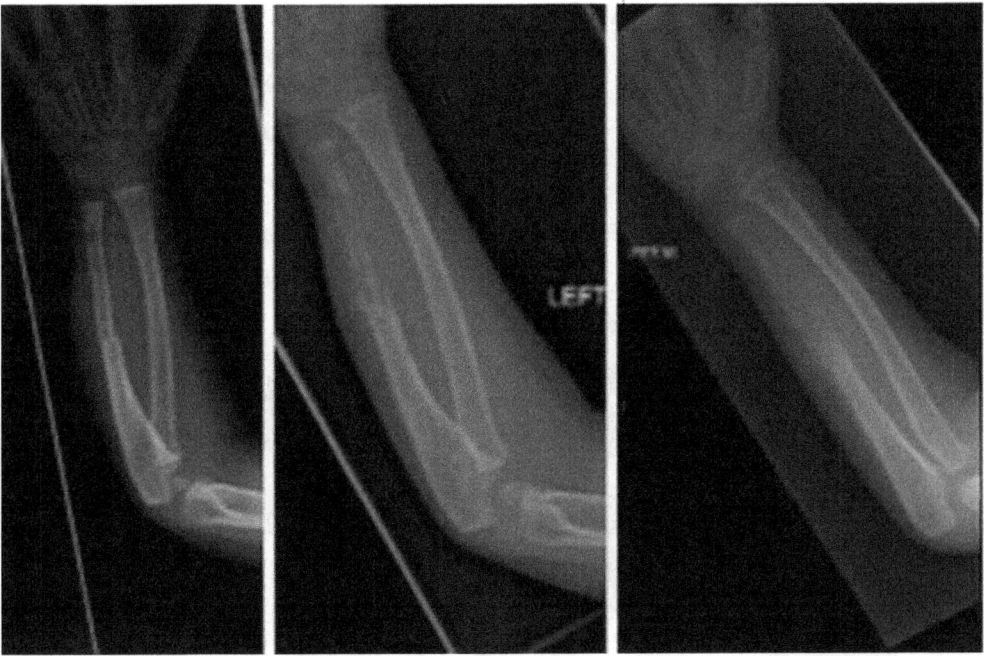

Fig. 1 Significant osteolytic process affected the left ulna with dissolution of part of the bone

Surgical technique

An Ilizarov fixator (Smith & Nephew Orthopaedics Ltd, Warwick, UK) was used. The ulnar osteotomy was performed percutaneously by pre-drilling the bone prior to attaching the frame. The level for the osteotomy was the proximal metaphysis just distal to the coronoid process. Initially, the Ilizarov fixator was set up for external transport, with a proximal half ring, a half ring for bone transport and a distal complete ring using the elevator method. The osteotomy was then completed with an osteotome after attachment of the frame. Within the first 2 weeks of treatment, the transport wire pulled through the osteopenic bone, necessitating revision. At the time of revision, the treatment was converted to an internal bone transport construct. We secured the bone transport segment with a 1.5-mm transport wire by threading the wire through a 3.5-mm cannulated screw, positioned perpendicular to the long axis of the bone (Fig. 2). The transport wire exited at the level of the wrist and was mounted to a slotted rod distraction device (Fig. 3).

The distraction started 5 days post-operatively at a rate of 0.75 mm/day. There were no complications in the immediate post-operative period. During the final stages of the bone transport, the patient received a course of oral antibiotics for a pin site infection. During the bone transport, radiographs were taken every 2 weeks in order to monitor new bone formation. After 3 months, the ulnar defect was effectively bridged and consolidated during the following 2 months (Fig. 3). The frame was removed when corticalisation of

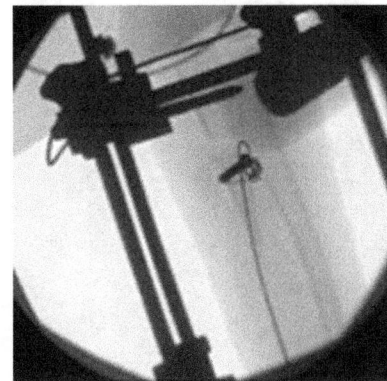

Fig. 2 Bone transport segment is secured on a traction wire by threading the latter through a 3.5-mm cannulated screw positioned perpendicular to the long axis of the bone

three out of four cortices was evident on radiographs. During the procedure to remove the frame, the docking site was assessed and stabilised using a small fragment plate; eventually, this was also removed 11 months later (Fig. 4).

The patient had supervised elbow and hand therapy throughout the treatment to maintain function. Initially, passive range-of-movement exercises were undertaken, and eventually, as the pain decreased, active exercises were encouraged. At the final follow-up, 30 months after the initial presentation, the patient remained pain-free and was able to undertake her usual daily activities without restrictions. She had equal range of movement to the contralateral arm, with mildly increased ulnar deviation at the left wrist; the latter was completely pain-free.

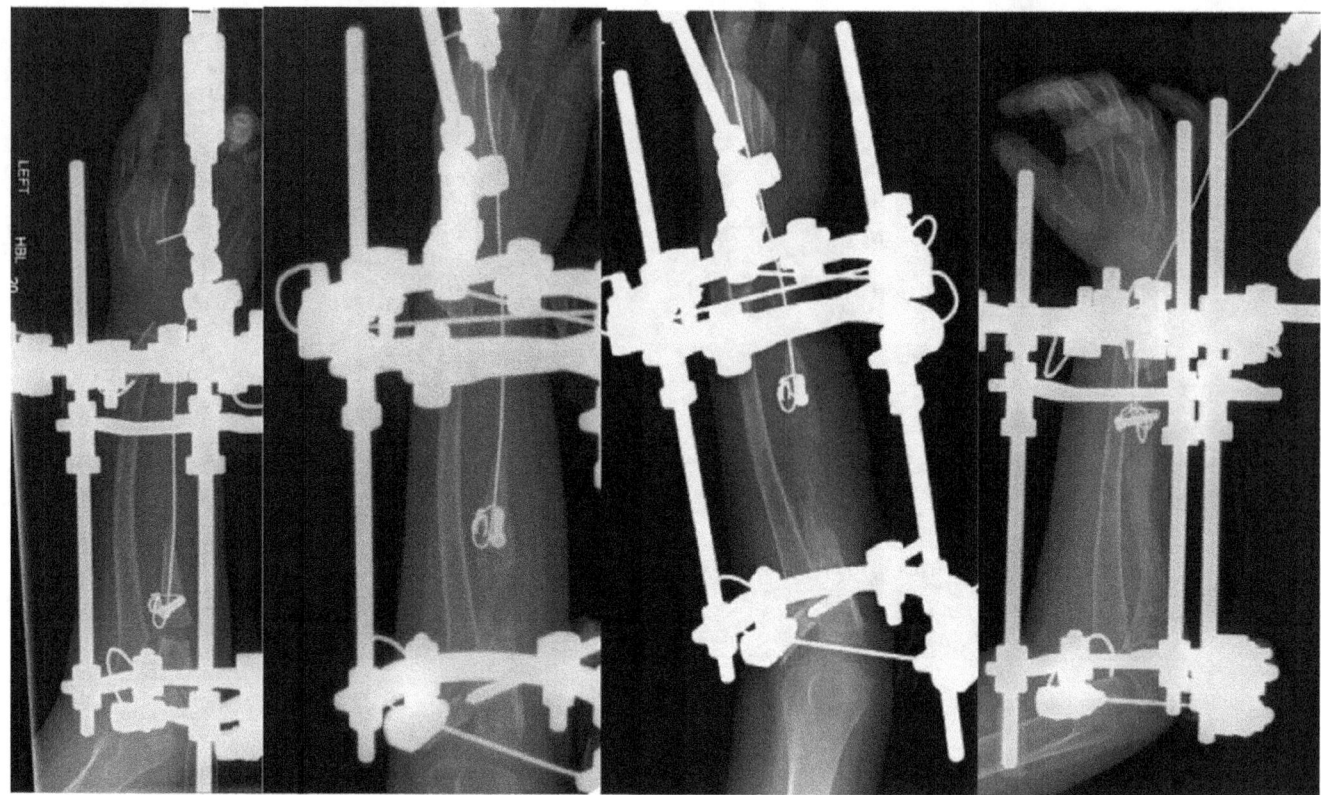

Fig. 3 Ulnar defect was bridged and consolidated during the course of the treatment

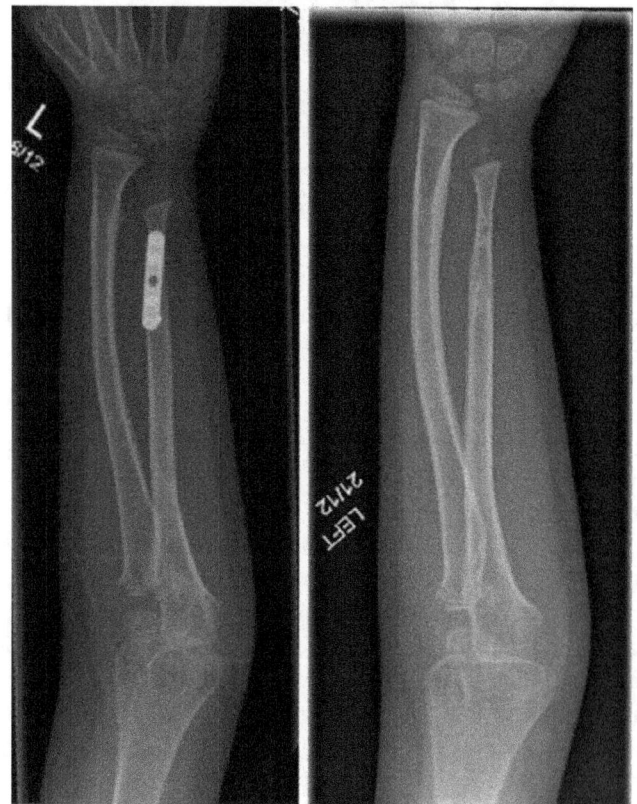

Fig. 4 Fixation of the docking site (*left*) and the end result (*right*)

Discussion

Bone transport can be internal or external; in the former, the transport segment is pulled by a construct that is inside the limb exiting distally, whereas during the latter, the bone segment is attached to a transport ring, with the construct moving through the soft tissues. The main advantage of the internal technique is that it eliminates the risk of transection of important structures, such as nerves. The main difficulty is the secure fixation of the internal transport construct to the bone transport segment, particularly if this is small and osteopenic.

Commonly used methods for the fixation of the internal bone transport segment include olive wires or flexible cables; both run the risk of "cheese wiring" through the bone transport segment. The use of a cannulated screw–wire construct proved effective in providing a secure mounting point in this case where the transport segment was osteoporotic and an external transport wire had cut out. Figure 5 depicts the cannulated screw technique, the two most commonly used techniques to secure the bone segment during internal bone transport and the external bone transport technique.

Potential alternative options for the treatment of a segmental ulnar bone loss, as in this case, include a vascularised bone graft or the creation of a one-bone forearm [3,

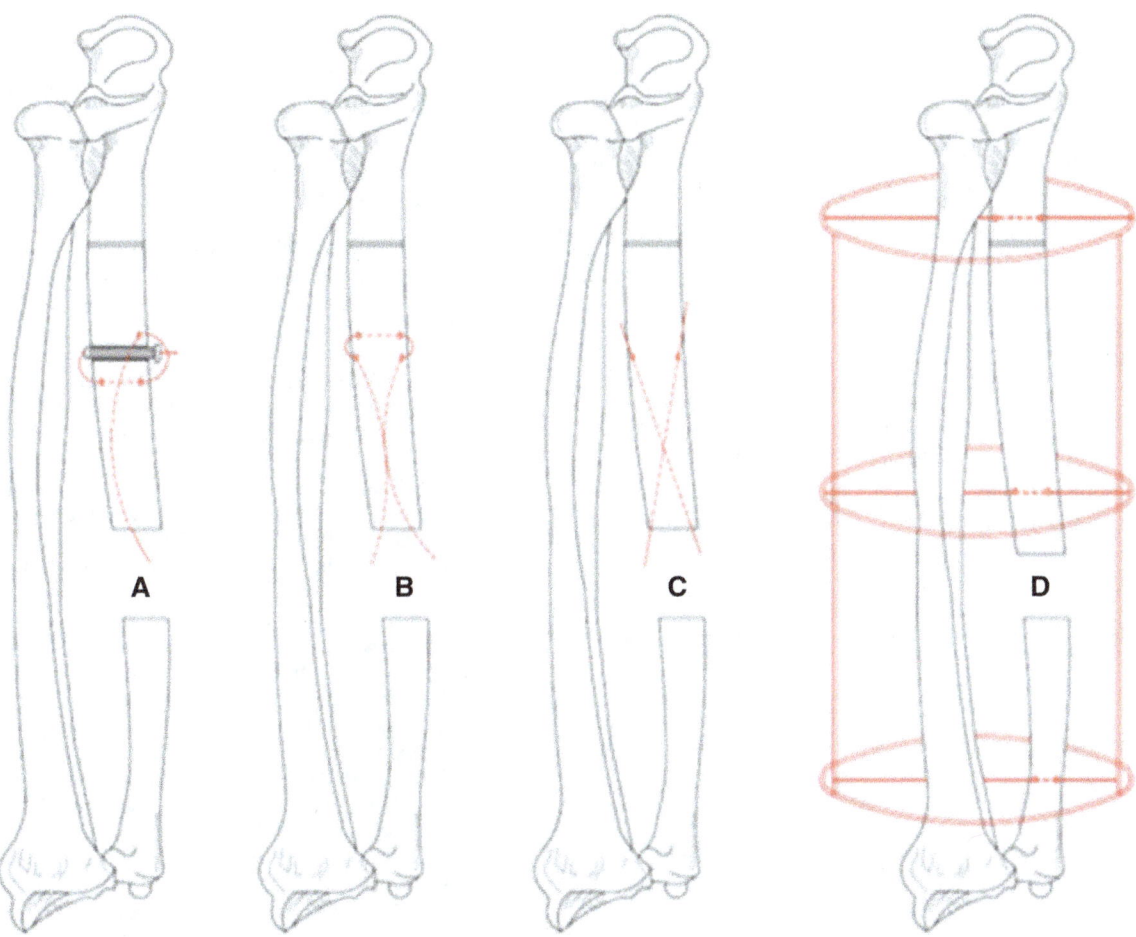

Fig. 5 Forearm model for bone transport [**a**, **b** and **c**, internal bone transport (**a** the cannulated screw technique, **b** the flexible cable technique, **c** the olive wire technique). **d** external bone transport]

4]. The latter can be accomplished by medial translocation of the radius to place it in continuity with the ulna. It can be associated with an increased incidence of complications and should probably be considered as a last resort option [5]. Vascularised bone grafts usually consist of a fibular segment, but radial and humeral grafts can also be used. The bone is vascularised, remains viable and also has structural strength. The disadvantages of this technique are substantial and include significant complexity, risk of failure of the vascular anastomosis, risk of non-union to the host bone and morbidity of the donor site. A comparison of this method with bone transport in the femur revealed superior results with the latter method [6].

PVL is an exoprotein with increased toxicity to immune cells. It was first described in 1932 and is secreted in approximately 2 % of *S. aureus* infections [7, 8]. PVL-secreting *S. aureus* infections are more aggressive, usually affect the soft tissues and can be complicated by secondary infections such as necrotising haemorrhagic pneumonia [9]. PVL-secreting *S. aureus* osteomyelitis in children is a rare entity with a limited number of reports in the literature

[10, 11]. Our patient developed a localised infection with a significant concomitant osteolysis and an almost complete dissolution of part of the ulnar diaphysis. We believe that this was a result of the significant virulence of the pathogen, which is in agreement with previous reports [10].

After a lengthy treatment, our patient enjoys a very functional, painless and infection-free arm. Nevertheless, there is still a residual relative discrepancy in the length of the radius and ulna (Fig. 4). We believe that this is a result of the proximal migration of the distal ulnar, whilst it was not in continuity with the rest of the shaft. In addition, although the osteomyelitic process appeared to be strictly diaphyseal, it may have had an indirect effect on the distal ulnar physis affecting its growth potential.

Patients with a discrepancy in the length of the radius and ulna are at risk of developing symptoms from the adjacent joints. In particular, a shorter ulna predisposes the patient to the risk of subluxation or dislocation of the radial head [12]. Such a deformity has not occurred in this case, and the patient has remained asymptomatic, precluding the need for further treatment. Nevertheless, the patient will continue to be followed up until skeletal maturity. Options for future treatment will depend on whether the discrepancy is progressive or stable and include radial epiphysiodesis with or without further ulnar lengthening, potentially employing the same treatment principles. Such intervention could accomplish a congruent distal radio-ulnar articulation, but would be prone to the risks associated with major limb reconstruction surgery.

Conclusions

The technique we present here offers an alternative mounting option for bone transport. We found this technique particularly useful in the treatment of bone loss secondary to infection, where previous treatment and prolonged immobilisation had led to osteopenia.

Acknowledgments We would like to thank Ms Nathmya Saffarini for the original diagrams in Fig. 5.

Financial support None of the authors received financial support for this study.

Informed consent Informed consent was obtained from the family of the child in this case.

References

1. Tsuchiya H, Tomita K (2003) Distraction osteogenesis for treatment of bone loss in the lower extremity. J Orthop Sci 8:116–124
2. Rigal S, Merloz P, Le Nen D et al (2012) Bone transport techniques in posttraumatic bone defects. Orthop Traumatol Surg Res 98:103–108
3. Olekas J, Guobys A (1991) Vascularised bone transfer for defects and pseudarthoses of forearm bones. J Hand Surg Br 16:406–408
4. Allende C, Allende BT (2004) Posttraumatic one-bone forearm reconstruction: a report of seven cases. J Bone Joint Surg Am 86(2):364–369
5. Jacoby SM, Bachoura A, Diprinzio EV et al (2013) Complications following one-bone forearm surgery for posttraumatic forearm and distal radioulnar instability. J Hand Surg Am 38:976–982
6. Song HR, Kale A, Park HB et al (2003) Comparison of internal bone transport and vascularised fibular grafting for femoral bone defects. J Orthop Trauma 17:203–211
7. Panton PN, Valentine FCO (1932) Staphylococcal Toxin. Lancet 1:506–508
8. Holmes A, Ganner M, McGuane S et al (2005) *Staphylococcus aureus* isolates carrying Panton-Valentine leukocidin genes in England and Wales: frequency, characterisation and association with clinical disease. J Clin Microbiol 43:2384–2390
9. Prevost G, Mourey D, Colin A et al (2001) Staphylococcal pore-forming toxins. Curr Top Microbiol Immunol 257:53–58
10. Bocchini CE, Hulten KG, Mason EO et al (2006) Panton-Valentine Leukocidin Genes are associated with enhanced inflammatory response and local disease in acute haematogenous *Staphylococcus aureus* osteomyelitis in children. Pediatrics 117:433–440
11. Sdougkos G, Chini V, Papanastasiou DA et al (2007) Methicillin-resistant *Staphylococcus aureus* producing Panton-Valentine leukocidin as a cause of acute osteomyelitis in children. Clin Microbiol Infect 13:651–654
12. Hill RA, Ibrahim T, Mann HA et al (2011) Forearm lengthening by distraction osteogenesis in children: a report of 22 cases. J Bone Joint Surg Br 93:1550–1555

25

Functional outcome of knee arthrodesis with a monorail external fixator

Alfred Cyril Roy[1] · Sandeep Albert[1] · Mohamad Gouse[1] · Dan Barnabas Inja[1]

Abstract Several methods for obtaining knee arthrodesis have been described in the literature and world; over, the commonest cause for arthrodesis is a failed arthroplasty. Less commonly, as in this series, post-infective or traumatic causes may also require a knee fusion wherein arthroplasty may not be indicated. We present salient advantages along with the radiological and functional outcome of twenty four patients treated with a single monorail external fixator. All patients went on develop fusion at an average of 5.4 months with an average limb length discrepancy of 3 cm (1.5–6 cm). Improvements in functional outcome as assessed by the lower extremity functional score (LEFS), and the SF-36 was significant ($p = 0.000$). Knee arthrodesis with a single monorail external fixator is a reasonable single-staged salvage option in patients wherein arthroplasty may not be the ideal choice. The outcome, though far from ideal, is definitely positive and predictable.

Keywords Knee arthrodesis · External fixator · Tuberculous arthritis · Post-septic sequelae · Post-traumatic sequelae

Introduction

Knee arthrodesis, performed since 1900, is achieved by various methods. Whilst the earliest recorded knee fusion, performed by Prof. Albert of Vienna, was for a flail knee in poliomyelitis, the most common indication today is a failed knee arthroplasty. In the developing world, knee arthrodesis is often performed for sepsis or for arthritis after tuberculosis or trauma.

Since 1948 [1], external fixators have been utilized to achieve compression across the fusion site. The use of larger diameter radially preloaded half pins has improved fixation and stability. The technique of knee arthrodesis with a monolateral fixator has been described using dynamic axial fixator (DAF, Orthofix SRL, Verona, Italy). The same type of device has been used to bridge bone defects [2]. In this series, we used a monorail external fixator to achieve fixation and compression across the knee for arthrodesis in patients with either post-traumatic or post-septic sequelae (Figs. 1, 2).

Methodology

Patients who underwent knee arthrodesis for various indications from January 2007 to January 2013 were in included in the study for analysis. Hospital records, clinical photographs, radiographs and follow-up radiographs were analysed, and the functional outcome at final follow-up was recorded. The SF-36 and the LEFS (lower extremity functional score) were utilized for pre-operative and final functional outcome assessment.

✉ Sandeep Albert
sandeepalbertor@gmail.com

Alfred Cyril Roy
alfredroy@cmcvellore.ac.in

Mohamad Gouse
gousemohamad@yahoo.com

Dan Barnabas Inja
injadan@gmail.com

[1] Department of Orthopedics Unit-1, CMC, Vellore, India

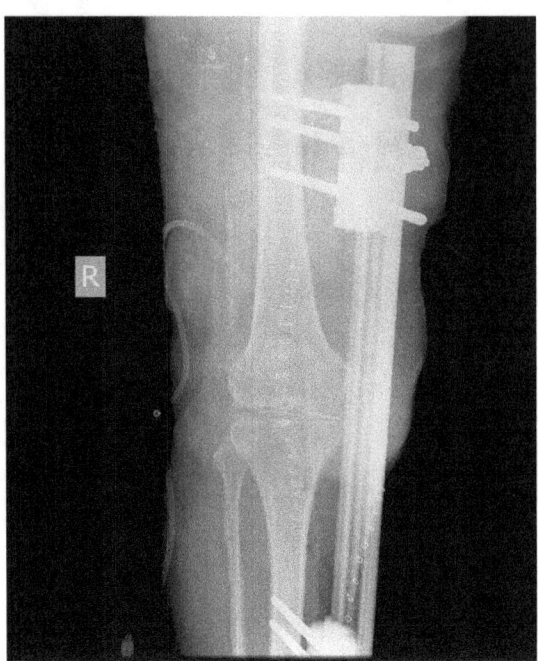

Fig. 1 Immediate post-operative antero-posterior plain radiographs showing knee arthrodesis performed with an anterior monorail fixator

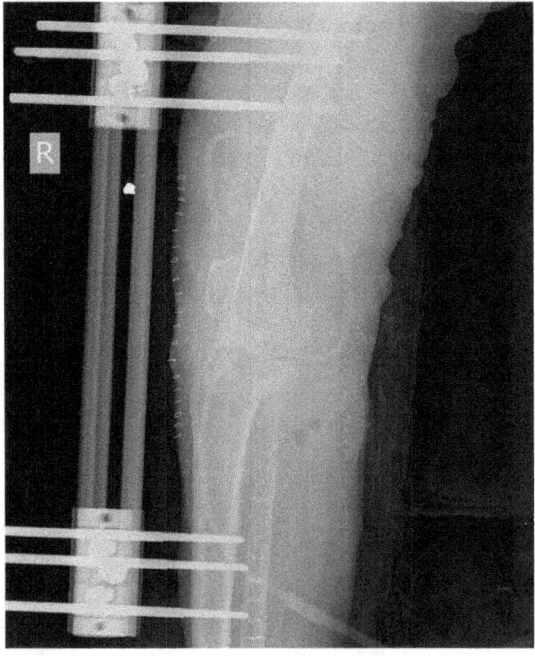

Fig. 2 Immediate post-operative lateral plain radiograph showing knee arthrodesis performed with an anterior monorail fixator

Pre-operative planning and operative technique

Pre-operative planning included a review of the patient's diagnosis, prior surgical procedures around the knee, the soft tissue condition and the presence of deformities or arthritis in other lower limb large joints. Radiographs were

analysed to assess deformity, bone defects and for planning resection margins. The target alignment in arthrodesis of the knee was neutral rotation, flexion of 10–15 degrees and valgus of 7–10 degrees. The patient was positioned supine. A radiolucent table and a tourniquet were used in all the cases. The knee joint was approached through an anterior incision which was modified depending on prior scars. The patella was reflected laterally and either resected or its articular surface removed for the main body to be used as graft to augment fusion. The joint was debrided thoroughly with near total excision of all granulation and granulomatous tissue, inflamed synovium and eburnated cartilage. The distal femur and proximal tibia were then cut appropriately till bleeding surfaces of cancellous bone were encountered. The tibia was cut with a mild posterior and lateral slope to allow for flexion and valgus alignment.

When the Orthofix monorail was employed anteriorly, the most proximal pin was inserted in the distal diaphysis of the femur ensuring central placement in the sagittal plane. The cut surfaces were then opposed to coapt bleeding surfaces of cancellous bone. The most distal pin on the tibial diaphysis was inserted along the sagittal plane just medial to the tibial crest. This ensured a slight valgus alignment and allowed for central and bicortical placement of the intervening pins. Such placement of the pins ensured positioning of a straight monorail across a slightly valgus knee. All pins (with a minimum of three on either side) were affixed to a single clamp. This facilitated compression when a compression device was utilized in the monorail. When the undersurface of the patella was prepared, the patella was allowed to fall back over the site of fusion with wound closure. Fixation with a screw or pin was not routinely required. Excision of the patella was done in a few cases to simplify closure in a scarred limb with poor soft tissue conditions. The wound was lavaged prior to closure under drains. An adequate distance between the rail and the skin allowed for wound closure and post-operative wound care. This was crucial as with the knee in flexion the monorail fixator was brought closer to the skin anteriorly. At the same time care was taken to avoid having the rail too far from the soft tissue thereby reducing biomechanical stability. There were occasions when additional soft tissue procedures were performed; medial or lateral gastrocnemius flaps served as work horses for defects surrounding the knee. Patients were encouraged to bear weight as tolerated. Partial weight bearing with support was continued for at least 3 months. Radiographs were obtained every 6 weeks for the first 3–6 months. The patients were educated and taught pin site care. Bridging trabeculae and sclerosis with blurring of the cut edges at the fusion site were signs of adequate fusion at which time the patient was usually able to ambulate full weight bearing without support. Frame removal was not routinely preceded by dynamization (Figs. 3, 4).

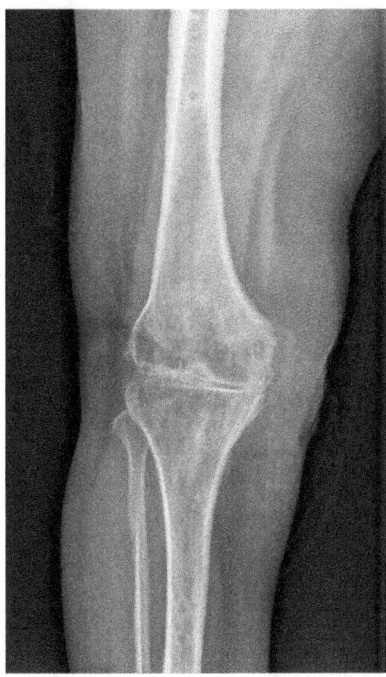

Fig. 3 Antero-posterior plain radiograph at seven months with consolidation at the arthrodesis site

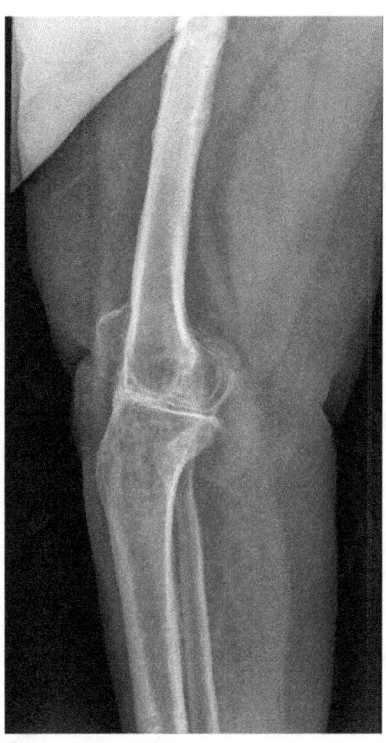

Fig. 4 Lateral plain radiograph at seven months showing good consolidation at the arthrodesis site

Results

This study was approved by the institutional review board (IRB no – 8538). The patient demographic data are listed in Table 1. The majority of patients were labourers from agrarian communities. The mean age was 42 years (19–68 years). Articular tuberculosis and other infective sequelae were the majority of causes. Nineteen of the 24 patients had undergone more than one prior surgical procedure including joint debridement, synovectomy or prior fixation for complex trauma. All patients described chronic debilitating pain and deformity affecting function at presentation. Six of 24 patients had wound complications which were managed with a medial or lateral gastrocnemius flap. All 24 patients went on to sound union with no additional intervention. The time to union was 5.4 months on average (4–7 months). None required an additional procedure to augment union. Fourteen of 24 patients were able to return to their pre-injury occupation after frame removal. The average limb length discrepancy was 3 cm (1.5–6 cm). This discrepancy was significantly higher in patients presenting with post-traumatic sequelae as compared to post-infective (5.5 cm vs. 2 cm). The average final valgus alignment was 7 degrees (2–11 degrees.) Nearly all patients had pin site issues especially in the proximal pins which settled with pin site care and oral antibiotics and a few had local antibiotic injections. None of the patients required exchange or revision of pins. The mean pre-operative and post-procedure LEFS and SF scores are given

in Table 2. Both the LEFS and SF-36 scores showed significant improvement in the time of frame removal ($p = 0.000$; Fig. 5).

Discussion

A failed arthroplasty is the most common indication for knee arthrodesis. However, post-traumatic and post-infective sequelae, including tuberculosis, are still encountered in developing countries. In the current era where knee arthroplasty is the dominant treatment for end-stage knee pathologies, combined with heightened patients' expectations and awareness, arthrodesis as a salvage procedure is often overlooked or even frowned upon. However, arthrodesis may be preferable for certain patients; this would include the patient's age, occupation and the presence of localized infection. For the younger patient, fusion is a good alternative to staged reconstructive procedures and may be cost effective giving the patient an early return to occupation. In this series, the mean age was 42 years (19–68) with most patients involved in agricultural or hard manual labour where a total knee replacement was not the preferred solution.

The presence of constant disabling pain with deformity and infection for many of these patients had a direct bearing on function as shown by the low pre-operative

Table 1 Patient demographic data

S. no	Age/sex	Host type	Diagnosis	No. of previous surgery index
1	20/M	A	Post-trauma	0
2	40/F	A	Pyogenic	1
3	45/M	A	Pyogenic	2
4	29/M	A	Tuberculosis	2
5	41/M	A	Post-trauma	2
6	68/M	B	Pyogenic	0
7	24/M	A	Post-trauma	2
8	58/M	A	Post-trauma	1
9	33/M	A	Tuberculosis	2
10	48/M	B	Pyogenic	2
11	43/M	A	Tuberculosis	0
12	56/M	A	Post-trauma	2
13	22/M	A	Tuberculosis	0
14	46/M	B	Pyogenic	2
15	69/F	B	Pyogenic	2
16	50/M	A	Tuberculosis	1
17	34/M	B	Tuberculosis	0
18	50/M	B	Tuberculosis	1
19	26/M	A	Tuberculosis	1
20	60/M	B	Pyogenic	1
21	51/M	A	Pyogenic	1
22	28/M	A	Post-trauma	1
23	57/M	A	Post-trauma	2
24	19/M	A	Post-trauma	1

Table 2 Pre- and post-scores

Variable	Pre-op	Post-op	p value
LEFS	39	64	0.000
SF			
Mental	32	51	0.000
Physical	33	43	0.000

LEFS and SF-36 scores. A joint debridement along with the stability achieved with compression through the monorail device, coupled with appropriate antimicrobial/antituberculous therapy, provides a conductive environment for fusion. Decrease in pain and improved stability after fusion resulted in an improvement in functional outcome.

Various studies have described the use of external fixators [1, 3, 9, 10], cannulated screws [4], intramedullary devices and other internal fixation (with and without bone graft) [5] for knee fusion. A majority of patients included in these studies included patients who underwent knee fusion following failed or infected knee arthroplasty. The outcomes have varied from 86 to 96 % [6–8] fusion

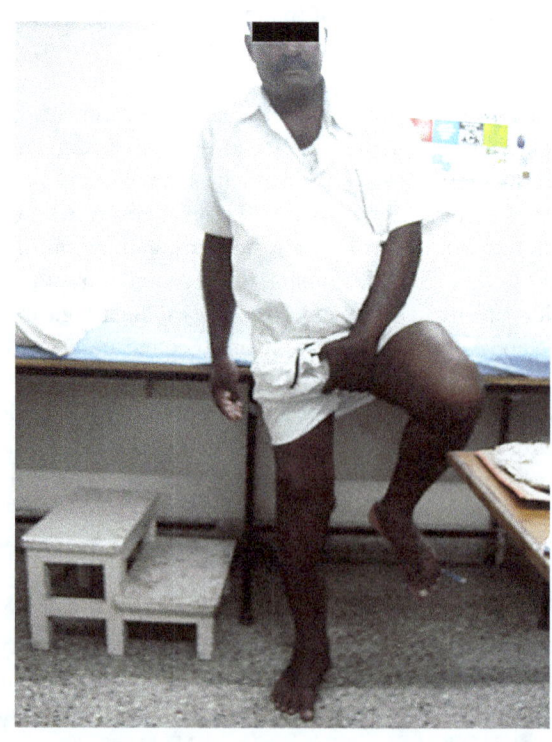

Fig. 5 Functional outcome at four years post-knee arthrodesis with an anterior monorail fixator

success. Corona et al. and Eralp et al. [9, 10] have also used monolateral external fixation in patients with failed total knee arthroplasty and had union success in 81–100 %. In this series, all patients achieved sound union at final follow-up and most of them returned to their previous occupation. The monorail fixator had the added advantage of patient comfort when compared with bulkier ring external fixators and obviated the need for plaster application as required with the Charnley's compression device.

Comparison of these data with other study groups was not possible due to patients in this study having had a failed arthroplasty and the average age lower. The outcome parameters in other studies were restricted to assessing limb alignment, length discrepancy and time to fusion. We have further quantified outcome with pre- and post-fusion scores.

Despite the disadvantages of an external fixator, the anterior rail had certain distinct advantages: it performs like a tension band when the limb is loaded; and the ease of application and improved patient comfort in the fixation period. All patients went on to stable fusion which was reflected on their improved scores and clinical outcomes.

Conclusion

A single anterior rail is a reliable method of obtaining knee fusion for post-infective and post-traumatic sequelae. The technique described offers a single-stage salvage procedure and enables an earlier return to work and occupation. It is a viable alternative over staged reconstructive procedures or complex arthroplasty for certain individuals.

Acknowledgments The authors would like to thank Professor Vinoo Mathew Cherian for his help and support with this study.

Informed consent Informed consent was obtained from all individual participants included in the study.

References

1. Charnley J, Lowe HG (1958) A study of the end-results of compression arthrodesis of the knee. J Bone Joint Surg Br 40:633–635
2. Conway J (2003) Arthrodesis of the knee using biplanar external fixation. Read at the Annual Meeting of the Limb Lengthening and Reconstruction Society
3. Brooker AF, Hansen NM (1981) The biplane frame: modified compression arthrodesis of the knee. Clin Orthop 160:163–167
4. Lim HC, Bae JH, Hur CR, Oh JK, Han SH (2009) Arthrodesis of the knee using cannulated screws. J Bone Joint Surg Br 91(2):180–184
5. Stiehl JB, Hanel DP (1993) Knee arthrodesis using combined intramedullary rod and plate fixation. Clin Orthop 294:238–241
6. Lonner JH, Hershman S, Mont M, Lotke PA (2000) Total knee arthroplasty in patients 40 years of age and younger with osteoarthritis. Clin Orthop 380:85–90
7. Gill GS, Chan KC, Mills DM (1997) 5- to 18-year follow-up study of cemented total knee arthroplasty for patients 55 years old or younger. J Arthroplasty 12(1):49–54
8. Mont MA, Lee CW, Sheldon M, Lennon WC, Hungerford DS (2002) Total knee arthroplasty in patients </=50 years old. J Arthroplasty 17(5):538–543
9. Corona PS, Hernandez A, Reverte-Vinaixa MM, Amat C, Flores X (2013) Outcome after knee arthrodesis for failed septic total knee replacement using a monolateral external fixator. J Orthop Surg 21(3):275–280
10. Eralp L, Kocaoğlu M, Tuncay I, Bilen FE, Samir SE (2008) Knee arthrodesis using a unilateral external fixator for the treatment of infectious sequelae. Acta Orthop Traumatol Turc 42(2):84–89

26

Internal fixation of shaft humerus fractures by dynamic compression plate or interlocking intramedullary nail: a prospective, randomised study

Mir G. R. Wali · Asif N. Baba · Irfan A. Latoo · Nawaz A. Bhat · Omar Khurshid Baba · Sudesh Sharma

Abstract Compare the results of internal fixation of shaft of humerus fractures using dynamic compression plating (DCP) or antegrade interlocking intramedullary nail (IMN). Fifty patients with diaphyseal fracture of the shaft of the humerus and fulfilling the inclusion criterion were randomly assigned to one of the two groups. Twenty-five patients were managed with closed antegrade interlocking intramedullary nail, and 25 underwent open reduction and internal fixation using dynamic compression plating. The mean age of patients with IMN fixation was 37.28 years (SD 12.26) and 37.72 years (SD 12.70) for those who underwent plating. Road traffic accident was the most common mode of injury in both groups. There was a statistically significant difference between the two groups with respect to duration of hospital stay, operative time and blood loss. There was no significant difference between the two groups in terms of union or complications. The functional assessment at the end of 1 year between the two groups did not show any significant difference in outcome. Antegrade interlocking IMN and DCP fixation are comparable when managing diaphyseal shaft of humerus fractures with respect to union rates and complications. Although shoulder related complications are more in the IMN group, however, it is associated with shorter hospital stay, lesser operative time and less blood loss. This makes interlocking IMN an effective option in managing these fractures.

Keywords Shaft humerus · Fracture · Intramedullary nailing · Plating

Introduction

Fractures of the shaft of humerus are relatively common, representing 1–3 % of all fractures [1, 2]. Humerus shaft fractures are unique among all long bone fractures in having very good results with non-operative methods like hanging cast, functional brace, Velpeau dressing, coaptation splint and abduction cast [3–5]. Good functional outcomes in these fractures are partly due to the tolerance of malunion in humerus. However, all fractures are not amenable to conservative methods. The indications for operative treatment of the humeral shaft fractures include open fractures, segmental fractures, pathological fractures, fractures associated with vascular injuries, bilateral humerus fractures, polytrauma, radial nerve palsy after fracture manipulation, neurological loss after penetrating injuries, fractures with unacceptable alignment and failure of conservative treatment [2]. Non-operative treatment requires a long period of immobilization, which carries a risk of prolonged shoulder joint stiffness and inconvenience for the patient [6, 7]. Furthermore, non-union after conservative treatment of these fractures does occur in up to 10 % of the cases, and treatment of this condition can be very difficult [8–10].

There is a growing interest in treating even simple humeral shaft fractures by surgical modalities in order to avoid these problems and to allow earlier mobilization and rapid return to work [11, 12]. The usual operative methods

M. G. R. Wali · A. N. Baba (✉) · I. A. Latoo · N. A. Bhat · O. K. Baba
Department of Orthopedics, Government Medical College, Srinagar, Srinagar, India
e-mail: drasifbaba@yahoo.co.in

S. Sharma
Department of Orthopedics, Government Medical College, Jammu, Jammu, India

involve the use of dynamic compression plate (DCP) or interlocking nail (ILN). Plate and screw fixation has traditionally been the preferred method and remains the gold standard for surgical management [13]. Use of the plate, however, requires extensive dissection and is complicated by the proximity of the radial nerve and the risk of mechanical failure in osteopenic bone. As a result of recent technical advances and success associated with nailing in other long bone fractures, there is a growing interest in the use of the humeral intramedullary nail for treating this fracture. ILN is a less invasive procedure with improved biomechanics and load-sharing feature of the implant. Fractures managed with ILN have better chances of union, as the surgery does not involve periosteal stripping and reaming produces act as an autograft. This benefit, however, comes at the cost of shoulder problems. We hypothesized that fractures managed by interlocking nailing would have faster union rates, less surgical time, shorter hospital stay, but more shoulder problems.

We compare the results of fixation of the humerus shaft fractures using either DCP or antegrade ILN with respect to hospital stay, blood loss, union time, functional results and complications associated with the procedure.

Materials and methods

A prospective, randomized, comparative study of the management of acute humeral shaft fractures by antegrade interlocking nail fixation and dynamic compression plating was conducted in the Department of Orthopaedics, Government Medical College, Jammu. An informed consent was obtained from all the patients and approval of the hospital ethical committee was sought. Fifty consecutive shaft humerus fracture patients, presenting to the hospital and fulfilling the inclusion criterion were randomly assigned to either ILN group (Group A) or DCP group (Group B). All skeletally mature patients with displaced fractures of humeral shaft, <3-week-old trauma, and requiring surgery were included. Skeletally immature patients, pathological fractures, compound fractures, associated neurovascular injuries, segmental fractures, radial nerve injury following closed reduction, non-cooperative patients and patients with other pathologies of the upper extremities were excluded. However, patients with pre-operative radial nerve injury were included in the study (except those where radial nerve palsy developed following manipulation). None of the patients necessitated intra-operative change in the procedure.

After complete pre-operative assessment and anaesthetic clearance, patients were randomized to receive either dynamic compression plating or interlocking nail, for definitive fracture fixation. AO classification system was used to classify the fractures. All surgeries were performed by surgeons (SS and MGR), familiar with both the procedures. In the plating group (group B), fixation was done with 4.5-mm dynamic compression plates using appropriate surgical techniques, depending on the fracture configuration. Transverse or short oblique fractures were stabilized by axial compression, while in the spiral or oblique fractures interfragmentary lag screw fixation was done, followed by application of plate in the neutralization mode. Anterolateral or posterior approach was used, depending upon the fracture configuration and the surgeon preference. Fixation of at least six cortices, preferably eight cortices, both proximal and distal to the fracture was obtained in every patient.

In group A (ILN), commercially available reamed antegrade interlocking nails (Nebula Surgicals, Gujarat, India) were used. The nails had a 5° bend in the proximal part. The nail was used because of the easy availability and economy. The nail had two screws proximally and two distally. One proximal screw was oriented transversely and the other obliquely, while one distal screw was directed anteroposteriorly and the other transversely. A 4–5 cm incision, lateral to the acromion, was made to facilitate the splitting of the deltoid muscle. The posterior margin of the greater tuberosity was exposed by retracting the supraspinatus tendon. The entry hole was made with an awl. The canal was gradually enlarged by reaming after insertion of a guide pin. During reaming, cortical contact at fracture site was ensured to prevent radial nerve injury. After passing the nail in the canal, fracture site was inspected under image intensifier to avoid distraction at the fracture site. The distal screws were fixed by the freehand technique. To prevent damage to the neurovascular structures, the entry holes were visualized by image intensifier followed by stab incision and blunt dissection to the bone. The proximal screws were fixed by the target device.

The blood loss was calculated from a modification of the Gross formula given below [14]:

Blood loss = Blood volume$[Hct(i) - Hct(f)]/Hct(m)$

where blood volume = body weight (kgs) $\times$ 70 ml/kg; $Hct(i)$, $Hct(f)$ and $Hct(m)$ were the initial, final and mean (for final and initial) haematocrits, respectively.

Post-operative radiographs were checked to know the adequacy of reduction and any iatrogenic complication. Post-operatively the limb was placed in an arm sling and pendulum and elbow movements were allowed on the second post-operative day. Patients were discharged once they became comfortable, wound was healthy and the patient was afebrile. Patients were followed up at 2, 6, 12, 24, 36 weeks and final follow-up at 52 weeks. On each follow-up, the patients were examined clinically to check for signs of infection, pain, range of motion of elbow and shoulder, neurovascular status and any other complication. Radiological assessment using plain radiographs was done to know the status of union of the fracture, alignment, hardware problems and any malunion. The functional results at the end of 1 year were assessed using the American Shoulder and Elbow Surgeons (ASES) score for 13 activities of daily living requiring the shoulder and elbow movement with each activity carrying a maximum of 4 points. Radiological union was defined as the presence of bridging callus in two planes (AP and lateral). Union was defined as fracture healing within 4 months, delayed union as no signs of union 4–6 months of injury and non-union as no signs of union after 6 months. Rodríguez–Merchán criteria were used to assess the final results [15]. This criterion includes the assessment of shoulder and elbow range of movement, pain and disability. When the criteria fall in different categories, the lower category is used to classify the outcome (Table 1). The results were analysed statistically using the SPSS 16.0 software with the Student's t test. The value of alpha was set to 0.05. The sample size was calculated after a literature review of previous similar studies.

Results

In our study, 25 patients of fracture shaft of humerus were treated with antegrade ILN and 25 more cases underwent DCP fixation. The ILN group comprised 21 male and 4 female patients with mean age of 37.28 years (SD 12.26), while the DCP group had 20 males and 5 females having mean age of 37.72 years (SD 12.70) (p value > 0.05). In the ILN group, 16 patients (64 %) had AO type A fracture, 6 (24 %) had AO type B and 3 (12 %) patients had AO type C fracture. The pattern was similar in DCP group with 17 patients (68 %) having type A, 6 (24 %) patients type B and 2 (8 %) patients had type C fracture. In our study, both the groups were comparable with respect to the level of fracture. Majority of the fractures in both the groups were in the middle third of the shaft of humerus. However, the next commonly involved level in DCP group was distal third (24 %) of shaft, compared with ILN group, where next commonly involved level was proximal third (24 %) of shaft.

Road traffic accident (RTA) was the most common mode of injury in majority of patients in both the groups, followed by fall from height and direct trauma to arm. In the DCP group, 18 patients (72 %) had RTA, 5 (20 %) had fall from height and two patients sustained direct trauma to arm. In the nailing group, 19 patients had RTA, 4 had fall from height and two sustained direct trauma to arm. The most common associated injuries were other long bone

Table 1 Criteria for evaluating functional results (Rodríguez–Merchán)

Rating	Elbow range of movement	Shoulder range of movement	Pain	Disability
Excellent	Extension 5° flexion 130°	Full range of movement	None	None
Good	Extension 15° flexion 120°	<10 % loss of total range of movement	Occasional	Minimum
Fair	Extension 30° flexion 110°	10–30 % loss of total range of movement	With activity	Moderate
Poor	Extension 40° flexion 90°	>30 % loss of total range of movement	Variable	Severe

Table 2 Associated injuries

	Other long bone fractures	Head injury	Chest trauma	Pelvis injury	Abdominal injury
DCP group	2	2	1	1	0
ILN group	4	1	2	1	1

fractures, followed by head injury, pelvic trauma and chest injury (Table 2). The mean interval between admissions to surgery was 6.12 days (SD 3.67) in the ILN group and 11.88 days (SD 3.29) in the DCP group, the difference between the two being statistically significant (p value < 0.05). In the DCP group, 17 patients were operated using the anterolateral approach and remaining 8 patients with the posterior approach. The average operating time in the ILN group was 50.8 min (SD 6.87) and 66.2 min (SD 8.07) in the DCP group, the difference again being statistically significant (p value < 0.05). The average blood loss in the ILN group was 140 ml (range 90–550), while the average loss in DCP group was 310 ml (range 160–880), the difference being statistically significant. The duration of hospital stay was 8.76 days in ILN group and 14.56 days in the DCP group, the finding again being statistically significant. The mean fluoroscopy time in the interlocking group was 4.6 min, while fluoroscopy was not used in the plating group.

Most of the fractures united within 16 weeks in both the groups (Figs. 1, 2, 3, 4, 5). Union was defined as the presence of bridging callus in two planes and the absence of pain and movement at fracture site. Three patients in nailing group and two in plating group had delayed union and united between 4 and 6 months. Two patients in ILN group (8 %) and two patients (8 %) in the DCP group did not show signs of union till 6 months (Table 3). One patient in nailing group had iatrogenic

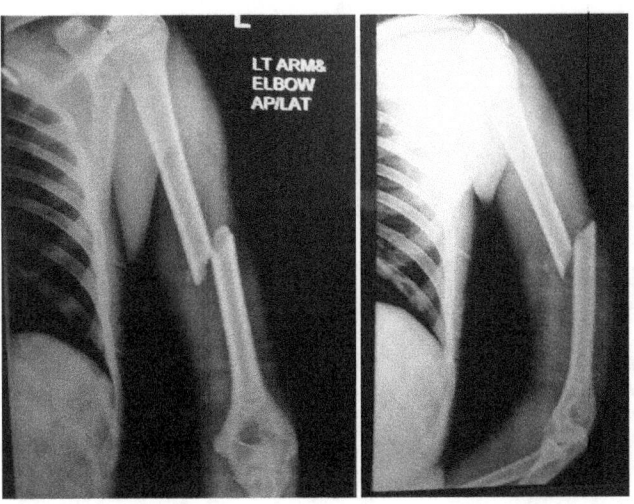

Fig. 1 AP and lateral radiographs of a fracture shaft of humerus in the middle third

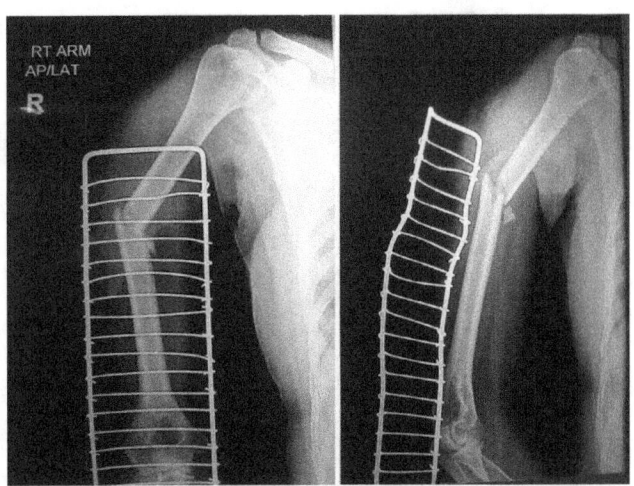

Fig. 3 AP and lateral radiographs of fracture middle third of the shaft of humerus

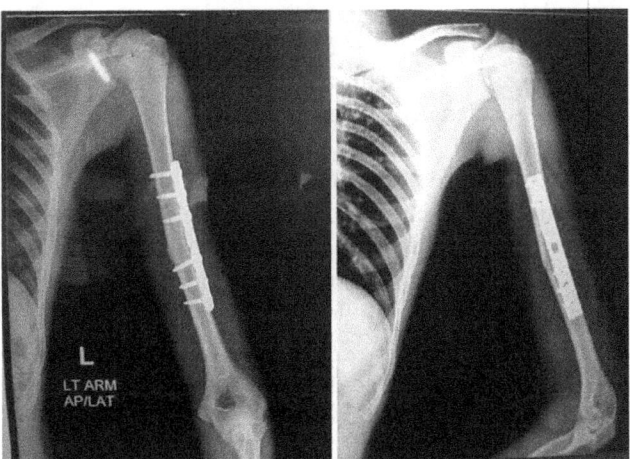

Fig. 2 AP and lateral radiographs of the fracture in Fig. 1 shows solid union with DCP after 9 months

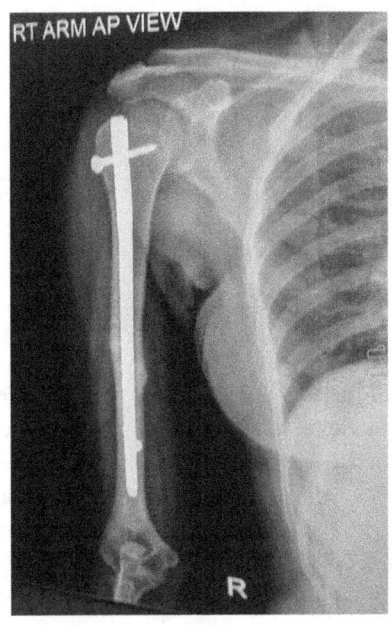

Fig. 4 AP view of fracture shows good union with IMN

comminution at the fracture site with distraction at the fracture site. Both patients in the nailing group underwent nail removal and plating with bone grafting, and the two patients in DCP group underwent bone grafting as a secondary procedure. All the fractures went on to eventual union. The mean duration of union in remaining patients in ILN group was 13.60 (SD 4.32) weeks and in DCP group was 15.2 (SD 5.65) weeks. Although average union time in ILN group was 1.6 weeks earlier than DCP group, the finding was not statistically significant (p value 0.376).

Pre-operative radial nerve palsy was seen in two patients in ILN group and one patient in DCP group. The radial nerve was explored only in the DCP group and found intact. All the three patients completely recovered. Two patients in plating group developed post-operative

radial nerve injury. One of the patients agreed for exploration, and the radial nerve was found stuck beneath the plate. One patient in the ILN group developed iatrogenic comminution at the site of nail entry, but this did not affect the final outcome. No patient in the plating had hardware failure in the form of plate bending or screw backout.

In the ILN group, shoulder stiffness was the most common complication occurring in 4 patients (16 %). Of these, stiffness resolved with physiotherapy in three patients and one patient continued to have stiffness. One patient in ILN group had severe shoulder impingement due to the protruding nail which required removal of the nail

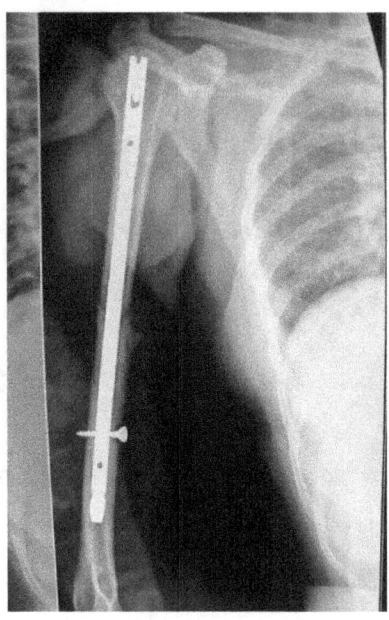

Fig. 5 Lateral view of fracture shaft of humerus shoes uniting fracture with the orientation of distal screw

Table 3 Time to union (weeks)

	Up to 8	8–12	13–16	17–24	>24
IMN ($n = 25$)	5	9	6	3	2
Plating ($n = 25$)	2	10	9	2	2

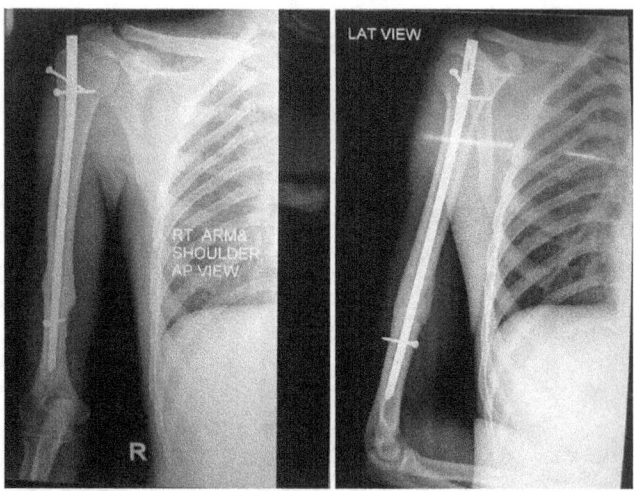

Fig. 6 AP and lateral view of a united fracture shows proximal protrusion of the nail

after achieving union (Fig. 6). This was one of the earliest cases in the series, and despite using C-arm, we were not able to appreciate the protrusion. One patient each, in both the groups, had elbow stiffness, while one patient in the plating group developed shoulder stiffness. One patient in nailing group developed superficial infection at the nail entry site which resolved with antibiotics. Two patients (8 %) in the plating group developed superficial infection which was resolved with antibiotics, and one patient developed deep infection which required serial debridement and antibiotics. Three patients in the nailing group and four in the plating group required repetition of operation (Table 4).

The functional assessment after 1 year of surgery using the ASES score did not reveal any significant difference between the two groups. ASES score in the ILN group was 43.2 and in the DCP group was 44.1. The final evaluation of ILN patients done with the Rodríguez–Merchán criteria revealed excellent results in 7 (28 %), good in 13 (52 %), fair in 3 (12 %) and poor in 2 patients. Results were similar in the DCP with excellent result in 8 (32 %), good in 13 (52 %), fair in 2 and poor in 2 patients.

Discussion

Humerus fracture is unique amongst the long bone fractures in its tolerance of less than anatomical reduction. Shortening up to 3 cm, rotation <30° and angulation up to 20° are considered acceptable [16]. Due to this fact, most of the humerus fractures are still managed conservatively and have good functional results. The most common indication of operative intervention is inability to achieve acceptable reduction, followed by associated vascular lesions, open fractures, radial nerve palsy, polytrauma patients, floating elbow and pathological fractures [17]. The preponderance of the fracture in young males, commonly in third and fourth decade of life, was seen in our series, as has been reported by other similar studies [18]. Road traffic accident is the most common mode of injury, especially in younger patients.

In the past, open reduction and plating was the preferred method of operative intervention, and still continues to remain the gold standard. However, conventional plating technique involves an extensive surgical approach for open reduction of fracture and is theoretically associated with increased risk of radial nerve injury and more blood loss. The excellent result of intramedullary interlocking nails in tibia and femur fractures has stimulated interest in applying the same methods in humerus fractures. Intramedullary nails are subjected to smaller bending loads than plates because they are closer to the mechanical axis than the usual plate position on the external surface of the bone. Intramedullary nails can also act as load-sharing devices in fractures with cortical contact. Moreover, the stress shielding commonly seen with plates and screws is minimized with intramedullary nails. Intramedullary nailing in humerus fractures is a less invasive procedure which

Table 4 Post-operative complications

	Superficial infection	Deep infection	Radial nerve palsy	Comminution at fracture site	Shoulder stiffness	Elbow stiffness	Delayed union	Non-union
IMN	1	0	0	0	4	1	3	2
DCP	2	1	2	1	1	1	2	2

maintains the biology and gives a good, stable fixation. It is also assumed to result in quicker union, less blood loss and less chances of radial nerve injury. However, controversy still exists over the best method of fixation. Ooyung et al. [19] in a meta-analysis of ten studies comparing the results of plating versus nailing concluded that both achieve similar results in humerus fractures, but plating was associated with reduced shoulder problems.

Union rates in our study were comparable between the two groups, non-union being seen in 8 % in ILN and 8 % in DCP group. Similar rates of non-union have been observed in most of the studies [20, 21]. Non-union in the DCP group is usually due to extensive soft tissue dissection or malreduction and is often associated with implant failure. Even though the effect of reaming might facilitate bone healing, non-union has been reported in 0–9 % of cases [22, 23] managed with reamed intramedullary nails. Non-union in ILN usually results from distraction at the fracture site as humerus seems to be less forgiving than tibia or femur in this aspect. Non-union in both groups was managed by open reduction and plating with bone graft, as has been suggested in the literature [24]. The time to achieve union in our study was less in ILN than in plating group, although not statistically significant. Denies et al. [25] also reported earlier union in nailing, probably due to the less invasive nature of the procedure and the maintenance of the fracture haematoma. Changulani et al. [26] also reported earlier union in nailing with a statistically significant difference.

Whether to use reamed or unreamed nails is still a controversial topic. The advantages of reaming include the significant increase in the blood flow to the muscles and surrounding soft tissues, and this increase persists for up to 6 weeks. The increase in soft tissue blood flow may increase the cortical blood flow and thus more chances of union. Further, the cost of reamed nails is less, which is an advantage for developing nations, like ours. The disadvantage of reaming is the chances of radial nerve injury, especially when there is a gap at the fracture site. Further, some studies have shown extensive heat necrosis from nailing in small diameter canals. Reaming in small diameter canals may lead to distraction at the fracture site.

Infection, iatrogenic radial nerve palsy and hardware failure are most important complications associated with plating. We had higher rates of infection and iatrogenic

radial nerve palsy in the plating group, as has been seen by Changulani et al. [26]. However, in a meta-analysis, Bhandari et al. [27] did not show higher risks of infection or radial nerve palsy with plating. Radial nerve is at a definite risk in plating, with special precautions being taken to prevent nerve from coming beneath the plate. Although radial nerve injury after nailing is rare, the risk can be further minimized by ensuring accurate reduction of the fracture (no gap) before passage of the reamers or the nail and by avoiding reaming in areas of comminution where the nerve is closely apposed to the bone.

Impairment of shoulder function is the main drawback of interlocking nailing. Shoulder pain in these patients may be related to violation of the rotator cuff, prominent nail end, adhesive capsulitis or unknown causes [27, 28]. We had shoulder problems in 20 % of our patients. One patient with protruding nail required a second surgery for the removal of implant. Chao et al. [28] also reported three patients with proximal protrusion of the nail. This usually arises from not pushing the nail distal enough, possibly from fear of producing a distal fracture, or from migration of an unlocked nail. We suggest assessing the length accurately before passing the nail and using C-arm till the procedure ends. Similar findings have been reported by many studies [28, 30, 31]. However, Flinkilla in an analysis of shoulder from different studies reported similar shoulder scores in both nailing and plating groups, with plating having better abduction and flexion [32]. We had intraoperative comminution at fracture site in one patient where the medullary canal was narrow which resulted in distraction at fracture site and eventually resulting in non-union. Introduction of large reamers or nail into a narrow canal can result in comminution at fracture site which are usually undisplaced fissures not requiring fixation. The incidence of this complication has decreased from 6 to 1.8 % due to introduction of newer nail designs [33]. Re-operation rates were similar between the two groups as has been seen by Denies et al. [25]. However, Bhandari et al. [27] reported more re-operations in the nailing group. Indications of re-operation in plating are union problems, hardware failure and revision for radial nerve palsy while the nailing patients it is for union problems, removal of protruding implant and management of preoperative fracture. A disadvantage of nailing is the need of fluoroscopy for the procedure and the associated risks to the surgeon and the theatre personnel. The fluoroscopy time reported by us is comparable to that reported in the literature and seen for other long bone fractures. To overcome this, expandable nails have come into the market which require less extensive use of fluoroscopy.

In our study, nailing was superior to plating with respect to the average post-operative stay of the patients and operating time. The main reason for the longer stay in the plating group in our study was because of the longer delay in surgery in the plating patients. This was due to our tendency to do DCP only when the swelling had completely subsided. In contrast, ILN does not need rigorous subsidence of the swelling. Most of our patients belonged to far-off places where sterile-dressing facilities were not readily available and thus tended to stay till the operative wound was deemed clean. ILN patients had an edge due to their smaller surgical wounds and so were discharged earlier. The shorter stay, with a less invasive method, such as closed nailing, is of great advantage in developing countries where the orthopaedic hospital beds are limited and resources are scarce. For the same reason, the less operating time reported by us is also advantageous. Chao et al. also had shorter operative time in ILN, although the difference was not significant, while Chaudhary et al. had shorter operative time in the plating group [29, 34]. ILN was also associated with significantly decreased blood loss than plating, as has been seen in most of the studies [29]. Although this difference is statistically significant, but in the clinical settings, this difference is marginal.

The ASES score and the final outcome in our series did not show any significant advantage of one method over the other. Some studies have shown plating to be more effective, while others have found better results with nailing [35, 36]. However, the meta-analysis of different randomized and quasi-randomised controlled trials comparing the two failed to find any significant difference between the two with respect to ASES scores [37].

The most important factors in obtaining fracture healing are anatomical reduction, stable fixation and adequate blood supply. Although internal fixation with DCP may result in a better reduction, it also carries a more extensive soft tissue dissection with risk of radial nerve lesion and infection. ILN provides secure and rigid fixation with less soft tissue damage and maintaining the biology. Although ILN is associated with relatively increased incidence of shoulder complications, it has definite advantages in terms of shorter hospital stay, less blood loss and shorter operative time, which are of immense importance in the developing countries with limited resources.

We conclude that antegrade locked intramedullary nailing is an effective alternative to plating in shaft humerus fractures as it has comparable results in terms of union rate and complications. In addition, it has the added advantage of lesser operative time and shorter hospital stay, both of which have a distinct advantage in those centres in developing countries which have the facility of fluoroscopy.

References

1. Brinker MR, O'Connor DP (2004) The incidence of fractures and dislocations referred for orthopaedic services in a capitated population. J Bone Joint Surg Am 86:290–297
2. Schemitsch EH, Bhandari M (2001) Fractures of the diaphyseal humerus. In: Browner BD, Jupiter JB, Levine AM, Trafton PG (eds) Skeletal trauma, 3rd edn. WB Saunders, Toronto, pp 1481–1511
3. Bohler L (1965) Conservative treatment of fresh closed fractures of humerus. J Trauma 5:464–468
4. Sarmiento A, Zagorski JB, Zych DO, Latta LL, Capps CA (2000) Functional bracing for the treatment of fractures of humeral diaphysis. J Bone Joint Surg Am 82:478–486
5. Koch PP, Gross DF, Gerber C (2002) The results of functional (Sarmiento) bracing of humeral shaft fractures. J Shoulder Elbow Surg 11:143–150
6. Rommens PM, Verbruggen J, Broos PL (1995) Retrograde locked nailing of humeral shaft fractures. A review of 39 patients. J Bone Joint Surg Br 77:84–89
7. Ulrich C (1996) Surgical treatment of humeral diaphyseal fractures. In: Flatow E, Ulrich C (eds) Humerus. Butterworth-Heinemann, Oxford, pp 128–143
8. Foulk DA, Szabo RM (1995) Diaphyseal humeral fractures; natural history and occurrence of nonunion. Orthopaedics 18:333–335
9. White WL, Mick GM, Mick CA, Brooker AF Jr, Weiland AJ (1987) Non union of humeral shaft. Clin Orthop 219:206–213
10. Jupiter JB, Vandec M (1998) Ununited humeral diaphysis. J Shoulder Elbow Surg 7:644–653
11. Heim D, Herkert F, Hess P, Regazzoni P (1993) Surgical treatment of humeral shaft fractures-the Basal experience. J Trauma 35:226–232
12. Robinson CM, Bell KM, Court-Brown CM, McQueen MM (1992) Locked nailing of humeral shaft fractures; experience in Edinburg over a two-year period. J Bone Joint Surg 74B:558–663
13. Paris H, Tropiano P, Clouet D'orval B, Chaudet H, Poitout DG (2000) Fractures of the shaft of the humerus: systematic plate fixation. Anatomic and functional results in 156 cases and a review of the literature. Rev Chir Orthop Reparatrice Appar Mot 86:346–359
14. Gross JB (1983) Estimating allowable blood loss: corrected for dilution. Anesthesiology 58(3):277–280
15. Rodríguez-Merchán EC (1995) Compression plating versus hackethal nailing in closed humeral shaft fractures failing non-operative reduction. J Orthop Trauma 9:194–197
16. Papasoulis E, Drosos GI, Ververidis AN et al (2010) Functional bracing of humeral shaft fractures. A review of clinical studies. Injury 41:e21–e27
17. Hoang-Kim A, Goldhahn J, Hak DJ (2012) Humeral shaft fractures. In: Bhandhari M, Gandhi R, Petrisor BA, Swiontkowski M (eds) Evidence-based orthopedics, 1st edn. Willey, Hoboken
18. Tsai CH, Fong YC, Chen YH, Hsu CJ, Chang CH, Hsu HC (2009) The epidemiology of traumatic humeral shaft fractures in Taiwan. Int Orthop 33:463–467
19. Ouyang H, Xiong J, Xiang P, Cui Z, Chen L, Yu B (2013) Plate versus intramedullary nail fixation in the treatment of humeral shaft fractures: an updated meta-analysis. J Shoulder Elbow Surg 22:387–395
20. Bell MJ, Beauchamp CG, Kellam JK, McMurtry RY (1985) The results of plating humeral shaft fractures in patients with multiple

Internal fixation of shaft humerus fractures by dynamic compression plate or interlocking intramedullary...

187

injuries. The Sunnybrook experience. J Bone Joint Surg Br 67:293–296

21. Ingman AM, Waters DA (1994) Locked intramedullary nailing of humeral shaft fractures. Implant design, surgical technique and clinical results. J Bone Joint Surg 76-Br:23–29

22. Fernandez FF, Matschke S, Hulsenbeck A, Egenolf M, Wentzensen A (2004) Five years' clinical experience with the undreamed humeral nail in the treatment of humeral shaft fractures. Injury 35:264–271

23. Sanzana ES, Dümmer RE, Castro JP, Díaz EA (2002) Intramedullary nailing of humeral shaft fractures. Int Orthop 26:211–213

24. McKee MD, Miranda MA, Riemer BL et al (1996) Management of humeral nonunion after the failure of locking intramedullary nails. J Orthop Trauma 10:492–499

25. Denies E, Nus S, Sermon A, Broos P (2010) Operative treatment of humeral shaft fractures. Comparison of plating and intramedullary nailing. Acta Orthop Belg 76:735–742

26. Changulani M, Jain UK, Keswani T (2007) Comparison of the use of the humerus intramedullary nail and dynamic compression plate for the management of diaphyseal fractures of the humerus. A Randomized controlled study. Intl Orthop 31:391–395

27. Bhandari M, Devereaux PJ, McKee MD, Schemitsch EH (2006) Compression plating versus intramedullary nailing of humeral shaft fractures: a meta-analysis. Acta Orthop 77:279–284

28. Brumback RJ, Bosse MJ, Poka A, Burgess AR (1986) Intramedullary stabilization of humeral shaft fractures in patients with multiple trauma. J Bone Joint Surg 68:960–970

29. Chao T-C, Chou W-Y, Chung J-C, Hsu C-J (2005) Humeral shaft fractures treated by dynamic compression plates, Ender nails and interlocking nails. Int Orthop 29:88–91

30. Chapman JR, Henley MB, Agel J, Benca PJ (2000) Randomized prospective study of humeral shaft fracture fixation: intramedullary nails versus plates. J Orthop Trauma 14:162–166

31. Raghavendra S, Bhalodiya HP (2007) Internal fixation of fractures of the shaft of the humerus by dynamic compression plate or intramedullary nail: a prospective study. Indian J Orthop 41:214–218

32. Flinkkilä T, Hyvönen P, Siira P, Hämäläinen M (2004) Recovery of shoulder joint function after humeral shaft fracture: a comparative study between antegrade intramedullary nailing and plate fixation. Arch Orthop Trauma Sur 124:537–541

33. Stannard JP, Harris HW, McGwin G Jr et al (2003) Intramedullary nailing of humeral shaft fractures with a locking flexible nail. J Bone Joint Surg 85-Am:2103–2110

34. Chaudhary P, Karn NK, Shrestha BP, Khanal GP et al (2011) Randomized controlled trial comparing dynamic compression plate versus intramedullary interlocking nail for management of humeral shaft fractures. Health Renaissance 9:61–66

35. McCormack RG, Brien D, Buckley RE, McKee MD, Powell J, Schemitsch EH (2000) Fixation of fractures of the shaft of the humerus by dynamic compression plate or intramedullary nail: a prospective, randomised trial. J Bone Joint Surg 82-B:336–339

36. Lin J (1998) Treatment of humeral shaft fractures with humeral locked nail and comparison with plate fixation. J Trauma 44:859–864

37. Kurup H, Hossain M, Andrew JG (2011) Dynamic compression plating versus locked intramedullary nailing for humeral shaft fractures in adults. Cochrane Database Syst Rev 15(6): CD005959. doi:10.1002/14651858

27

Midterm results of Ilizarov hip reconstruction for late sequelae of childhood septic arthritis

Mahmoud A. El-Rosasy · Mostafa A. Ayoub

Abstract The management of hip instability as a consequence of septic arthritis in childhood is difficult. Ilizarov hip reconstruction is a double-level femoral osteotomy with the objective of eliminating hip instability, through a proximal valgus–extension–derotation osteotomy and a distal varization–lengthening osteotomy for mechanical axis correction and equalization limb length. Ilizarov hip reconstruction was performed for 16 adult patients with complaints of hip pain, leg-length discrepancy, limping, reduced activity and limited abduction of the hip as a result of childhood septic arthritis. Their ages ranged from 19 to 32 years (mean 23.2 ± 4.2). Ilizarov external fixator was used in all cases. At the time of last follow-up that ranged from 60 to 132 months (mean 85.6 ± 23.5), the Harris hip score (HHS) showed excellent functional outcome in two cases (12.50 %), good in 13 cases (81.25 %) and fair in one case (6.25 %). There was no poor functional outcome in any case. Preoperatively, the mean HHS was 56.18 points, and at the time of last follow-up, it improved to a mean of 84.62 points. Pain subsided in all patients, the Trendelenburg sign became negative in all but three (19 %) patients, no patient had limb-length discrepancy, and the alignment of the extremity was reestablished in all cases. No additional operations were required. Ilizarov hip reconstruction is a valuable and durable solution for the late sequelae of childhood septic arthritis of the hip presenting in adult patients.

Keywords Hip joint · Septic arthritis · Ilizarov · Pelvic support osteotomy

M. A. El-Rosasy (✉) · M. A. Ayoub
Department of Orthopaedic Surgery, Faculty of Medicine,
Tanta University Hospital, University of Tanta, Al-Geish Street,
Tanta, Egypt
e-mail: elrosasym@yahoo.com

Introduction

The late sequela of septic arthritis of the hip in childhood is a complex problem. The symptoms are a limp, with or without pain, limb-length discrepancy, deformity and hip stiffness. The management of this problem in young adults is controversial. Arthrodesis of the hip joint offers a stable, painless but immobile hip joint, which makes sitting on a chair and in public transportation difficult and can render difficulties with perineal hygiene. Moreover, conversion of a fused hip into total hip arthroplasty is challenging and has some higher risks, and this is not the ideal choice for young patients due to the increased activity and the need for frequent revisions [1–5].

The pelvic support osteotomy (PSO) was described to solve the problem of hip instability by transferring body weight to the femoral shaft through a proximal valgus osteotomy [6]. Although this osteotomy can provide sufficient pelvic support, it results in lateralization of the limb and did not address limb-length discrepancy [7]. Ilizarov added a second, more distal varus femoral osteotomy for lengthening to restore the overall alignment of the lower limb [8].

This study presents our midterm (minimum 5-year follow-up) results of the Ilizarov hip reconstruction (IHR) procedure using the Ilizarov external fixator in adult patients who have a unilateral hip disorder after septic arthritis of the hip.

Materials and methods

Sixteen adult patients constitute the cohort of this retrospective study. The ages range from 19 to 32 years (mean 23.2 ± 4.2 years). There are nine males and seven female patients. The inclusion criteria were a unilateral hip

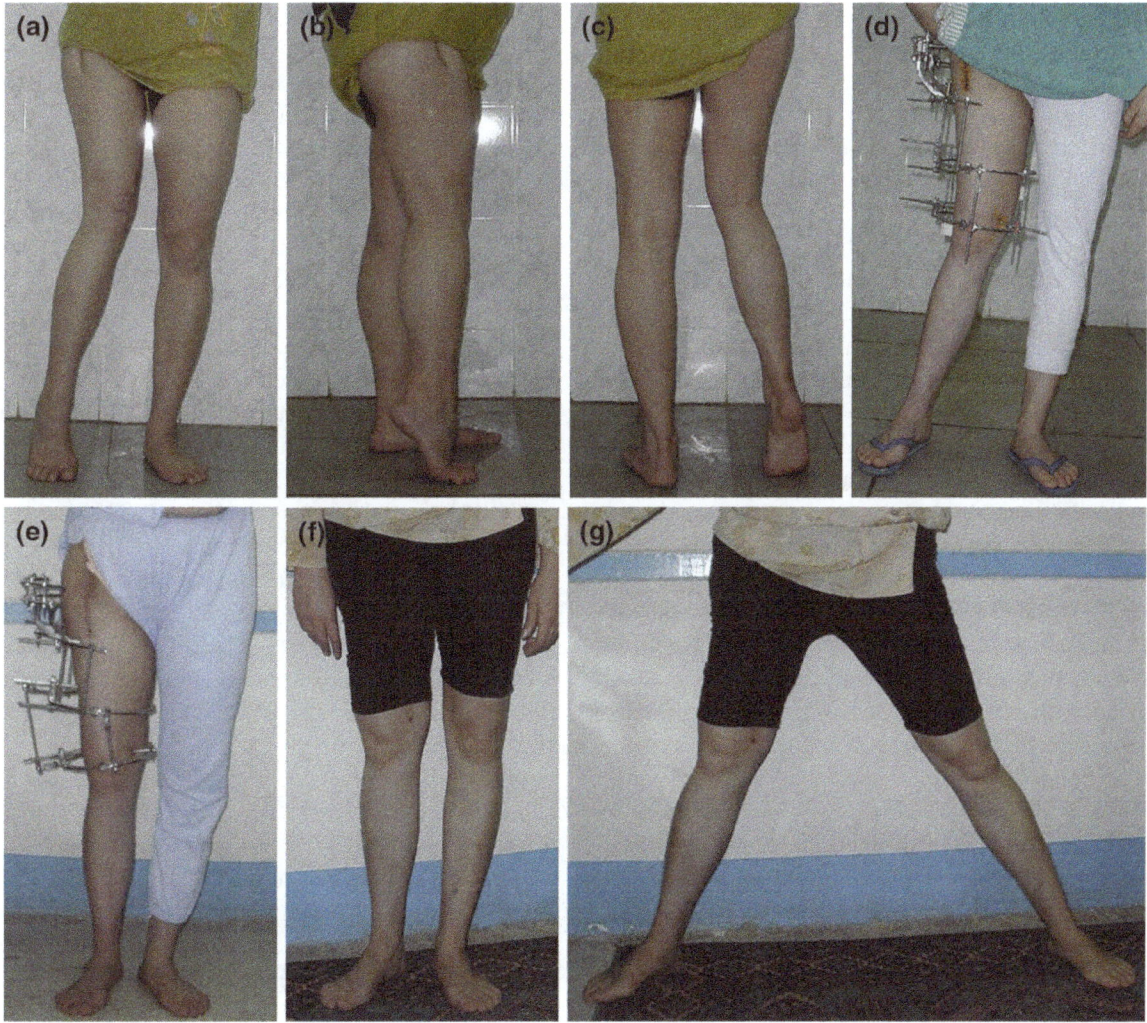

Fig. 1 a–c Preoperative clinical photographs of a 32-year-old female patient with sequelae of septic arthritis in childhood affecting the right hip joint. The patient had flexion, adduction, internal rotation deformities and an apparent limb-length discrepancy of 12 cm. **d** Postoperative photograph shows the applied Ilizarov frame, valgus of the lower limb due to the proximal osteotomy and reduction in the limb-length discrepancy to 4 cm. **e** Photograph after 4 cm lengthening and correction limb alignment by varus angulation at the distal osteotomy. **f, g** Follow-up photographs show the functional outcome

insufficiency after septic arthritis of the hip in childhood and with a minimum postoperative follow-up of 5 years.

The presenting symptoms were a limp (with or without pain), leg-length discrepancy, deformity, hip stiffness and, in some, difficulty with marital relationship (Fig. 1a). Surgery in all cases was performed by the first author and data collection and evaluation at final follow-up by the second author who was not involved in surgery.

Preoperative evaluation

This included a general assessment of the medical status and patient's expectations from the treatment. Local examination was done to record the presence of pain, scars of previous surgery, sinuses, fixed pelvic obliquity and fixed contractures of the hip, limb-length discrepancy (by the block method) and the neurological, muscle strength and vascular status of the lower limb.

Plain radiographs were obtained for the lumbosacral spine (to detect fixed scoliotic deformity), pelvis and hip joints. A CT scan of the pelvis and both hip joints was obtained for better evaluation of the hip joint regarding the location of the femoral head relative to the acetabulum and presence of fibrous or bony ankylosis of the joint.

Procedure

The procedure was performed with the patient in the supine position. An adductor tenotomy was performed through a medial approach. Mobilization of the damaged hip was performed by undoing the ankylosis through a limited anterolateral approach to the hip and under image intensifier, where the remnants of the femoral head were removed piecemeal using a bone rongeur. The affected limb was then maximally adducted over the other limb so that the upper part of the femur was seen parallel to the lateral wall of the pelvis on the affected side and abutting against the ischium; that point of abutment was marked as the site of the proximal osteotomy. With the limb maximally adducted, half pins were inserted in the proximal femur perpendicular to the sagittal plane of the patient's body and parallel to the horizontal plane. A fixation block consisting of one small and one large arch from the Ilizarov system was attached to these pins. The limb was then abducted back to the neutral position, and a preconstructed Ilizarov frame was then applied to the femur distal to the proposed proximal osteotomy with the pins inserted perpendicular to the axis of the distal femur. The proximal osteotomy was performed percutaneously using a drilling and osteotome method. Holding both the proximal block and the distal part of the frame, the osteotomy was manipulated to affect a derotation–extension–valgus osteotomy but with care to avoid excessive displacement and loss of bone contact. The proximal and distal parts of the frame were connected using threaded rods and oblique supports. The level of the distal osteotomy was determined preoperatively so that the mechanical axis of the lower limb passes through the acetabulum and the knee joint line of the knee remains horizontal. The distal osteotomy was performed percutaneously.

Postoperative management and follow-up

The patient was mobilized after postoperative pain had subsided. The patient was encouraged to mobilize the lower limb joints and bear weight as tolerated. The amount of limb lengthening needed was estimated using the block method; in the assessment, an awareness of the fixed pelvic obliquity was maintained so as not to overestimate the actual discrepancy (there is an adduction contracture present frequently). Distraction of the distal osteotomy was started after 5–7 days at a rate of 1 mm per day until the limb-length discrepancy was corrected. Thereafter, hinges were built into the external fixator to gradually move the distal segment into varus until the knee joint line was horizontal (Fig. 1b–d). After consolidation of the osteotomies, the frame was removed without anesthesia (as an outpatient procedure usually). No cast was applied. Figure 2 demonstrates the procedure radiologically and the follow-up result.

Evaluation of results

The results were recorded from the patients' notes. Clinical and radiological assessments and subsequent data analysis

and calculation of scores were performed at the time of last follow-up by the second author. The functional outcome was graded using the Harris hip score (HHS). This has a total of 100 points: Pain receives 44 points; function, 47 points (activities of daily living have 14 points and gait 33 points); range of motion, 5 points; and deformity, 4 points. A total score below 70 points is considered a poor result; 70–79, a fair result; 80–89, a good result; and 90–100, an excellent result [9].

The follow-up radiographs were assessed for orientation of the knee joint line and restoration of the overall mechanical axis of the lower limb, such that extension of the mechanical axis of the tibia and distal femur should pass through the acetabulum with a horizontal knee joint-orientation line.

Statistical analysis was done using SPSS version 11.0.1 for Windows (SPSS Inc., Chicago, IL, USA). The one-sample t test was used for dependent variable mean comparison, and one-way analysis of variance (ANOVA) test and its nonparametric equivalent, the Kruskal–Wallis test, were used for variables that were small and not normally distributed. A p value ≤ 0.05 was considered to be statistically significant.

Results

There were 16 patients with ages ranging from 19 to 32 years (mean 23 ± 4.2 years). There were nine (56 %) male and seven (44 %) female patients. The right side was affected in nine (56 %) cases and the left side in seven (44 %) cases. A fixed flexion deformity of the hip was present in all cases and ranged from 20 to 45° (mean $32.8 \pm 7.9°$). A fixed adduction contracture of the hip was present in eleven cases (69 %) and ranged from 10 to 25° (mean $16.8 \pm 5.1°$). A fixed internal rotation deformity was present in eight cases (50 %) and ranged from 5 to 15° (mean $10.6 \pm 3.2°$). Preoperative limb-length discrepancy was present in all cases and ranged from 3 to 12 cm (mean 5.6 ± 2.3 cm); after release of the ankylosis and fixed contractures, this shortening when reassessed (postoperatively and prior to the start of lengthening) was found to have a mean 2.8 (as measured clinically by the block method, Table 1). The surgical release of the ankylosis of the hip joint improved the apparent preoperative LLD significantly ($p \leq 0.001$).

Limb lengthening was performed in all cases through the distal femoral osteotomy to address the residual limb shortening. The mean external fixator time (the time spent in the external fixator) was 4.6 ± 0.97 months. The mean external fixator index (the time in external fixation divided by the lengthening in months/cm) was 1.6 ± 0.24.

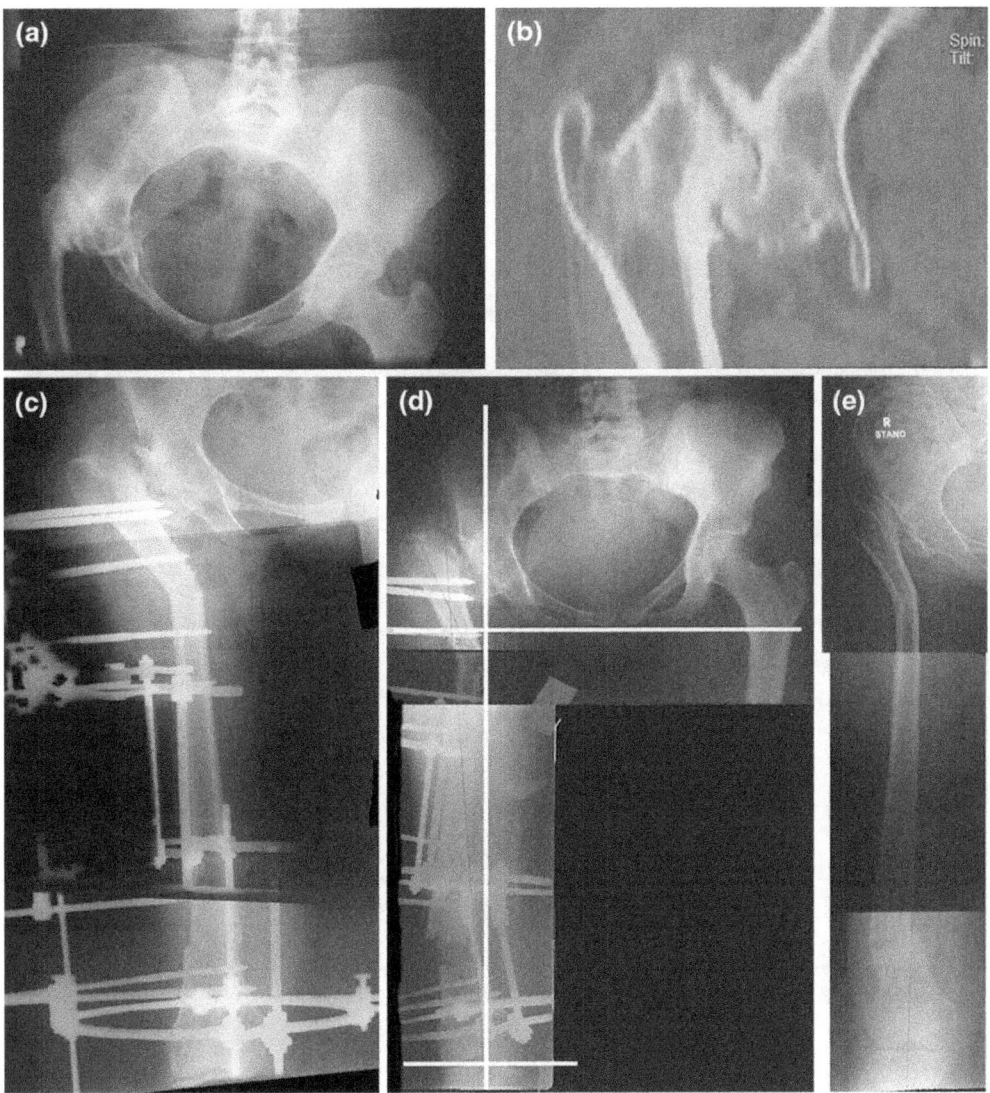

Fig. 2 a, **b** Preoperative plain radiograph and CT scan show destruction of the femoral head and acetabulum and fibrous ankylosis as a result of septic arthritis of the right hip in childhood. The radiograph shows evidence of hip adduction, flexion (non-visualized obturator foramen) and internal rotation (non-visualized lesser trochanter). **c**, **d** Radiographs during treatment show the proximal and distal osteotomies, lengthening and varus through the distal osteotomy. The knee joint-orientation line is horizontal and proximal extension of the mechanical axis of the distal femur passes through the acetabulum. **e** Follow-up radiograph shows the consolidated osteotomies and maintained alignment

The follow-up period ranged from 60 to 132 months (mean 85.6 ± 23.5). At the time of last follow-up, the HHS showed an excellent functional outcome in two cases (12.50 %), good in 13 cases (81.25 %) and fair in one case (6.25 %). There was no poor functional outcome. Preoperatively, the mean HHS was 56.18 ± 7.41 points, and at the time of last follow-up, it improved to a mean of 84.62 ± 4.19 points (Table 2). Improvement in the functional outcome was statistically significant ($p \leq 0.001$). The functional outcome was noted to be significantly better:

1. in male than female patients;
2. when the apparent LLD was less than 6 cm;
3. when the distal femoral lengthening was less than 3 cm; and
4. when the external fixator time was 4 months maximally (Table 3).

Pain subsided in all patients and the Trendelenburg sign became negative in all but three (19 %) patients. None had a limb-length discrepancy (as measured clinically by the block method), and the alignment of the extremity was reestablished in all cases.

Superficial pin tract infections occurred in all cases and were managed by frequent pin site care and oral

Table 1 Preoperative demographic data of the patients

No.	Age (years)	Sex	Side	Fixed hip deformities			LLD (cm)	
				Flexion	Adduction	Internal rotation	Preoperative	Postoperative
1	19	Male	Left	40°	15°	10°	8	2.5
2	32	Female	Right	45°	25°	15°	12	4
3	20	Male	Left	30°	20°	0°	6	3
4	19	Male	Left	20°	15°	0°	4	2
5	22	Male	Right	35°	10°	0°	5	2
6	21	Female	Right	40°	15°	10°	7	4
7	24	Female	Right	25°	0°	5°	4	2.5
8	30	Male	Left	30°	0°	0°	4	2
9	19	Male	Left	30°	20°	0°	3	2
10	20	Female	Right	35°	15°	10°	5	3
11	24	Female	Right	45°	25°	15°	8	4
12	30	Male	Left	20°	0°	0°	4	3
13	26	Female	Right	25°	0°	0°	4	2.5
14	23	Male	Right	40°	0°	0°	6	4
15	20	Male	Right	30°	10°	10°	5	3
16	22	Female	Left	35°	15°	10°	4	2
Range	19–32			20°–45°	10°–25°	5°–15°	3–12	2–4
Mean ± SD	23.2 ± 4.2			32.8 ± 7.9	16.8 ± 5.1	10.6 ± 3.2	5.6 ± 2.3	2.8 ± 0.8

LLD limb-length discrepancy

Tables 2 Results of treatment

No.	Limb lengthening (cm)	External fixator time (months)	External fixator index	Harris hip score		Follow-up (months)
				Preoperative	Postoperative	
1	2.5	4	1.6	50	85	124
2	4	6	1.5	45	85	132
3	3	4	1.3	60	88	100
4	2	3.5	1.7	65	90	64
5	2	4	2	55	84	72
6	4	6	1.5	68	88	100
7	2.5	3.5	1.4	65	88	64
8	2	4	2	60	85	70
9	2	4	2	56	80	86
10	3	5	1.6	50	84	66
11	4	6	1.5	45	75	122
12	3	4	1.3	60	92	70
13	2.5	5	2	60	85	78
14	4	6	1.5	45	80	90
15	3	5	1.6	60	82	60
16	2	3.5	1.7	55	83	72
Range	2–4	3.5–6	1.3–2	45–68	75–92	60–132
Mean ± SD	2.8 ± 0.79	4.6 ± 0.97	1.6 ± 0.24	56.18 ± 7.41	84.62 ± 4.19	85.6 ± 23.5

antibiotics. No cases of deep infection or neurovascular injury occurred as a result of this treatment. At the time of last follow-up, three patients complained of lurch while walking; however, no additional procedures were required. No cases of regenerate fracture were encountered in this study.

Table 3 Factors affecting clinical outcome

Factors		Harris hip score				Statistical analysis	
Group	Subgroup	Excellent	Good	Fair	Total	Statistical value	p value
Age groups	18–20	1	5	0	6	4.433*	0.066
	21–30	1	7	1	9		
	31–40	0	1	0	1		
Gender	Males	2	7	0	9	3.603**	0.2
	Females	0	6	1	7		
Initial LLD	Less than 6 cm	2	8	0	10	3.167*	0.115
	6–10 cm	0	4	1	5		
	More than 10 cm	0	1	0	1		
Distal femoral lengthening	Less than 3 cm	1	7	0	8	4.194**	0.2
	3 cm or more	1	6	1	8		
External fixator time	Up to 4 months	2	7	0	9	3.603**	0.2
	More than 4 months	0	6	1	7		

LLD limb-length discrepancy

* *F* value of one-way analysis of variance test

** *H* value of Kruskal–Wallis test

Discussion

A resection arthroplasty of the hip joint (Girdlestone) has been described for alleviation of pain and improvement in hip function, but this arthroplasty produces an unstable joint, limb-length discrepancy and functional disability [10]. The pelvic support osteotomy (PSO) was introduced to improve hip stability by directly transferring the body weight to the distal femur and to relieve pain by offloading the stump of the femoral head [6, 11, 12]. The aim of the PSO is to support the pelvis on the femur, reduce lumbar lordosis and increase the distance of the greater trochanter from the pelvis, which in turn tensions the gluteus medius muscle and reduces the Trendelenburg limp [7, 8]. Milch described a similar angulation osteotomy with the addition of femoral head resection in patients with anterior dislocation who had developed arthrosis [6]. A shortcoming of the original PSO is the abducted position of the lower limb places high stresses on the knee joint, and it does not address the limb-length discrepancy [8].

Ilizarov added another distal osteotomy to restore the orientation of the knee and ankle joint lines in the coronal plane and to allow femoral lengthening while maintaining the advantages of the proximal osteotomy in lateralizing and displacing the greater trochanter and, in so doing, increasing the efficiency of the abductor muscles [8]. A successful Ilizarov hip reconstruction (IHR) reduces limp through abolishing the Trendelenburg lurch (due to elimination of any further adduction between the femur and the pelvis which then prevents pelvic drop during the single stance phase of gait), equalizes limb length and facilitates a more energy-efficient gait through the stability provided to the hemipelvis [7, 11–17]. In Ilizarov hip reconstruction, the mechanical axis of the lower limb should, ideally, go upward as an extension of the normal mechanical axis of the tibia (from the center of the ankle to the center of the knee joint) through the original acetabulum perpendicular to the horizontal line of the pelvis (line connecting top of both iliac crests). The proximal part of the femur should lie parallel to the lateral wall of the pelvis so that in performing the Trendelenburg test, the pelvis rests on the proximal femur with zero-degree adduction and so produces the negative Trendelenburg sign.

It is recommended that the hip joint should be mobile or the femoral head absent for a successful PSO. In this cohort, we performed a resection of the femoral head remnants to produce mobilization of the hip joint; this procedure also served to correct the fixed contractures of the hip joint and reduce that component of limb shortening arising from joint contractures. This increased range of movement then allowed for maximum adduction of the limb prior to performing the more proximal osteotomy.

Hip pain was present in all patients in this cohort. This had reduced postoperatively. The mean preoperative limb-length discrepancy of 5.6 ± 2.3 cm (range 3–12) was reduced substantially after hip resection and mobilization and required a reestimation of the required limb lengthening. In all patients, the limb-length discrepancy was corrected through the distal osteotomy. Due to the muscle bulk of the thigh, the distal femoral osteotomy, which included a varus correction, did not produce a clinically visible deformity.

The HHS improved significantly compared with the preoperative values. Several other studies have confirmed the beneficial effects of the Ilizarov hip reconstruction using clinical and imaging studies and through gait analysis. The improvement in HHS after IHR has been attributed to the increased hip abductor muscle mass after

PSO (documented with MRI studies) and the decreased joint reaction forces (as confirmed by gait analysis parameters) [7, 13, 17, 18].

In a biomechanical study, Inan et al. [19] showed a distal and lateral translation osteotomy of the greater trochanter after a traditional PSO increases the length of the abductor moment arm more than that obtained by traditional PSO alone. In our study, a residual lurching gait was present in three cases (18.7 %) and was clinically significant in one patient (6.2 %). This positive Trendelenburg sign may be attributed to: (1) weakness of hip abductors due to long-standing disuse; (2) pressure atrophy of the tissues inter-posed between the angulated proximal femur and the lateral wall of the pelvis which subsequently permits some of adduction and a return of the positive Trendelenburg sign. Some authors recommend an overcorrection of the proxi-mal osteotomy (about 15° of additional valgus) in antici-pation of this loss of support in maximum adduction, but it is our opinion that there may be some unpredictability in the functional results and patient's satisfaction after this increased valgus angulation.

The main adverse effect of Ilizarov hip reconstruction osteotomy is the altered anatomy of the proximal femur in both sagittal and frontal planes which would increase the difficulty of a future total hip replacement (THR). How-ever, Thabet et al. [5] have reported a successful THR 15 years after a PSO and concluded that the altered anat-omy of the proximal femur after PSO did not preclude the subsequent THR; however, the THR can be tricky and careful attention to the surgical details is necessary to achieve a successful outcome.

In the light of these midterm results, we conclude that the Ilizarov hip reconstruction is a valuable and durable solution for the late sequelae of childhood septic arthritis of the hip.

References

1. Baghdadi T, Saberi S, Sobhani Eraghi A, Arabzadeh A, Mar-dookhpour S (2012) Late sequelae of hip septic arthritis in chil-dren. Acta Med Iran 50(7):463–467
2. Forlin E, Milani C (2008) Sequelae of septic arthritis of the hip in children: a new classification and a review of 41 hips. J Pediatr Orthop 28(5):524–528
3. Manzotti A, Rovetta L, Pullen C, Catagni MA (2003) Treatment of the late sequelae of septic arthritis of the hip. Clin Orthop Relat Res 410:203–212
4. Hunka L, Said SE, MacKenzie DA, Rogala EJ, Cruess RL (1982) Classification and surgical management of the severe sequelae of septic hips in children. Clin Orthop Relat Res 171:30–36
5. Thabet AM, Catagni MA, Guerreschi F (2012) Total hip replacement fifteen years after pelvic support osteotomy (PSO): a case report and review of the literature. Musculoskelet Surg 96(2):141–147
6. Milch H (1941) The "pelvic support" osteotomy. J Bone Joint Surg Am 23(3):581–595
7. Rozbruch SR, Paley D, Bhave A, Herzenberg JE (2005) Ilizarov hip reconstruction for the late sequelae of infantile hip infection. J Bone Joint Surg Am 87(5):1007–1018
8. Ilizarov GA (1992) Transosseous osteosynthesis. Springer, Berlin
9. Harris WH (1969) Traumatic arthritis of the hip after dislocation and acetabular fractures: treatment by mold arthroplasty. An end result study using a new method of result evaluation. J Bone Joint Surg Am 51:737–755
10. Oheim R, Gille J, Schoop R, Mägerlein S, Grimme CH, Jürgens C, Gerlach UJ (2012) Surgical therapy of hip-joint empyema. Is the Girdlestone arthroplasty still up to date? Int Orthop 36(5):927–933
11. Cheng JC, Lam TP (1996) Femoral lengthening after type IVB septic arthritis of the hip in children. J Pediatr Orthop 16(4):533–539
12. Gürsu S, Demir B, Yildirim T, Er T, Bursali A, Sahin V (2011) An effective treatment for hip instabilities: pelvic support oste-otomy and femoral lengthening. Acta Orthop Traumatol Turc 45(6):437–445
13. El-Mowafi H (2005) Outcome of pelvic support osteotomy with the Ilizarov method in the treatment of the unstable hip joint. Acta Orthop Belg 71(6):686–691
14. Marimuthu K, Joshi N, Sharma CS, Bhargava R, Meena DS, Bansiwal RC, Govindasamy R (2001) Ilizarov hip reconstruction in skeletally mature young patients with chronic unstable hip joints. Arch Orthop Trauma Surg 131(12):1631–1637
15. Mahran MA, Elgebeily MA, Ghaly NA, Thakeb MF, Hefny HM (2001) Pelvic support osteotomy by Ilizarov's concept: is it a valuable option in managing neglected hip problems in adoles-cents and young adults ? Strategies Trauma Limb Reconstr 6(1):13–20
16. Mandar A, Tong XB, Song SH, Park YE, Hong JH, Lee H, Song HR (2012) Pelvic support osteotomy for unstable hips using hybrid external fixator: case series and review of literature. J Orthop Sci 17(1):9–17
17. Kocaoglu M, Eralp L, Sen C, Dinçyürek H (2002) The Ilizarov hip reconstruction osteotomy for hip dislocation: outcome after 4–7 years in 14 young patients. Acta Orthop Scand 73(4):432–438
18. Inan M, Alkan A, Harma A, Ertem K (2005) Evaluation of the gluteus medius muscle after a pelvic support osteotomy to treat congenital dislocation of the hip. J Bone Joint Surg Am 87(10):2246–2252
19. Inan M, Mahar A, Swimmer T, Tomlinson T, Wenger DR (2004) Changes in the lengths of the gluteus medius and gluteus mini-mus muscles with trochanteric transfer following pelvic support osteotomy: a biomechanical study. Acta Orthop Traumatol Turc 38(1):67–70

28

Proximal humeral reconstruction using nail cement spacer in primary and metastatic tumours of proximal humerus

Zile Singh Kundu · Paritosh Gogna ·
Vinay Gupta · Pradeep Kamboj · Rohit Singla ·
Sukhbir Singh Sangwan

Abstract Limb salvage surgery for malignant tumours of proximal humerus is an operative challenge, where the surgeon has to preserve elbow and hand functions and retain shoulder stability with as much function as possible. We treated 14 consecutive patients with primary malignant or isolated metastasis of proximal humerus with surgical resection and reconstruction by nail cement spacer. There were 8 females and 6 males, with a mean age of 28.92 years (range 16–51 years) and a mean follow-up of 30.14 months (range 12–52 months). The diagnosis was osteosarcoma in 8 patients, chondrosarcoma in 4 patients and metastasis from thyroid and breast carcinoma in 1 patient each. One of our patients had radial nerve neuropraxia, 1 developed inferior subluxation and 3 developed distant metastasis. Two patients died of disease and one developed local recurrence leading to forequarter amputation, leaving a total of 11 patients with functional extremities for assessment at the time of final follow-up which was done using the Musculoskeletal Tumour Society (MSTS) score. Though we were able to preserve the elbow, wrist and hand functions in all patients, the abductor mechanism, deltoid muscle and axillary nerve were not salvageable in any of cases. The mean MSTS score at the time of final follow-up was 19.09. Thus, proximal humeral reconstruction using nail cement spacer is a technical simple, cost-effective and reproducible procedure which makes it a reliable option in subset of patients where the functions around the shoulder cannot be preserved despite costlier prosthesis.

Z. S. Kundu · P. Gogna (✉) · V. Gupta · P. Kamboj ·
R. Singla · S. S. Sangwan
Department of Orthopaedics and Rehabilitation, PGIMS,
2/11-J Medical Enclave, Rohtak 124001, Haryana, India
e-mail: paritosh.gogna@gmail.com

Keywords Proximal humerus · Tumours · Limb salvage · Nail cement spacer

Introduction

The proximal humerus is a relatively common location for primary and metastatic tumours of bone in adults. Limb salvage surgery, instead of amputation, has become treatment of choice as it offers both functional and cosmetic advantages [1]. Various techniques have been advocated for reconstruction of skeletal defects after limb salvage. The options for reconstruction include osteoarticular allograft, allograft-prosthesis composite, free vascularized fibula graft, cement nail spacers, a sling procedure with a vascularized fibular graft, claviculo-pro-humerus and endoprosthetic replacement of the proximal humerus [1–10]. Every procedure has its own set of pros and cons, and there is no consensus on the gold standard procedure. The optimum method of reconstruction of the proximal humerus remains controversial as the function of the shoulder joint can only be restored partially as a result of various degrees of muscle loss during resection of tumour [6].

Radical removal is a principal of tumour surgery, but as much functionality as possible should be retained. These conditions often conflict, so a compromise has to be reached. When the proximal end of the humerus has to be resected, it becomes important to reconstruct it in order to give functional mobility to the upper limb. The most important issues of limb salvage surgery of proximal humerus are to maximize local control of the tumour, to preserve both elbow and hand functions and to improve shoulder stability and with as much function possible [4–8]. After resection of a malignant bone tumour of the proximal humerus, we used a nail cement spacer for limb salvage [7, 8]. The aim of this study was to evaluate the functional outcome of limb salvage surgery using nail cement spacer after wide resection of primary malignant and metastatic tumours of proximal humerus.

Patients and methods

We retrospectively reviewed the hospital record for patients with primary malignant and metastatic tumours of the proximal humerus who were operated at our orthopaedic oncology wing between January 2005 and December 2009. There were a total of 31 patients with tumour involving the proximal humerus (metastasis $n = 5$), (primary sarcomas $n = 26$). Only those patients were included in the study in which the magnetic resonance imaging (MRI) revealed invasion of the rotator cuff or abductor mechanism with the possibility of obtaining a safe surgical margin without resecting the glenoid (Malawar classification of shoulder girdle resections type IB) [11]. Excluded from the study were patients with neurovascular bundle involvement supplying to the distal part of extremity, extensive pulmonary metastasis, soft tissue sarcomas or tumours of the clavicle, scapula or proximal part of the humeral diaphysis which did not involve the humeral head. Fourteen patients (metastasis $n = 2$), (primary sarcomas $n = 12$), fulfilled the inclusion criteria and formed the patient cohort; all these patients were managed by limb-sparing tumour excision surgery with resection of the proximal humerus and reconstruction with antibiotic bone cement [gentamycin–polymethylmethacrylate (PMMA)]-coated Kuntscher's nail spacer. Before surgery, all patients underwent staging studies, including plain radiographs and MRI of the limb, contrast enhanced computerized tomography (CECT) scans of the chest and whole-body isotope bone scan. None of the patients had distant metastasis at the time of operation. MRI was used to define the extent of the lesion, the involvement of the soft tissues, its relation to the neurovascular bundle and the level of involvement of the bone. Preoperative histopathological diagnosis was obtained by core needle biopsy. The diagnosis was osteosarcoma in 8 patients, chondrosarcoma in 4 patients and 2 patients had single metastasis from thyroid and breast carcinoma, respectively. The primary goal of surgery was complete wide excision of the tumour, with preservation of the limb. Tumours were classified according to the Enneking's staging system. All patients with osteosarcoma were treated with the appropriate (neo) adjuvant chemotherapy using the appropriate treatment protocols. Chondrosarcomas were treated by surgical resection only, and those with metastasis were treated with wide resection along with adequate treatment of primary and appropriate chemotherapy as per hospital protocol.

We retrospectively analysed all medical records for patient characteristics, age at diagnosis, diagnosis, surgical treatment and approach, duration of follow-up, integrity of abductor mechanism, humeral resection length measured from the tip of the greater tuberosity, resection margins, adjuvant treatment, postoperative complications, oncological parameters including overall survival, and local or systemic relapse.

The lesions were approached by way of an extended deltopectoral anterolateral incision, the exact position of which was determined by the site of biopsy and the location and extent of the tumour. Previous biopsy tracts were incorporated into the incision and were completely excised. All were transarticular resections, leaving the glenoid intact. The glenohumeral joint was disarticulated by dividing the long head of biceps as well as the tendinous portion of the rotator cuff. The tendons of pectoralis major, latissimus dorsi, teres major and the long head of biceps were detached. A cuff of normal soft tissue was retained around the proximal humerus so as to complete the 'wide excision'. Meticulous dissection was carried out, and an intraarticular proximal humerus with the humeral diaphysis was isolated at least 2.5 cm from the most distal part of the lesion (as determined by MRI) and cut using an oscillating saw. Marrow from remaining distal humeral diaphysis was sent for frozen section evaluation.

Once the tumour was excised, haemostasis was achieved. The glenoid and remaining humerus were prepared to accept the implant. The humeral canal was reamed to accept the intramedullary nail. Depending upon the length of humerus resected, Kuntscher's nail antibiotic cement (PMMA) spacer was prepared, moulding the semisolid cement around the nail to provide the shape and volume of resected humerus. At the proximal end, cement was moulded to provide the shape of humeral head. The distal end of nail inserted into the reamed intramedullary canal which was filled with cement for better fixation. The longest possible nail was used to construct the spacer. The cement head made at proximal end was abutted into the glenoid. Soft tissue reconstruction was completed mainly through crossed suture and reattachment of the residual muscles around the shoulder girdle to provide static stability. The residual muscles were anchored to the nail spacer with the help of four to six sutures passed through holes made in cement before setting when it was solid and mouldable, using braided non-absorbable No. 2 Ethibond suture. Soft tissue and skin were sutured over a negative suction drain. Postoperatively the arm was placed in an arm chest bandage. Stitches were removed after 3 weeks, and the hand, wrist and elbow were mobilized. After 6–8 weeks, the sling was removed and passive mobilization began. They were then followed up at regular intervals and were assessed for local control, function and complications related to the implant. Functional assessment at the time of final follow-up was done using the Musculoskeletal Tumour Society (MSTS) functional scores [12].

Results

There were 8 females and 6 males. The mean age at the time of surgery was 28.92 years (range 16–51). The mean follow-up was 30.14 months (range 12–52 months). The mean length of resected bone was 12 cm (range 9–15). The details of the patients profile and the final outcome is given in Table 1. All resection margins were histologically free of disease on intraoperative frozen sections and final analysis. The abductor mechanism, deltoid muscle and axillary nerve were not salvageable in any of the 14 cases. There were no major intraoperative complications (neurovascular) and no superficial or deep infections. One patient had postoperative radial nerve neuropraxia, which recovered in 5 months, and another patient developed inferior subluxation of the proximal humeral head associated with a dragging sensation and paraesthesia due to shoulder instability. Ten patients remained free from disease till final follow-up. One of the patients with osteosarcoma had a local recurrence after 26 months of follow-up and underwent forequarter amputation. One patient with osteosarcoma had lung metastasis and died 16 months after surgery, and another patient with breast carcinoma had lung and brain metastasis and died 12 months after operation. A patient with chondrosarcoma was diagnosed to have a lung metastasis after 20 months of surgery. The

patient is not willing for any further surgical intervention but is still under follow-up at 24 months.

There was no case of cement implant loosening, implant failure or fracture. Wrist and fine movements of the hand were preserved in all patients, although elbow extension was limited in 3 cases in the early postoperative months which gradually improved to almost full extension with physiotherapy. All the patients were able to perform their day-to-day activities and routine work (hand and face washing, eating, lifting a cup and other household works). Functional data were available for 11 patients with functional extremity at the time of final follow-up (Table 1). The mean MSTS score was 19.09 (range 15–23) with the mean overall functional rating of 63.63 % (range 50–6.67 %). With regard to pain, emotional acceptance and manual dexterity, the results were rated as satisfactory with a score of 3.0 points or more in 11 patients.

Discussion

For high-grade malignant tumours of the shoulder girdle, limb salvage surgery rather than amputation has become treatment of choice in last few decades as it offers both functional and cosmetic advantages. Limb salvage is socially and emotionally easier for patients to accept than amputation. Most replacements of the proximal humerus act as functional spacers rather than as an articulating reconstruction. The optimum method of reconstruction of the proximal humerus remains controversial as the function of the shoulder joint can only be restored partially as a

Table 1 Demographic profile of the patients and the functional outcome

S. No.	Age/sex	Diagnosis	Pathological fracture	Stage	Complications	MSTS score	Metastasis	Latest status	Follow-up (in months)
1	28/F	Osteosarcoma	No	IIB	–	20	–	CDF	48
2	17/M	Osteosarcoma	No	IIB	–	19	–	CDF	30
3	32/F	Chondrosarcoma	No	IIB	–	23	–	CDF	52
4	16/F	Osteosarcoma	No	IIB	–	19	–	CDF	32
5	51/F	Chondrosarcoma	No	IIB	–	16	–	CDF	40
6	44/F	Metastasis from thyroid	Yes	–	–	18	–	CDF	36
7	22/M	Osteosarcoma	No	IIB	–	–	Lung	DOD	16
8	20/F	Osteosarcoma	No	IIB	Radial nerve neuropraxia	21	–	CDF	18
9	17/M	Osteosarcoma	No	IIB	Local recurrence	–	–	DF	26
10	48/M	Chondrosarcoma	No	IB	–	15	Lung	AWD	24
11	34/F	Chondrosarcoma	No	IIB	Inferior subluxation	18	–	CDF	36
12	18/M	Osteosarcoma	Yes	IIB	–	19	–	CDF	28
13	16/M	Osteosarcoma	No	IIB	–	22	–	CDF	24
14	42/F	Metastasis from breast	No	–	–	–	Lung, brain	DOD	12

M male, *F* female, *CDF* continuous disease free, *DF* disease free, *DOD* died of disease, *AWD* alive with disease

result of various degrees of muscle loss during resection of tumour [6].

When evaluating a reconstruction technique, the factors which need to be considered include the ease of the procedure, its morbidity, complications, functional outcome and durability. In the past, the wide resection with no reconstruction at all was done and healing occurred by fibrosis. However, a salvaged flail shoulder may result in traction neuropathy and reduced function of the hand, forearm and elbow, due to mechanical instability [13].

Shoulder arthrodesis after resection requires graft augmentation, which is further fraught with the risk of fatigue fractures or failure of fixation [14]. The use of the avascular strut allograft is often limited by the available length of the resection, risk of non-union, fracture and infection, besides the fear of disease transmission. Vascularized fibular grafts specifically require microsurgical expertise and entail longer operating times and increased blood loss without an improved functional outcome. Further, it adds morbidity to the normal limb [4]. Free fibular graft from contralateral leg in the presence of extensive dissections, especially if it is resected for more than 12 cm, may lead to fracture and failure of incorporation of graft and, even if it survives, will take a very long time to heal with poor functional outcome [7, 15]. Endoprosthesis is the most common mode of reconstruction nowadays, but its high cost (more than 2,000 US $) is the major limiting factor in many parts of the world. Furthermore, in extra-compartmental bone tumours of the proximal humerus, the rotator cuff has to be resected (Malawer resection type IB) [11]. Shoulder function is directly related to the restoration of

rotator cuff function. If this proves to be impossible, the patient ends up with an unstable joint and unsatisfactory function with compromised active positioning of the hand and poor lifting ability. With resection of deltoid muscle, rotator cuff and axillary nerve, the prosthesis replacement has to overcome failure of humeral fixation, superior head migration and lack of muscle insertion, finally acting as a passive spacer [7, 16]. Although newer techniques and prosthesis are coming up to meet the deficiencies, it further adds to the cost and requires expertise [16, 17].

The choice of reconstruction technique should be based on the extent of the resection and the need of the patient. Most authors agree that after reconstruction of extensive proximal humeral lesions, the shoulder function is compromised [6]. Stability at the proximal end of the reconstruct ensures good hand and elbow function. Although little function is restored to the shoulder, such reconstructions provide a stable fulcrum for function of the elbow and hand and prevent pain related to traction on the neurovascular bundle. Reconstructing these defects using this cement K-nail spacer is an inexpensive (the implant with cementation costs less than US $100) and effective method, which gives adequate shoulder and arm stability and ensures excellent hand and elbow function (Figs. 1, 2). Furthermore, the operative time is short, and the procedure is less technically demanding [7]. The complications in bone graft incorporation due to the use of adjuvant chemotherapy and radiotherapy leading to a delay in postoperative rehabilitation are avoided with this metallic implant–cement spacer. This method offers immediate distal fixation and early administration of radiotherapy in

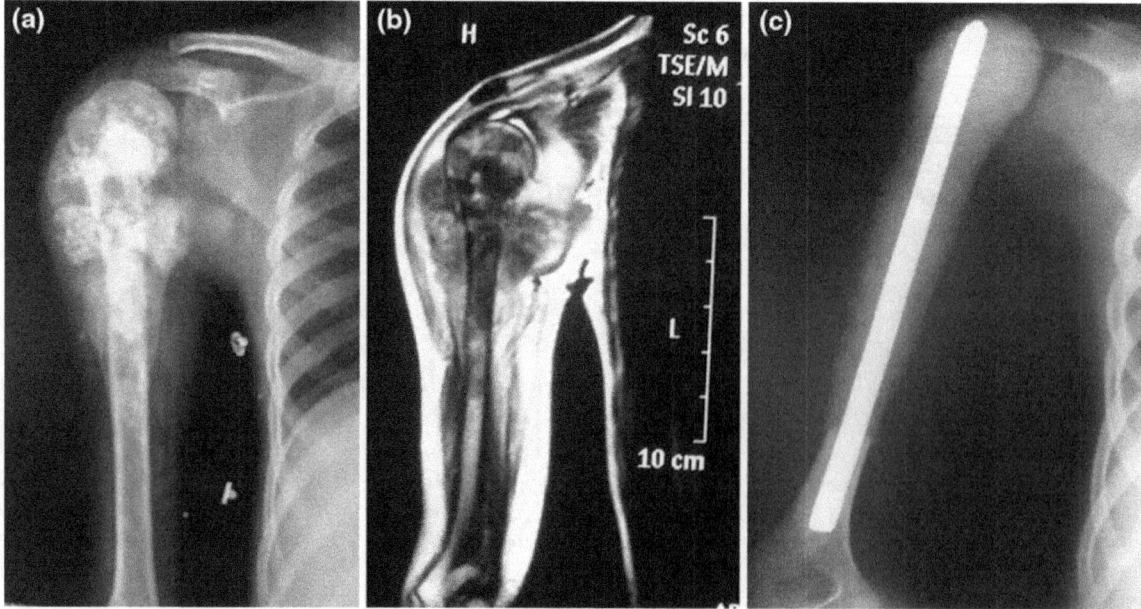

Fig. 1 **a** Preoperative X-ray of osteosarcoma after neo-adjuvant chemotherapy. **b** MRI showing the extent in the soft tissue and in the medullary canal **c** Postoperative X-ray showing the Kuntscher's nail cement spacer after subtotal resection of the humerus

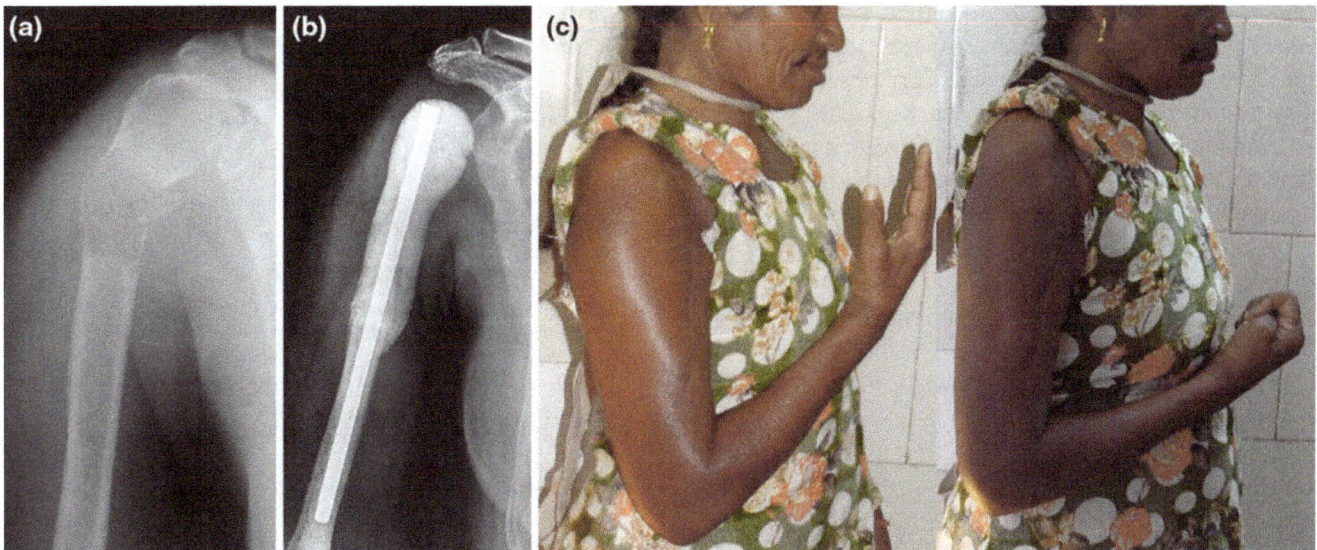

Fig. 2 a Metastasis from thyroid preoperative X-ray. **b** Postoperative X-ray showing the Kuntscher's nail cement spacer. **c** Good flexion of elbow and hand movements

immediate postoperative period if required [8]. Unlike the lower limb, which is subject to variable stresses and loading, the upper limb faces relatively less intense biomechanical forces, and this could be the reason why none of our reconstructs needed revision so far. The use of antibiotic cement provides higher concentration of local antibiotic and helps in combating local infection. Extensive resections may often compound the problem if the remaining distal stump of bone is very small. This K-nail cement spacer with intramedullary nail can be used even in these cases with shorter lengths. Even endoprosthesis needs a definite amount of residual host bone for adequate fixation of the stem after resection, and this is a limiting factor to their use in such cases [11]. Reconstructing these defects using custom-made plates has been advocated, but the number of screws through the distal fragment is limited with the risk of implant failure [10].

The 14 patients who had reconstruction with a functional spacer generally fared well from a reconstructive standpoint. One of the problems related to these spacers was subluxation of spacer from glenoid fossa. Van de sande et al. [18] compared the outcomes after transarticular tumour resection and proximal humeral reconstructions using allograft-prosthesis composite ($n = 10$), osteoarticular allograft ($n = 13$) or a modular tumour prosthesis ($n = 14$) over a mean follow-up of 10 years. There was one case of subluxation in osteoarticular group, one case of dislocation in modular prosthesis group and 3 cases of subluxation and 1 case of dislocation in allograft-prosthesis composite group. Scotti et al. [19] in there series of 40 cases of proximal humeral metastasis managed with endoprosthetic reconstruction reported superior dislocation of

the humeral head in 3 cases. The subluxation/dislocation rate in the present series is much lower than that reported with other procedures. This could be attributed to the use of proline mesh, which we applied around the spacer in all our cases. Ioannou et al. [20] in their study to evaluate the postoperative outcomes of reconstructive surgery for malignant and aggressive benign tumours of proximal humerus identified that that stabilization of the prosthesis with the use of mesh avoids instability. Marulanda et al. [21] also advocated the use of a synthetic vascular mesh for proximal humerus reconstruction. In their study of 16 patients with proximal humerus replacements reconstructed with a synthetic mesh, with a follow-up ranging from 13 to 43 months, there was not even a single case of shoulder dislocation. The present study also supports the evidence in favour of mesh reconstruction for proximal humerus reconstruction which reduces subluxation/dislocation and facilitates soft tissue attachment and reconstruction after tumour resection.

There was one case of neuropraxia in the current series. Bickel et al. [22] reported 13 transient nerve palsies in there series of 134 patients who underwent limb-sparing resection for tumours around shoulder girdle. Though loosening of the cemented stem of the modular spacer within the humeral canal was not seen in our series, one should be vigilant enough to look for these changes clinicoradiologically as there may be pain and resorption at the junction of the reconstruct and the humerus.

The functional, psychological, emotional and cosmetic results were acceptable to all our patients and were better than those that have been reported after amputation and use of external prostheses [13]. Furthermore, this spacer can be converted to other available options at any time. If the patient has financial constraints, expected survival time is short (metastasis) and only moderate orthopaedic oncology infrastructure is available; then, the Kuntscher's nail and cementation method is an acceptable treatment. The final decision of the procedure is influenced by patient's age, functional condition, stage of tumour, degree of soft tissue involvement and available expertise and experience of the surgeon. Cemented Kuntscher's nail spacer offers a cost-effective limb salvage procedure with preservation of elbow and hand. The low cost of the implant makes it a good alternative option of treatment in these selected indications.

References

1. Marcove RC, Lewis MM, Huvos AG (1977) En bloc upper humeral interscapulo-thoracic resection. The Tikhoff–Linberg procedure. Clin Orthop Relat Res 124:219–228
2. Frassica JF, Sim FH, Chao EY (1987) Primary malignant bone tumours of the shoulder girdle: surgical technique of resection and reconstruction. Am Surg 53:264–269
3. Gebhardt MC, Roth YF, Mankin HJ (1990) Osteoarticular allografts for reconstruction in the proximal part of the humerus after excision of a musculoskeletal tumour. J Bone Joint Surg [Am] 72:334–345
4. Wada T, Usui M, Isu K, Yamawaki S, Ishii S (1999) Reconstruction and limb salvage after resection for malignant bone tumour of the proximal humerus: a sling procedure using a free vascularised fibular graft. J Bone Joint Surg (Br) 81:808–813
5. Hsu RWW, Wood MB, Sim FH, Chao EYS (1997) Free vascularised fibular grafting for reconstruction after tumour resection. J Bone Joint Surg (Br) 79:36–42
6. Rödl RW, Gosheger G, Gebert C, Lindner N, Ozaki T, Winkelmann W (2002) Reconstruction of the proximal humerus after wide resection of tumours. J Bone Joint Surg (Br) 84:1004–1008
7. O'Connor MI, Sim FH, Chao EY (1996) Limb salvage for neoplasms of the shoulder girdle. Intermediate reconstructive and functional results. J Bone Joint Surg Am 78:1872–1888
8. Shin KH, Park HJ, Yoo JH, Hahn SB (2000) Reconstructive surgery in primary malignant and aggressive benign bone tumour of the proximal humerus. Yonsei Med J 41:304–311
9. Kumar D, Grimer RJ, Abudu A, Carter SR, Tillman RM (2003) Endoprosthetic replacement of the proximal humerus: long-term results. J Bone Joint Surg Br 85:717–722
10. Puri A, Gulia A (2011) An inexpensive reconstruction method after resection in tumours of the proximal humerus with extensive involvement of the diaphysis. Int J Shoulder Surg 5:44–46
11. Malawer MM, Meller I, Dunham WK (1991) A new surgical classification system for shoulder girdle resections. Analysis of 38 patients. Clin Orthop Relat Res 267:33–44
12. Enneking WF, Dunham W, Gebhardt MC, Malawar M, Pritchard DJ (1993) A system for functional evaluation of reconstructive procedures after surgical treatment of tumours musculoskeletal system. Clin Orthop Relat Res 286:241–246
13. De Wilde L, Van Ovost E, Uyttendaele D, Verdonk R (2002) Limb-sparing technique in tumour surgery of the proximal humerus. Rev Chir Orthop 88:373–378
14. Bilgin SS (2012) Reconstruction of proximal humeral defects with shoulder arthrodesis using free vascularized fibular graft. J Bone Joint Surg Am 94:941–948
15. Enneking WF, Eady JL, Burchardt H (1980) Autogenous cortical bone grafts in the reconstruction of segmental skeletal defects. J Bone Joint Surg Am 62:1039–1058
16. De Wilde L, Sys G, Julien Y, Van Ovost E, Poffyn B, Trouilloud P (2003) The reversed delta shoulder prosthesis in reconstruction of the proximal humerus after tumour resection. Acta Orthop Belg 69:495–500
17. Griffiths D, Gikas PD, Jowett C, Bayliss L, Aston W, Skinner J et al (2011) Proximal humeral replacement using a fixed-fulcrum endoprosthesis. J Bone Joint Surg Br 93:399–403
18. Van de Sande MA, Dijksatra PD, Taminiau AH (2011) Proximal humerus reconstruction after tumour resection: biological versus endoprosthetic reconstruction. Int Orthop 35(9):1375–1380
19. Scotti C, Camnasio F, Peretti GM, Fontana F, Fraschini G (2008) Modular prostheses in the treatment of proximal humerus metastases: review of 40 cases. J Orthop Traumatol 9(1):5–10
20. Ioannou M, Papanastassiou J, Athanassiou AE, Ziras N, Kottakis S, Demertzis N (2009) Surgical options in cases of tumorous destruction of the proximal humerus: twenty-one patients followed from 4–9 years. J BUON 14(1):57–61
21. Marulanda GA, Henderson E, Cheong D, Letson GD (2010) Proximal and total humerus reconstruction with the use of an aortograft mesh. Clin Orthop Relat Res 468(11):2896–2903
22. Bickels J, Wittig JC, Kollender Y, Kellar-Graney K, Meller I, Malawer MM (2002) Limb-sparing resections of the shoulder girdle. J Am Coll Surg 194(4):422–435

29

Cytotoxic agents are detrimental to bone formed by distraction osteogenesis

Fergal P. Monsell · James Ralph Barnes ·
M. C. Bellemore · L. Biston · Allen Goodship

Abstract Distraction osteogenesis can be used to replace segmental bone loss when treating malignant bone tumors in children and adolescents. These patients often receive cytotoxic chemotherapy as part of their treatment regimen. The effect of cytotoxic drugs on the cellular processes during distraction osteogenesis and the structural and mechanical properties of regenerate bone is unknown. We therefore used a rabbit model of distraction osteogenesis to determine that cytotoxic agents had a detrimental effect on regenerate bone formed by this technique. We administered adriamycin and cisplatinum to 20 rabbits using two different simulated chemotherapy regimens. All rabbits underwent an osteotomy at 12 weeks of age. Distraction osteogenesis began 24 h later at a rate of 0.75 mm a day for 10 days, followed by 18 days without correction to allow for consolidation. Regenerate bone was assessed using plain radiographs, bone densitometry, and mechanical testing. Peri-operative chemotherapy decreased the mechanical properties of the regenerate with regard to yield strain (3.7×10^{-2} vs. 5.2×10^{-2}) and energy at yield (2.73×10^7 vs. 3.92×10^7). Preoperative chemotherapy in isolation reduced bone mineral density (0.38 vs. 0.5 g/cm^2), bone mineral content (0.24 vs. 0.36 g), and volumetric bone mineral density (0.57 vs. 0.65 g/cm^2) with no alterations in the mechanical properties. Conclusions: Preoperative chemotherapy appears to decrease the volume of regenerate bone, without affecting structural integrity, suggesting that the callus formed is of good quality. The converse appears true for peri-operative chemotherapy.

Keywords Osteogenesis · External fixator · Cytotoxic · Chemotherapy · Rabbit · Tibia · Bone tumor

F. P. Monsell (✉) · J. R. Barnes
Department of Paediatric Orthopaedic Surgery, Bristol Royal Hospital for Children, Paul O'Gorman Building, Upper Maudlin Street, Bristol BS2 8BJ, UK
e-mail: fergal.monsell@uhbristol.nhs.uk

J. R. Barnes
e-mail: jamesralphbarnes@yahoo.co.uk

M. C. Bellemore
Department of Orthopaedic Surgery, Royal Alexandra Hospital for Children, Sydney, Australia

L. Biston
Prince of Wales Medical Research Institute and Faculty of Medicine, University of New South Wales, Sydney, Australia

A. Goodship
Institute of Orthopaedics and Musculoskeletal Science UCL, Royal National Orthopaedic Hospital, Stanmorem, London, UK

Introduction

The treatment of malignant bone tumors in children and adolescents has improved over the last four decades as a result of progress in many disciplines. The development of potent cytotoxic agents has been of fundamental importance and initially involved a multiagent approach [8, 17, 27, 28]. Subsequently, a regimen using only two agents (adriamycin and cisplatinum) not only produced equivalent 15-year disease-free survival (DFS) and overall survival (OS) [4, 35], but that there was also only a 9 % rate of local recurrence [34]. This decreased rate of local recurrence has allowed limb-sparing surgery to be used more frequently after tumor excision.

The use of endoprostheses in the reconstruction of the distal femur has been reported to give good or excellent functional results in 83 % of patients, with a 10 year survivorship of 77 % [3, 26]. Even in patients with substantial growth remaining, expandable and adjustable prostheses have shown satisfactory functional outcomes in 71 % of patients, assessed using the American Musculoskeletal Tumor Society (AMSTS) functional rating system [6, 10, 32].

Reconstruction using extensive allograft has also been described for treating osteogenic and Ewing's sarcoma but is associated with 77 % complication rate (other than a limb-length discrepancy) and 54 % rate of allograft fracture [1, 20]. Reconstruction with microvascular-free fibular grafts has also been reported with decreased fatigue fracture and nonunion compared to allograft and an AMSTS of good or excellent in 85 % of patients [11, 23, 33].

Distraction osteogenesis is a surgical technique sometimes used to regenerate bone, equalize limb lengths, and replace segmental bone loss [5, 12–15]. Tsuchiya et al. [37] also reported a decreased external fixation index (34 days/cm vs. 40 days/cm) and good or excellent functional results in 89 % of patients when using this technique compared to bone transport when reconstructing extensive defects (average 8.4 cm) after excising skeletal tumors [36]. Distraction osteogenesis relies on the ability of the body to generate enough bone to not only fill the defect left by tumor excision, but also to be robust enough to allow the individual to weight bear. Any interruption to these cellular processes could have a detrimental effect on new bone formation, which in turn could lead to failure through the regenerate bone. To date, we do not know the effect of a multiagent chemotherapy regimen on these processes, and this study was designed to address the deficiencies in the literature.

The questions we aimed to address in our study were as follows:

1. Do cytotoxic agents affect the structural properties of new bone formed by distraction osteogenesis?
2. Do cytotoxic agents affect the mechanical integrity of regenerate bone?
3. Does the timing of chemotherapy influences this affect?

Materials and methods

Forty rabbits were divided equally and assigned on a random basis into two groups. Preoperative cycles of cisplatinum and adriamycin were used to simulate the clinical protocols reported by Malawer et al. [19] and pre- and postoperative cycles to simulate the cytotoxic regimen used by the European Osteosarcoma Intergroup [4, 35].

In the preoperative chemotherapy group, cisplatinum and adriamycin were administered in combination at 8 weeks of age, with a second infusion 14 days later at 10 weeks of age.

In the postoperative group, cisplatinum and adriamycin were administered in combination 10 days prior to and 4 days after the osteotomy, in order to standardize the interval between infusions at 14 days.

In both groups, the infusion was either an initial 1 mg/kg cisplatinum and 2 mg/kg adriamycin followed by a second infusion of 1 mg/kg cisplatinum and 4 mg/kg adriamycin or an identical volume of normal saline at identical points (Fig. 1).

We did not perform a priori power analysis as the literature was deficient, and no relevant data were available. This study should be regarded as a pilot and has generated an hypothesis that will form the basis of further research.

For all surgical procedures, animals were premedicated 30 min before with 10 mg/kg intramuscular ketamine (Parnell Laboratories Australia Pty Ltd, Alexandria, New South Wales, Australia), 4 mg/kg of xylazine (Ilium Xylazil-20; Troy Laboratories Pty Ltd, Smithfield, New South Wales, Australia), and 0.05 mg/kg of buprenorphine (Reckitt & Coleman Products Ltd, Hull, UK). General anesthesia was induced through a face mask using an enflurane (Abbott Australia Pty Ltd Botany, New South Wales, Australia) and a nitrous oxide/oxygen mixture. After each anesthetic, the animal was observed until alert and drinking before being returned to its cage.

Through an incision in the right groin, a 20-gauge intravenous cannula (Terumo Corporation, Tokyo, Japan) was inserted into the femoral vein and secured between two silk sutures providing a watertight seal. About 50 mL adriamycin/cisplatinum (intervention) or 50 mL normal saline (control) was infused over 2 h using an IVAC® syringe pump (ALARIS Medical Systems Australia, Pty Ltd Seven Hills, New South Wales, Australia). Two weeks later, a second infusion was administered using an identical approach through the left femoral vein.

The tibial osteotomy was performed at 12 weeks of age in an attempt to reproduce the stage of skeletal development equivalent to a human adolescent [16]. The right leg was shaved and prepared with chlorhexidine. A medial longitudinal skin incision was used with subperiosteal exposure of the tibia along its length. Three-millimeter external fixator pins (Orthofix, Bussolengo, Italy) were inserted 1.5 cm proximal and distal to the midtibial diaphysis using a standard jig and power drill. We determined the positions of the remaining two pins using the jig to create a standard configuration of pins accurately aligned along the length of the tibia. An M100 monolateral fixator (Orthofix) was then secured approximately 1.5 cm from the skin to accommodate for postoperative swelling. The osteotomy was performed by predrilling the diaphysis and completing the osteotomy with bone cutters.

Fig. 1 Illustration showing the chemotherapy regimens used

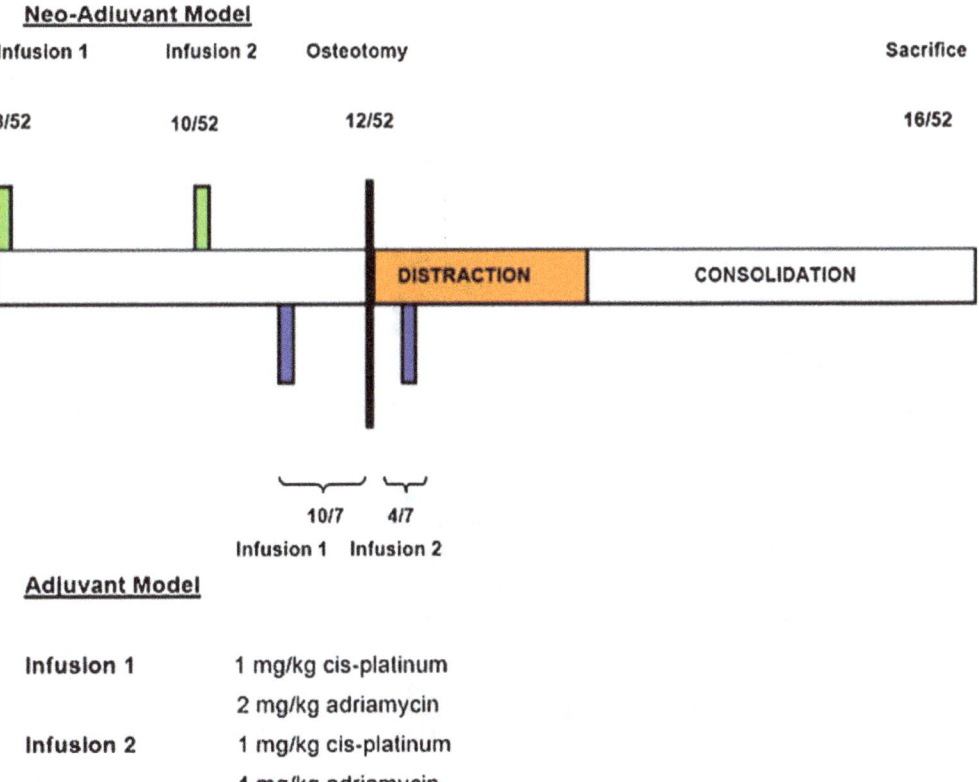

Neo-Adjuvant Model

| Infusion 1 | Infusion 2 | Osteotomy | | Sacrifice |

8/52   10/52   12/52   16/52

DISTRACTION   CONSOLIDATION

10/7   4/7
Infusion 1   Infusion 2

Adjuvant Model

Infusion 1	1 mg/kg cis-platinum
	2 mg/kg adriamycin
Infusion 2	1 mg/kg cis-platinum
	4 mg/kg adriamycin

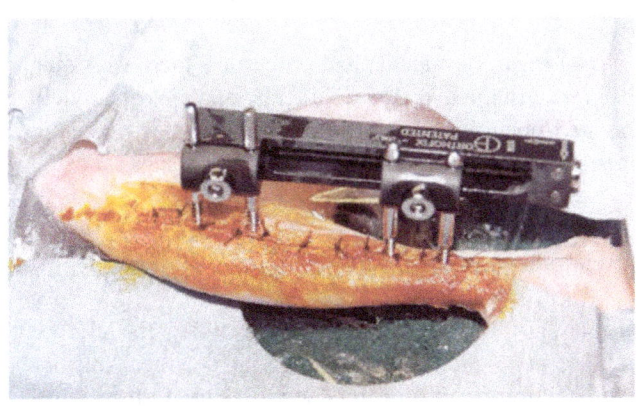

Fig. 2 Orthofix *M* 100 External fixator in situ after middiaphyseal tibial osteotomy

The wound was then closed with interrupted sutures (Fig. 2) and dressed with povidone-iodine ointment (Professional Disposables Inc, Orangeburg, NY, USA).

Distraction osteogenesis began 24 h after surgery. The fixator was distracted by a half turn every 12 h for 10 days, followed by a period of 18 days to allow the consolidation of the regenerate.

Animals in both arms of the study were euthanized. At 16 weeks of age, the right hind limb was disarticulated and aligned to produce consistent craniocaudal and mediolateral images with a Siemens (Erlangen, Germany) Multix H/UPH configuration with a focus to film distance of 100 cm and a 50-kV ($\pm$2 mV) and 4-mA exposure (Fig. 3). A single observer (FPM) assessed regenerate length, AP, and lateral alignment on the orthogonal images.

Bone density measurements were made using a total body dual-energy X-ray densitometer (DXA; LUNAR DPX; LUNAR Radiation Corp, Madison, WI, USA) and software designed for measuring small animals (LUNAR DPX, Small Animal Software Version 1.0; LUNAR Radiation Corp). The distance from the knee to the top of the callus and the height of the callus were measured and recorded. Each scan produced values for bone mineral density (BMD), bone mineral content (BMC), and volumetric bone mineral density (vBMD). vBMD was calculated assuming that the bone is an elliptical cylinder.

The area of the cross - section of bone
$$= \pi \times \frac{(\text{AP Bone Width})}{2} \times \frac{(\text{Lat Bone Width})}{2}.$$

The volume of the region V = Cross-sectional Bone Area $\times$ ROI Height

$$\text{Volumetric BMD}(g/cm^3) = \frac{BMC}{V}$$

The tibiofibular complex was embedded in the mounting block and placed in an Instron mechanical testing machine (Instron Corporation, Norwood, MA, USA). Similar to comparable studies [18], the tibia was loaded in compression to failure at a rate of 2 mm/min using a 10-kN

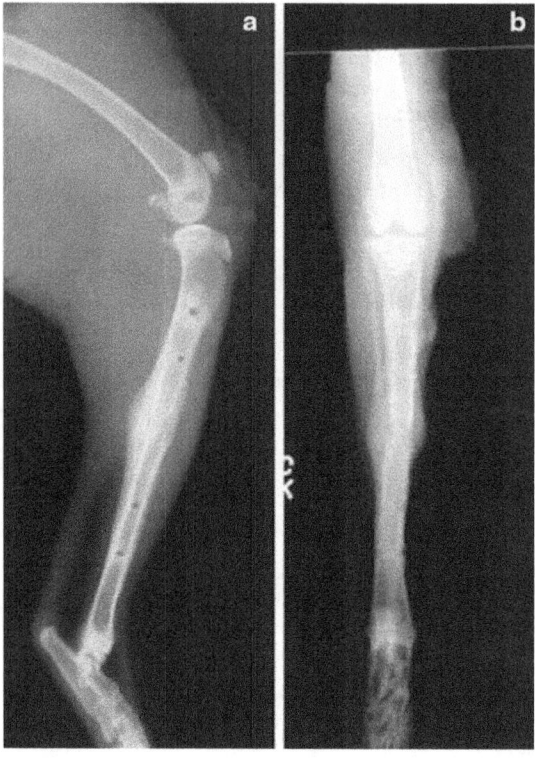

Fig. 3 a Lateral and **b** AP radiographs of the tibia after removal of the fixator. Note the elliptical callus formation, the limb alignment, and the distance between the osteotomy and the pin sites

load cell. The length of exposed bone (lo) was measured before compression testing. This was standardized during mounting, ensuring that the polyester resin covered the screw holes adjacent to the regenerate. It was assumed that the regenerate was elliptical, and the mean area was calculated from DXA measurements. The load/displacement data were transformed to produce stress/strain data using the following formula:

$$\frac{\text{Stress}}{\text{Strain}} = \frac{\text{Load/Area}}{\text{Displacement/l}_o}$$

The data were transferred to Easy Plot (Spiral Software, Maryland, USA), and stress strain curves were produced for each specimen.

After mechanical testing, the regenerates were decalcified and stained with hematoxylin and eosin. One assessor (JRB) ( ) blinded to the identity of each specimen was used to undertake histological examination of each slide (Fig. 4a, b). Cortical thickening was assessed by taking [3] separate measurements from the endosteal to the periosteal surface of the regenerate bone, and the mean thickness was calculated for each specimen and used for comparison. Modularization was determined by the trabecular bone volume. This is the relative volume of total cancellous bone occupied by trabeculae, expressed as a percentage

[25]. A Shapiro–Wilk test was used to confirm data produced by mechanical testing, and DEXA analysis was normally distributed, before an unpaired t test was used. The two-sided statistic with a 95 % confidence interval was used in each case.

For histological analysis, a Mann–Whitney U test was used to compare the histological parameters between intervention and control groups.

Results

Structurally, preoperative chemotherapy had a detrimental effect on BMD ($p < 0.01$), BMC ($p = 0.02$), and vBMD ($p = 0.04$; Table 1, data produced by DEXA analysis) compared with a control population.

We observed a reduction ($p = 0.97$) in the modulus of elasticity from 5.47 to 5.15 ($\times 10^3$), which would be expected, because the modulus/stiffness is dependent on the degree of mineralization (Table 2).

There was no difference in BMD, BMC, or vBMD in the peri-operative group compared with the control. Histologically, there was a trend for decreased cortical thickness in both chemotherapy groups compared with control populations, but these data were not statistically significant ($p = 0.06$ and 0.12; Table 3, data produced by histological assessment).

With regard to mechanical properties, there was a major difference in the average yield strain and energy at yield of the peri-operative group when compared to the control population (Table 2, data produced by mechanical testing).

Discussion

The aim of this study was to investigate the effects of multiagent cytotoxic agents on both the mechanical and structural properties of regenerate bone formed by distraction osteogenesis in a rabbit model. The clinical relevance of this work was to highlight the concerns with reconstruction of segmental defects after malignant bone tumor excision by distraction osteogenesis in the presence of cytotoxic chemotherapy. But the limitations of the study are clear and direct comparisons should not be made.

Interpretation of the clinical relevance of this work requires an analysis of the effect on the material and mechanical characteristics of the regenerate bone. The clinical issue is whether observed differences matter and are of sufficient concern to prevent reconstruction by this method.

Readers should be aware of the limitations of our study. First, the group sizes proved to be barely adequate to allow robust statistical analysis of the mechanical parameters, and future work should focus on a single specific area with

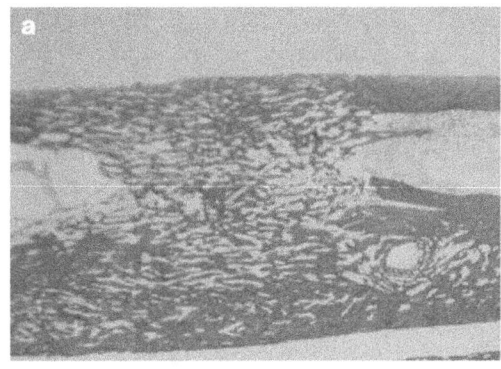 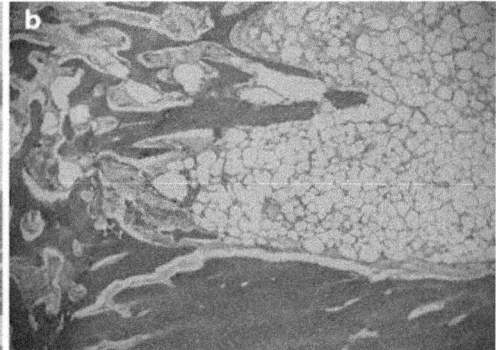

Fig. 4 a Hematoxylin and eosin stain (original magnification, × 4) showing consolidated regenerate bone at the tibial osteotomy site after distraction. **b** Hematoxylin and eosin (original magnification, × 10) showing medullary/regenerate interface showing partial modularization of the regenerate bone

Table 1 Data obtained from DXA

	Pre-operative group	Peri-operative group
Mean value of BMC (g)		
Intervention	0.24	0.23
Control	0.36	0.22
p value	0.02	0.79
Mean value of BMD (g/cm2)		
Intervention	0.38	0.4
Control	0.5	0.4
p value	<0.01	0.97
Mean value of vBMD (g/cm3)		
Intervention	0.57	0.67
Control	0.65	0.63
p value	0.04	0.34

Table 2 Data obtained from mehanical testing

	Pre-operative group	Peri-operative group
Mean modulus of elasticity (Pa)		
Intervention	5.88×10^8	5.65×10^8
Control	5.92×10^8	4.62×10^8
p value	0.97	0.32
Mean energy at yield		
Intervention	2.45×10^7	2.73×10^7
Control	3.14×10^7	3.92×10^7
p value	0.31	0.01
Mean yield stress		
Intervention	1.64×10^7	1.68×10^7
Control	1.63×10^7	1.89×10^7
p value	0.94	0.39
Mean yield strain		
Intervention	3.2×10^{-2}	3.7×10^{-2}
Control	3.7×10^{-2}	5.2×10^{-2}
p value	0.44	0.01
Mean energy at failure		
Intervention	4.92×10^7	5.25×10^7
Control	5.48×10^7	6.41×10^7
p value	0.59	0.27
Mean failure stress		
Intervention	1.95×10^7	1.89×10^7
Control	1.87×10^7	1.98×10
p value	0.71	0.67
Mean failure strain		
Intervention	4.7×10^{-2}	5.2×10^{-2}
Control	5.4×10^{-2}	6.4×10^{-2}
p value	0.41	0.11
Mean postyield energy		
Intervention	5.63×10^7	2.51×10^7
Control	2.34×10^7	2.48×10^7
p value	0.31	0.97

a larger number of animal pairs. Second, we used plain radiographs to assess the morphology of the regenerate and determine the alignment of the lengthened bone in two orthogonal (AP and lateral) planes; however, the accuracy of plain radiographs is limited. Third, DXA does not account for the spatial distribution and inherent material properties of the tissues. While DXA has been used in similar studies 18, alternative methods of assessment include peripheral quantified CT (pQCT) and single photon emission CT. pQCT would have offered a potentially superior method of assessment [21, 22] and should be considered as a method of assessment in future work. Fourth, the regimen chosen was rudimentary when compared to current multiagent regimens used in clinical practice. The purpose of this study was to investigate the effects of cytotoxic agents on osteogenesis in general and not the efficacy of a specific regimen.

Table 3 Histologiocal data

	Mean cortical thickness (mm)
Peri-operative chemotherapy	
Intervention	2.51
Control	3.81
p value	0.06
Postoperative chemotherapy	
Intervention	2.46
Control	3.12
p value	0.12

Decrease in weight has been identified in previous animal studies as an indicator of cytotoxic effect [38]. This effect is also seen in human clinical practice and is the result of several factors, including anorexia and a catabolic response to cytotoxic drugs. We demonstrated this difference in each experimental group, suggesting that the animals received clinically relevant amounts of cisplatinum and adriamycin. It was not possible to quantify the mechanism leading to this observation, because food and water were given ad libitum.

There were major differences noted in BMC, BMD, and vBMD with reduction in the preoperative chemotherapy group. This observation was likely to be a real effect and contradicts previous work [7] that did not demonstrate an alteration in DXA parameters after cisplatinum infusion. A possible explanation is that the addition of adriamycin has produced a more profound effect on regenerate mineralization, but more detailed comment is not possible from the data produced.

Failure occurs on the compression side of an eccentrically loaded bone, leading to progressive bending of regenerate, which is observed in clinical practice. This mode of failure is simulated by axial compression, which was considered most representative of the in vivo mode of failure. Previous studies [2, 24] have demonstrated a relationship between structural and mechanical properties of bone with this type of compression testing, and a simple uniaxial loading test provided a reproducible method of analysis for this experiment.

The experiment required reproducible longitudinal alignment of the bone during compression testing, and this was achieved using a mounting block. The mounting block consisted of two cylinders with an adjustable connector to accommodate variable bone lengths.

The lack of effect on the structural properties of regenerate is in agreement with Gravel et al. [9], even with the addition of cisplatinum.

The mechanism in which adriamycin and cisplatinum affect regenerate mineralization is not clear. The formation of regenerate bone involves a sequence of events, including neoangiogenesis [29], chondrocyte differentiation with expression of bone matrix proteins [31], and collagen I formation [39]. Adriamycin causes structural alterations in normal bone with reduction in cortical thickness, histological changes within the physeal plate, marrow hypoplasia [40], and specifically inhibits prolyl hydroxylation, leading to loss of stability of procollagen [30]. Cisplatinum causes histomorphometric changes in bone, including decreased volume of mineralized bone volume and decreased proportion of osteoblast-covered bone [7].

In the peri-operative group, there was no observed difference in bone mineralization, which concurs with previous work by Erhart et al. [7]. The power of these observations was however low, and this may represent a Type II error. The high power of the equivalent observations in the preoperative group is highly suggestive of a real effect, and the difference between groups may be spurious.

Of interest in the peri-operative group are the major differences in energy at yield and yield strain with difference in means of 30 % (energy at yield) and 29 % (yield strain) and appropriate statistical power. This is suggestive of a real effect and may have clinical implications, particularly because the main concern in human practice is of regenerate failure after fixator removal. The reduction in energy at yield after cytotoxic chemotherapy is likely to be clinically important and if translated into human practice may represent an increased risk of regenerate failure after limb reconstruction. This may require either prolonged fixator wear or external support after fixator removal; however, further research is required to quantify this. Definition of a chemotherapy regimen that would have a clinically irrelevant effect on the material properties of the regenerate is beyond the scope of this experiment.

It has been possible to develop a reproducible model of limb lengthening in this species. Bone is consistently formed in the distraction gap, and the overall alignment was satisfactory in all lengthened limbs. This model is suitable for future experiments investigating limb lengthening in the juvenile New Zealand white rabbit. We have observed that cytotoxic chemotherapy has a detrimental affect on bone formed in a lapine model of distraction osteogenesis. This should add a note of caution to the use of this technique for reconstruction in a clinical context, but this study is unable to address the effect of conventional chemotherapy regimens in human subjects.

Acknowledgments We would like to thank Mr Michael Parry MD. This work was funded by the Ingham foundation and the Financial Markets Foundation for Children.

References

1. Alman BA, De Bari A, Krajbich JI (1995) Massive allografts in the treatment of osteosarcoma and Ewing sarcoma in children and adolescents. J Bone Joint Surg Am 77(1):54–64
2. An HS, Xu R, Lim TH, McGrady L, Wilson C (1994) Prediction of bone graft strength using dual-energy radiographic absorptiometry. Spine 19(20):2358–2362
3. Bradish CF, Kemp HB, Scales JT, Wilson JN (1987) Distal femoral replacement by custom-made prostheses. Clinical follow-up and survivorship analysis. J Bone Joint Surg Br 69(2):276–284
4. Bramwell VH, Burgers M, Sneath R et al (1992) A comparison of two short intensive adjuvant chemotherapy regimens in operable osteosarcoma of limbs in children and young adults: the first study of the European Osteosarcoma Intergroup. J Clin Oncol 10(10):1579–1591
5. De Bastiani G, Aldegheri R, Renzi-Brivio L, Trivella G (1987) Limb lengthening by callus distraction (callotasis). J Pediatr Orthop 7(2):129–134
6. Eckardt JJ, Safran MR, Eilber FR, Rosen G, Kabo JM (1993) Expandable endoprosthetic reconstruction of the skeletally immature after malignant bone tumor resection. Clin Orthop Relat Res 297:188–202
7. Ehrhart N, Eurell JA, Tommasini M, Constable PD, Johnson AL, Feretti A (2002) Effect of cisplatin on bone transport osteogenesis in dogs. Am J Vet Res 63(5):703–711
8. Eilber F, Giuliano A, Eckardt J, Patterson K, Moseley S, Goodnight J (1987) Adjuvant chemotherapy for osteosarcoma: a randomized prospective trial. J Clin Oncol 5(1):21–26
9. Gravel CA, Le TT, Chapman MW. Effect of neoadjuvant chemotherapy on distraction osteogenesis in the goat model. *Clin Orthop Relat Res*. 2003(412):213-224. Epub 2003/07/03
10. Gupta A, Pollock R, Cannon SR, Briggs TW, Skinner J, Blunn G (2006) A knee-sparing distal femoral endoprosthesis using hydroxyapatite-coated extracortical plates Preliminary results. J Bone Joint Surg Br 88(10):1367–1372
11. Hsu RW, Wood MB, Sim FH, Chao EY (1997) Free vascularised fibular grafting for reconstruction after tumour resection. J Bone Joint Surg Br 79(1):36–42
12. Ilizarov GA. The tension-stress effect on the genesis and growth of tissues. Part I. The influence of stability of fixation and soft-tissue preservation. *ClinOrthopRelat Res*. 1989(238):249-281
13. Ilizarov GA. The tension-stress effect on the genesis and growth of tissues: Part II. The influence of the rate and frequency of distraction. *ClinOrthopRelat Res*. 1989(239):263-285
14. Ilizarov GA (1990) Clinical application of the tension-stress effect for limb lengthening. Clin Orthop Relat Res 250:8–26
15. Ilizarov GA, Ledyaev VI (1969) The replacement of long tubular bone defects by lengthening distraction osteotomy of one of the fragments. Clin Orthop Relat Res 1992(280):7–10
16. Kaweblum M, Aguilar MC, Blancas E et al (1994) Histological and radiographic determination of the age of physeal closure of the distal femur, proximal tibia, and proximal fibula of the New Zealand white rabbit. J Orthop Res 12(5):747–749
17. Link MP, Goorin AM, Miser AW et al (1986) The effect of adjuvant chemotherapy on relapse-free survival in patients with osteosarcoma of the extremity. N Engl J Med 314(25):1600–1606
18. Little DG, Smith NC, Williams PR et al (2003) Zoledronic acid prevents osteopenia and increases bone strength in a rabbit model of distraction osteogenesis. J Bone Miner Res 18(7):1300–1307 Epub 2003/07/12
19. Malawer M, Buch R, Reaman G et al (1991) Impact of two cycles of preoperative chemotherapy with intraarterial cisplatin and intravenous doxorubicin on the choice of surgical procedure for high-grade bone sarcomas of the extremities. Clin Orthop Relat Res 270:214–222
20. Mankin HJ, Gebhardt MC, Tomford WW (1987) The use of frozen cadaveric allografts in the management of patients with bone tumors of the extremities. Orthop Clin North Am 18(2):275–289
21. Markel MD, Chao EY (1993) Noninvasive monitoring techniques for quantitative description of callus mineral content and mechanical properties. Clin Orthop 293:37–45
22. Markel MD, Wikenheiser MA, Morin RL, Lewallen DG, Chao EY (1991) The determination of bone fracture properties by dual-energy X-ray absorptiometry and single-photon absorptiometry: a comparative study. Calcif Tissue Int 48(6):392–399
23. Moore JR, Weiland AJ, Daniel RK (1983) Use of free vascularized bone grafts in the treatment of bone tumors. Clin Orthop Relat Res 175:37–44
24. Ohyama M, Miyasaka Y, Sakurai M, Yokobori AT Jr, Sasaki S (1994) The mechanical behavior and morphological structure of callus in experimental callotasis. Biomed Mater Eng 4(4):273–281 Epub 1994/01/01
25. Recker RR. Bone histomorphometry: techniques and interpretation. Recker RR, editor. Boca Raton, FL: CRC Press; 1983
26. Roberts P, Chan D, Grimer RJ, Sneath RS, Scales JT (1991) Prosthetic replacement of the distal femur for primary bone tumours. J Bone Joint Surg Br 73(5):762–769
27. Rosen G (1985) Preoperative (neoadjuvant) chemotherapy for osteogenic sarcoma: a 10 year experience. Orthopedics 8(5):659–664
28. Rosen G, Marcove RC, Huvos AG et al (1983) Primary osteogenic sarcoma: eight-year experience with adjuvant chemotherapy. J Cancer Res Clin Oncol 106(Suppl):55–67
29. Rowe NM, Mehrara BJ, Luchs JS et al (1999) Angiogenesis during mandibular distraction osteogenesis. Ann Plast Surg 42(5):470–475 Epub 1999/05/26
30. Sasaki T, Holeyfield KC, Uitto J. Doxorubicin-induced inhibition of prolyl hydroxylation during collagen biosynthesis in human skin fibroblast cultures. Relevance to impaired wound healing. *J ClinInvest*. 1987;80(6):1735-1741
31. Sato M, Yasui N, Nakase T et al (1998) Expression of bone matrix proteins mRNA during distraction osteogenesis. J Bone Miner Res 13(8):1221–1231 Epub 1998/08/26
32. Schiller C, Windhager R, Fellinger EJ, Salzer-Kuntschik M, Kaider A, Kotz R (1995) Extendable tumour endoprostheses for the leg in children. J Bone Joint Surg Br 77(4):608–614
33. Shea KG, Coleman DA, Scott SM, Coleman SS, Christianson M (1997) Microvascularized free fibular grafts for reconstruction of skeletal defects after tumor resection. J Pediatr Orthop 17(4):424–432
34. Simon MA, Aschliman MA, Thomas N, Mankin HJ (1986) Limb-salvage treatment versus amputation for osteosarcoma of the distal end of the femur. J Bone Joint Surg Am 68(9):1331–1337
35. Souhami RL, Craft AW, Van der Eijken JW et al (1997) Randomised trial of two regimens of chemotherapy in operable osteosarcoma: a study of the European Osteosarcoma Intergroup. Lancet 350(9082):911–917
36. Tsuchiya H, Abdel-Wanis ME, Sakurakichi K, Yamashiro T, Tomita K. Osteosarcoma around the knee. Intraepiphyseal excision and biological reconstruction with distraction osteogenesis. *JBone Joint SurgBr*. 2002;84(8):1162-1166
37. Tsuchiya H, Tomita K, Minematsu K, Mori Y, Asada N, Kitano S. Limb salvage using distraction osteogenesis. A classification of the technique. *JBone Joint SurgBr*. 1997;79(3):403-411
38. Wanless RB, Anand IS, Poole-Wilson PA, Harris P (1987) An experimental model of chronic cardiac failure using adriamycin in the rabbit: central haemodynamics and regional blood flow. Cardiovasc Res 21(1):7–13

Permissions

List of Contributors

T. Monni, P. de Lange and C. H. Snyckers
Steve Biko Academic Hospital, Pretoria, Gauteng, South Africa Department of Orthopaedics, University of Pretoria, Pretoria, Gauteng, South Africa

F. F. Birkholtz
Private Practise, Netcare Unitas Hospital, Pretoria, Gauteng, South Africa

Alec Cikes, Étienne Trudeau-Rivest, Fanny Canet, Jonah Hébert-Davies and Dominique M. Rouleau
Hôpital du Sacré-Coeur de Montréal (HSCM), 5400 Gouin Ouest, Local C-2095, Montreal, QC H4J 1C5, Canada
Synergie-Medical Center, Rue du Grand-Pré 2B, 1007 Lausanne, Switzerland
University of Montreal, 2900 Boulevard Edouard-Montpetit, Montreal, QC H3T 1J4, Canada

Sherif Ahmed El Ghazaly and El-Hussein Mohamed El-Moatasem
Orthopedic Department, Al-Demerdash Hospital, Ain Shams University, Abbassia Square, Abbassia, 11381 Cairo, Egypt

Konstantin Horas
Bone Research Program, ANZAC Research Institute, University of Sydney, Gate 3 Hospital Road, Concord 2139, Australia

Reinhard Schnettler and Gerrit Maier
Department of Trauma Surgery/Laboratory of Experimental Trauma Surgery, Justus-Liebig-University, Rudolf- Buchheim-Str. 7, 35392 Giessen, Germany

Gaby Schneider
Institute of Mathematics, Goethe-University, Robert-Mayer- Str. 10, 60325 Frankfurt, Germany

Uwe Horas
Department of Orthopaedic and Trauma Surgery, Kliniken des Main-Taunus-Kreises GmbH, Kronberger Str. 36, 65812 Bad Soden, Germany

S. S. Madan, K. Robinson, P. D. Kasliwal, M. J. Bell, M. Saleh and J. A. Fernandes
Department of Trauma and Orthopaedic Surgery, Sheffield Children's NHS Foundation Trust, Western Bank, Sheffield S10 2TH, UK

Paul Dearden, Kathryn Lowery, Kevin Sherman and Hemant Sharma
Hull Royal Infirmary, Anlaby Road, Hull, UK

Vishy Mahadevan
Royal College of Surgeons, England, UK

Tatyana N. Varsegova, Natalia A. Shchudlo, Mikhail M. Shchudlo, Marat S. Saifutdinov and Mikhail A. Stepanov
Russian Ilizarov Scientific Center for Restorative Traumatology and Orthopaedics, 6, M.Ulyanova Street, Kurgan, Russian Federation 6640014

Narinder Kumar and Vyom Sharma
Military Hospital, Kirkee, Pune, Maharashtra 411020, India

Richard C. Barksfield, James Ralph Barnes and Fergal P. Monsell
Department of Paediatric Orthopaedic Surgery, Bristol Royal Hospital for Children, Paul O'Gorman Building, Upper Maudlin Street, Bristol BS2 8BJ, UK

Edgardo R. Rodriguez-Collazo
Department of Surgery, Presence Saint Joseph Hospital, 2900 N Lake Shore Dr., Chicago, IL 60657, USA

Maria L. Urso
Arteriocyte Medical Systems, 45 South St., Suite 3, Hopkinton, MA 01748, USA

Rasmus Elsoe, Søren Kold and Juozas Petruskevicius
Department of Orthopaedic Surgery, Aalborg University Hospital, Aalborg University, 18-22 Hobrovej, 9000 Aalborg, Denmark
Department of Orthopaedics, Aarhus University Hospital, Århus, Denmark

Peter Larsen
Department of Occupational Therapy and Physiotherapy, Aalborg University Hospital, Aalborg University, 18-22 Hobrovej, 9000 Aalborg, Denmark

Julian Fürmetz, Nikola Schuster, Florian Wolf and Peter H. Thaller
3D-Surgery, Department of General, Trauma and Reconstructive Surgery, Munich University Hospital LMU, Germany, Nußbaumstraße 20, 80336 Munich, Germany

Mohamed F. Mostafa, Yasser Y. Abed and Sallam I. Fawzy
Orthopedic Oncology Unit, Department of Orthopedic Surgery, Mansoura University Hospital, 36 Al-Gomhoria Street, Mansoura, Egypt

Valentino Coppa, Luca Dei Giudici and Antonio Gigante
Clinical Orthopaedics, Department of Clinical and Molecular Science, School of Medicine, Università Politecnica delle Marche, Via Tronto, 10/A, 60126 Ancona, Italy

Stefano Cecconi and Mario Marinelli
Clinic of Adult and Paediatric Orthopaedic, Azienda Ospedaliero-Universitaria, Ospedali Riuniti di Ancona, Ancona, Italy

Austin T. Fragomen
Weill Medical College, Cornell University, 535 East 70th Street, New York, NY 10021, USA
Hospital for Special Surgery, 535 East 70th Street, New York, NY 10021, USA

Fiona R. Fragomen
Hospital for Special Surgery, 535 East 70th Street, New York, NY 10021, USA

John Ham, Mark Flipsen, Marianne Koolen and Arnard van der Zwan
Orthopædic Department, Expertise Center MO, OLVG, Amsterdam, The Netherlands

Konrad Mader
Section Upper Extremity, Department of Orthopaedic, Trauma and Spine Surgery, Asklepios Klinik Altona, 22763 Hamburg, Germany
Berliner Freiheit 9, Aalto- Hochhaus 14/9, 28327 Bremen, Germany

Lalit Maini, Santosh Kumar, Sahil Batra and Rajat Gupta
Department of Orthopaedic Surgery, Maulana Azad Medical College and Associated Lok Nayak Hospital, New Delhi 110002, India

Sumit Arora
Department of Orthopaedic Surgery, Maulana Azad Medical College and Associated Lok Nayak Hospital, New Delhi 110002, India
C/o Mr. Sham Khanna, 2/2, Vijay Nagar, Delhi 110009, India

Yasser Elbatrawy
Department of Orthopedic Surgery and Traumatology, Al-Azhar University Hospital, Assiut, Egypt

Francesco Sala and Dario Capitani
Department of Orthopedic Surgery and Traumatology, Niguarda Hospital, Piazza Ospedale Maggiore 3, 20162 Milan, Italy

Giovanni Lovisetti and Salvatore Alati
Department of Orthopedic Surgery and Traumatology, Menaggio Hospital, Menaggio, CO, Italy

Ibrahim Elsayed Abdellatif Abuomira
Department of Orthopedic Surgery and Traumatology, Al-Azhar University Hospital, Assiut, Egypt
2 Nile Street, Sohâg, Egypt

J. A. D. van der Woude, S. Spruijt and B. T. J. van Ginneken
Limb Deformity Reconstruction Unit, Department of Orthopaedic Surgery, Maartenskliniek Woerden, Polanerbaan 2, 3447 GN Woerden, The Netherlands

R. J. van Heerwaarden
Centre for Deformity Correction and Joint Preserving Surgery, Kliniek ViaSana, Hoogveldseweg 1, 5451 AA Mill, The Netherlands

Mootaz F. Thakeb, Mahmoud A. Mahran and El-Hussein M. El-Motassem
The Department of Orthopedic Surgery, Ain Shams University, Cairo, Egypt

Anna C. Peek, Anna Timms, Kuen F. Chin, Peter Calder and David Goodier
Royal National Orthopaedic Hospital, Stanmore, UK

Levent Eralp
Department of Orthopaedics and Traumatology, Istanbul Faculty of Medicine, Istanbul University, 34390 Topkapi, Istanbul, Turkey

F. Erkal Bilen and Mehmet Kocaoglu
Department of Orthopaedics and Traumatology, Memorial Health Group, 34385 Okmeydani, Istanbul, Turkey

S. Robert Rozbruch
Hospital for Special Surgery, Limb Lengthening and Complex Reconstruction Service (LLCRS), Weill Cornell Medical College, Cornell University, 535 East 70th Street, New York, NY 10021, USA

Ahmed I. Hammoudi
Orthopedic Department, Faculty of Medicine, Al-Azhar University Hospitals, Nasr City, Cairo 11884, Egypt

Konstantinos Tsitskaris, Heledd Havard and Robert A. Hill
Department of Orthopaedics, Great Ormond Street Hospital for Children, London WC1N 3JH, UK

Paulien Bijlsma
Department of Orthopaedics, St Mary's Hospital and Hillingdon Hospital, London, UK

Alfred Cyril Roy, Sandeep Albert, Mohamad Gouse and Dan Barnabas Inja
Department of Orthopedics Unit-1, CMC, Vellore, India

M. G. R. Wali, A. N. Baba, I. A. Latoo, N. A. Bhat and O. K. Baba
Department of Orthopedics, Government Medical College, Srinagar, Srinagar, India

S. Sharma
Department of Orthopedics, Government Medical College, Jammu, Jammu, India

Mahmoud A. El-Rosasy and Mostafa A. Ayoub
Department of Orthopaedic Surgery, Faculty of Medicine, Tanta University Hospital, University of Tanta, Al-Geish Street, Tanta, Egypt

Zile Singh Kundu, Paritosh Gogna, Vinay Gupta, Pradeep Kamboj, Rohit Singla and Sukhbir Singh Sangwan
Department of Orthopaedics and Rehabilitation, PGIMS, 2/11-J Medical Enclave, Rohtak 124001, Haryana, India

M. C. Bellemore
Department of Orthopaedic Surgery, Royal Alexandra Hospital for Children, Sydney, Australia

L. Biston
Prince of Wales Medical Research Institute and Faculty of Medicine, University of New South Wales, Sydney, Australia

Allen Goodship
Institute of Orthopaedics and Musculoskeletal Science UCL, Royal National Orthopaedic Hospital, Stanmorem, London, UK

Index